W9-AGY-757

"It's rare that scientific acumen comes in the form of a great populist communicator. Garth Davis is that rare talent. An experienced surgeon not only immersed in peer-reviewed nutrition research but exuding the unique ability to expertly relate his knowledge and experience in a manner that connects, elucidates, and inspires everyday people to make quantum, sustainable improvements in their diet and lifestyles. *Proteinaholic* is a book for the ages. A book that once and for all dispels the nutritional myths that have rendered our prosperous nation sicker than ever. A book that will help you lose weight, keep it off, prevent lifestyle disease, and even reverse it. A book every health-conscious person should own and every doctor should prescribe their patients."

—Rich Roll, bestselling author of *Finding Ultra* and
The Plantpower Way

Proteinaholic hits the nail on the head, because we are a nation with an epidemic of tragic life-shortening diseases strongly promoted by the overconsumption of animal protein. Our obsession and addiction to animal products has lead us down the path to nutritional suicide, and this wake-up call from Dr. Davis is important to save lives."

—Joel Fuhrman, M.D., author of the *New York Times* bestsellers
Eat to Live, Eat to Live Cookbook, The End of Dieting,
The End of Diabetes, and *Super Immunity*

"A groundbreaking book from one of America's leading physicians, *Proteinaholic* will revolutionize your understanding of your body and how to keep it healthy. Garth Davis, M.D., is a medical visionary whose wisdom and wealth of experience have opened a powerful new pathway to the best of health."

—Neal D. Barnard, M.D., President, Physicians Committee for
Responsible Medicine, and Adjunct Associate Professor of Medicine,
George Washington University School of Medicine, Washington, DC

"Dr. Davis is in the 'trenches' applying science to patient care and a true expert. His experience and research is groundbreaking, and *Proteinaholic* is a must-read that will be the basis for reclaiming our health. This book will be in exam rooms in my clinic."

—Joel Kahn, M.D., F.A.C.C., Clinical Professor of Medicine,
Wayne State University School of Medicine, and author of
The Whole Heart Solution

"*Proteinaholic* documents the simple and easy-to-understand truth that billions of people have died, and that life on Planet Earth faces extinction as a direct consequence of product-promoting nutritional myths created and perpetuated by the egg, dairy, meat, poultry, and fish industries. Protein deficiency is unknown on any natural diet; protein poisoning is epidemic worldwide."

> —John McDougall, M.D., founder of the McDougall Program

"This is a book that will change lives. If you heed its wise and clear advice, your body will thank you for the rest of your life."

> —John Robbins, president of the Food Revolution Network and author of *Diet for a New America* and *The Food Revolution*

"Dr. Garth Davis has hit the nail on the head with this eye-opening look at America's most misunderstood macronutrient—protein. Read it, and rescue yourself before it's too late!"

> —Rip Esselstyn, health activist and bestselling author of *The Engine 2 Diet*

"A brilliant tour de force of how and why our 'addiction' to animal protein is killing us. This book just may save your life and make all of your moments healthier."

> —Robert Ostfeld, M.D., M.Sc., Director, Cardiac Wellness Program, and Associate Professor of Clinical Medicine, Montefiore Medical Center

"Exhaustively researched and fascinating."

> —*Publishers Weekly*

"Through extensive analysis of popular protein-pushing diet plans and meticulous assessment of nutritional research, Davis' passionate advocacy of a more healthful eating plan is also refreshingly transparent. Every claim and recommendation is fully annotated, making this reasoned and reasonable treatise a life-changer in the truest sense of the word."

> —*Booklist*

Protein aholic

HOW OUR OBSESSION WITH MEAT
IS KILLING US AND
WHAT WE CAN DO ABOUT IT

Garth Davis, M.D.
with Howard Jacobson, Ph.D.

HarperOne
An Imprint of HarperCollins*Publishers*

HarperOne

This book contains advice and information relating to health care. It should be used to supplement rather than replace the advice of your doctor or another trained health professional. If you know or suspect that you have a health problem, it is recommended that you seek your physician's advice before embarking on any medical program or treatment. All efforts have been made to assure the accuracy of the information contained in this book as of the date of publication. The publisher and the author disclaim liability for any medical outcomes that may occur as a result of applying the methods suggested in this book.

PROTEINAHOLIC. Copyright © 2015 by Garth Davis. All rights reserved. Printed in the United States of America. No part of this book may be used or reproduced in any manner whatsoever without written permission except in the case of brief quotations embodied in critical articles and reviews. For information, address HarperCollins Publishers, 195 Broadway, New York, NY 10007.

HarperCollins books may be purchased for educational, business, or sales promotional use. For information, please e-mail the Special Markets Department at SPsales@harpercollins.com.

HarperCollins website: http://www.harpercollins.com

FIRST HARPERCOLLINS PAPERBACK EDITION PUBLISHED IN 2016

Designed by Terry McGrath

Library of Congress Cataloging-in-Publication Data is available upon request.

ISBN 978–0–06–227931–6

18 19 20 LSC(C) 10 9 8 7 6 5 4

CONTENTS

PART IV The Proteinaholic Recovery Plan

PART ONE

Garth Davis, Proteinaholic

I'm Garth, and I'm a Proteinaholic

My name is Garth Davis, and I was a proteinaholic.

For many years, I obeyed what I'd been taught by the medical establishment, by my colleagues, and by the media: that each and every meal and snack had to contain a huge serving of my beloved protein. I would gulp down protein drinks whenever possible, and dive into big, thick steaks practically daily. Protein was my drug and, worse yet, it was my prescription. I actually pushed protein on my patients, encouraging them to do as I did.

I am happy to say that I have overcome this obsession with protein. This book is a detailed guide to my recovery. As you read through my journey you may think that I actually hate protein. In reality, how can you hate a macronutrient? Obviously we need protein. My concern is more with the fact that we no longer talk about food as food. Rather we are obsessed with breaking food down to its component parts and, in so doing, have developed an unhealthy obsession for one particular macronutrient. I am disturbed by the fact that protein has become a veritable nutritional rock star, omnipresent in our food and advertising like never before. We seemingly cannot get enough of protein, and this reality is leading us down a very dangerous road. In fact, "eat more protein" may be the worst advice that "experts" give to the public.

Whether you are seeing your doctor, nutritionist, or your trainer, protein is strongly advised. Should you happen upon a vitamin store you will be inundated with pills and concoctions boasting higher and higher protein contents. Even our grocery stores are pushing new and interesting food-type substances that are loaded with protein, while the produce aisles get smaller and less inviting. Why buy an apple when you can get high-protein cereal bars, high-protein drinks, even protein in your vodka. Do people really think vodka laced with protein is healthy? The answer is most certainly yes. As a recent *Wall Street Journal* article puts it, "Protein on a label has what researchers call a 'health halo effect.' People assume the product will give them energy or make them full." The article was appropriately entitled, "When the Box Says Protein, Shoppers Say I'll Take It." Most recently, a survey done by the International Food Information Council Foundation found that 63 percent of Americans are looking for protein foods when deciding what to eat, and a whopping 57 percent said they are trying to eat as much protein as possible!

Protein is everywhere. Big deal. So what is the problem? In a word: confusion. Some of us eat protein to lose weight, while others eat protein to gain weight. Ponder that paradox for a second. The same product sold to people to lose weight is relabeled and sold to others to gain weight! There are many who believe eating protein will make them healthier and help them live longer. And everybody seems to think protein will give them energy. Meanwhile, anyone who knows the basics of biochemistry or physiology will tell you that energy comes from carbs or fat, not protein. Possibly even more frightening is the fact that protein is one of the few food items that everyone seems to agree on. "Experts" argue about good fats and bad fats, or good carbs and bad carbs. This is very much part of the reason we are so confused about what to eat. But in protein we all seem to feel safe. No one would dare to argue that protein is bad for you.

Believe me, I am not writing this book because I dare to be different and buck the norm. I am not looking to be sensational, and I certainly hate to further confuse the public. However, given my experience, I am in a unique position to see that we have missed the forest for the trees. The fact is, our protein obsession is killing us and nobody seems to notice. This is not my opinion alone. I have done a tremendous amount of research to come to this controversial conclusion, and I will share with you what I have learned along the way. By the end of this book, you will see that the science shows that our protein obsession may be one of the main causes for the rise we are seeing in obesity, cancer, diabetes, hypertension, and heart disease. The United States is arguably the sickest first world country with the lowest life expectancy, and we eat more protein than any other country. Protein very well may be to blame for our poor health!

Before you dismiss me as a fearmonger, I want you to ask yourself this simple question, "Is all this protein making us healthier?" In all my years in medicine I have never, ever, seen a patient who was suffering from protein deficiency. I have searched the medical literature and cannot find a single case of protein deficiency in someone eating adequate calories. In fact, if you are getting adequate calories, I am not sure there is such thing as protein deficiency. So how did we get from eating adequate protein to be healthy to our current state of super physiologic doses, and is this making us healthier? When will we finally see that a healthy diet doesn't have to feature protein?

It's been said that we don't change when we see the light, but when we feel the heat. That's how I finally woke up. A couple of personal health scares shook me so profoundly that I began to doubt what I'd been taught about nutrition in medical school—and what my colleagues continued to advise. Instead, I began to do the research for myself.

I was shocked to discover that none of the elements of the Protein Gospel were even a little bit true:

- Protein is not the key to weight loss—in fact, animal protein is one of the biggest factors behind the obesity epidemic, and, in virtually every study, animal protein is correlated with weight gain.

- Animal protein is not one of the healthiest foods around—rather, it is strongly associated with diabetes, hypertension, heart disease, and cancer, the primary killers of our time.

- Plant-based protein not only exists—it's much better for you than animal protein and all plants contain more than enough to support every one of your health needs.

- A lower-protein (and low-fat) diet is the most effective way to lose weight, improve your health, and prevent future disease.

- Carbs, far from being the enemy, are (in their natural state) the source of human health, vitality, and vigor.

After years of intense research, I could come to only one conclusion: People whose diets are high in animal protein have significantly higher rates of chronic diseases: hypertension, cancer, diabetes, heart disease, and many, many others, including cataracts, diverticulitis, diverticulosis, inflammatory bowel disease, gall bladder disorders, gout, hypertension, irritable bowel syndrome, kidney stones, and rheumatoid arthritis. That's what we know for certain. In emerging research (not yet conclusive), higher animal protein consumption is linked to poor mood, loss of mental concentration, and dementia.

This conclusion is supported by virtually every large-scale scientific study: massive efforts that followed thousands of people over many years in multiple countries around the globe. Study after study kept turning up the same types of correlations between animal protein, saturated fat, obesity, and chronic illness. When scientists compared people who ate meat with people who didn't, the meat eaters were heavier, sicker, and more likely to die sooner. (I'll give you more detail in Part II, "How We Became Proteinaholics.")

Is Animal Protein Making You Sick?

So many of us—myself included—have spent years accepting our poor health as "normal." How many of these symptoms do you have?

1. Are you overweight?
2. Do you have high cholesterol?
3. Do you have irritable bowel syndrome?
4. Do you have hypertension?
5. Are you constipated?
6. Do you suffer from diarrhea?
7. Is your skin marked with acne?
8. Are you often tired or lacking energy?
9. Do you have brain fog—problems with memory, focus, concentration?
10. Do you get sick often?

These symptoms might be common, but they do not have to be a "normal" part of life. They indicate imbalances and disorders that animal protein is either causing or making worse. In most cases, they will start to resolve within two weeks and be gone in a month or two—once you start eating a plant-based diet.

But it's not just large-scale studies of human populations that support my conclusion—cutting-edge laboratory science has affirmed that clear biochemical mechanisms link animal protein to obesity, hypertension, heart disease, diabetes, and cancer, as well as many other disorders, and to a shorter life span generally. As I pored through one journal article after another, I identified the key elements of animal protein—including amino acids, heme iron, insulin growth factor 1 (IGF1), and N-nitroso compounds—that were implicated in decreased longevity, premature aging, and the chronic disorders that plague our time.

As if that weren't enough, human and animal studies all pointed in the same direction. In dozens of randomized controlled clinical trials, the gold standard in medical research, the more animal protein consumed, the worse the participants fared.

I reviewed thousands of original studies, and hundreds of meta-analyses and reviews. And all of my research kept pointing to the same conclusion: Consuming animal protein is linked to chronic disorders and premature death. Eating lots of fruits, vegetables, whole grains, and legumes is associated with staying healthy.

Protein Addiction

As the title of this book indicates, I think our society has a protein addiction. I want you to know that this isn't sloppy language that serves to trivialize "real" addictions; I mean it quite literally and intentionally.

Sure, proteinaholism is different from an alcohol or drug addiction, mostly in that it's socially sanctioned and doesn't cause instantaneous functional impairment. But our obsessive and mindless overconsumption of protein fits the pattern of addiction, and its health consequences—for individuals and society as a whole—are no less serious in the long term.

I realized protein was a true addiction through the many counseling sessions with my weight-loss patients that have occurred over the last several years. They usually go something like this:

ME: *So last time I asked you include more fruit and vegetables in your diet. Specifically we talked about having an apple for a snack, and starting dinner with a salad. How did that go?*

PATIENT: *I thought about it, but I realized if I ate the apple or the salad, I wouldn't have enough room for the protein.*

ME: *But we talked about this at length. You don't need so much protein. In fact, too much animal protein is the main reason you're in my office.*

PATIENT: *I know, but I'm scared of not getting enough protein.*

These patients panic when they even consider withdrawal. They cling to both the notion that protein is the King of Nutrients, and to the specific protein-rich animal foods that make up their daily intake. Asking them to deviate even a little causes them to respond much like an alcoholic whose friends suggest that he might be a bit out of control: "I don't have a problem. Leave me alone."

How Much Protein Are We Talking About?

Americans consume more protein than just about any other nationality: on average, according to the World Health Organization, around 130 grams per day (about 4.5 ounces). The National Health and Nutrition Survey estimates are lower: 102 grams per day for men and 70 grams per day for women.

Is that a lot or a little? Well, the recommended daily allowance (RDA) put out by the U.S. Department of Agriculture (USDA) is just 56 grams for men and 46 grams for women.

Remember, these figures are grams of protein—not servings of meat. When you consider that a 4-ounce hamburger patty—which is pretty small by American standards—has 20 grams of protein, and a 6-ounce steak—again, pretty small, especially here in Texas—has 70 grams of protein, you can see just how much more protein we are eating than the RDA recommended levels. Those single servings blow the highest RDA out of the water, and most of us are consuming portions like this at each meal.

Lots of my patients will add a small amount of chicken breast to a lunch salad (3.5 ounces at 30 grams of protein) and eat a "healthy-sized" burger for dinner (8 ounces of beef patty for 40 more grams). They've already exceeded the RDA for adult men by 14 grams, and we haven't even looked at breakfast, or snacks, or the cheese on the patty, the ranch dressing on the salad, or the protein bars and shakes that help us "round out" our nutritional needs.

Here's something else to consider: the RDA recommendations are actually optimal values, not minimal needs. Since some people require more protein than others, the USDA chose as their recommendation a value that assures adequate protein for 99 percent of the country. Based on the assumption that too much is safer than not enough (not true, as you'll see), they actually overestimated by a bit what almost everybody really needs. There's no real danger in that slight overadjustment, but when many Americans get *double* the RDA of protein, which itself is roughly double our true requirement, it becomes a big problem. (We'll go into this in more detail in Chapter 15, "How Much Protein Do We Need?")

To help you figure out where you are right now on the proteinaholic scale, here are a couple of sample menus and their protein values. The first is based on that National Health and Nutrition Survey, which found that U.S. men average 102 grams of protein each day.

- 2 large eggs (12 grams)

- 4 ounces of milk (for your coffee, tea, or cereal) (4 grams)

- 8-ounce hamburger patty (40 grams)

- 3½-ounce chicken breast (30 grams)

Does that sound like the way you eat? Or is your daily protein consumption more like this one, based on the World Health Organization finding of 130 grams protein/day?

- 2 large eggs (12 grams)

- 1 strip of bacon (3 grams)

- 4 ounces of milk (4 grams)

- 8-ounce hamburger patty (40 grams)

- 1 ounce of cheddar cheese (to make it a cheeseburger) (8 grams)

- 8-ounce fillet of salmon (48 grams)

During my proteinaholic days, I wouldn't have seen any problem with these menus or numbers. I didn't realize they far exceeded the U.S. government RDAs for protein. I didn't realize the RDAs were themselves inflated for most people. I didn't realize I was looking at a daily dose of animal protein high enough to be toxic.

If you had told me about our protein intake and the RDAs, I would probably have said something like, "Sure, we're eating a lot of protein! That's because it's such a healthy food—and that's why we Americans are the healthiest people in the world."

The Healthiest People in the World?

It turns out my American pride in our superior health was seriously misplaced. According to a 2013 survey sponsored by the National Institute of Health and conducted by the National Research Council and the Institute of Medicine, we are some of the unhealthiest people in the developed world (Woolf and Aron, 2013). We die at an earlier age, on average, than our European and Japanese counterparts. We have higher rates of obesity, heart disease, and diabetes. And we suffer from more cancers. Our medical advances have slightly reduced our cancer death rates—meaning, we get cancer more often, but stay alive longer due to aggressive treatment—but basically, if it's a war, cancer is winning.

The report concludes, " . . . the tragedy is not that the U.S. is losing a contest with other countries, but that Americans are dying and suffering from illness and injury at rates that are demonstrably unnecessary."

So we eat more protein, spend more money on health care, and are some of the unhealthiest people in the developed world. That doesn't prove that protein is the culprit, of course, but it's a staggering piece of circumstantial evidence, especially when you look at the countries who are thriving and discover that they eat very little protein. The longest-lived people in the world get an average of 10 percent of their total calories from protein. Our average is as high as 15 to 20 percent, and of course, if you're on a high-protein diet—Atkins, Paleo, or the diets recommended by many of my colleagues, and formerly by me—that figure goes up to 40 or 50 percent.

Compare that to the inhabitants of the island of Okinawa. They consume the vast majority of their calories in the form of rice and yams, those supposed "high-carb killers," and get just 7 percent of their calories from protein. They live longer than Americans, have among the world's highest percentage of centenarians (people who live to one hundred), and have far lower rates of obesity. Their old people are vigorous, active, and full of life. Only when Okinawans move to the United States does their health decline—or when they start eating at the U.S.-style fast-food restaurants that have begun to colonize their island.

We'll look at more of the where the world's healthiest people live—and what they eat—in Chapter 4. Even though this data doesn't strictly "prove" that excess animal protein causes disease, it's awfully suggestive. And it definitely contradicts the low-carb narrative that only through high-protein and high-fat diets can we possibly be healthy.

Do You Have to Go Vegan When You Recover from Proteinaholism?

In a word, no. Just because I'm a vegan doesn't mean you have to be one. I do happen to think that the healthiest possible choice, both for our health and our environment, is to be a vegan—someone who consumes no animal protein whatsoever—and when you've finished reading this book, you may also.

However, to get the benefit of this book, you don't have to go full-on vegan. Rather than becoming "anti animal protein," I'd rather you take a stand "pro fruits and vegetables." That is, the vast majority of the calories you consume should come from fresh, whole fruits and veggies; nuts and seeds; beans of all types; and whole, unrefined grains. By focusing on the healthy and delicious plant-based options, you automatically crowd the animal protein off your plate without obsessing over it.

And if you're currently a proteinaholic, as I was, and as most of my patients are when they first come to see me, please take a deep breath and keep an open mind. As you'll discover in the coming pages, plant foods contain all the protein you need, plus a boatload of other good things: antioxidants, anti-inflammatories, vitamins, minerals, and other micronutrients. As long as the vast majority of your calories come from plants, you're on the right track. (I'll share my suggestions for what to eat in Chapter 16 and17, which includes a sample meal plan with accompanying recipes.)

The key message here is not "zero meat" but rather "more plants." More than 100 percent dietary purity, I want you to shift your overall dietary pattern. Once you've read through the evidence, you can draw your own conclusions and make your own decisions as to how far you want to go. While evidence suggests that the closer you get to 100 percent, the better you'll feel and healthier you'll become, the slightly imperfect diet you follow is infinitely better than the perfect diet you won't stick with.

Breaking Through the Protein Myths

We'll explore and explode these myths in depth in Part III. For now, here's an overview of proteinaholic myths and the facts that contradict them.

MYTH: A diet high in carbohydrates causes diabetes.
FACT: Carbs do not cause not diabetes. Meat and fat do. Yes, you read that right. Carbs don't cause diabetes—not even sugar causes diabetes unless consumed in excess. It's meat that leads to insulin resistance and rising insulin levels, a syndrome that is the number one precursor to diabetes and a major contributor to obesity.

MYTH: A high-carbohydrate diet predisposes you to heart disease.
FACT: Carbs do not cause heart disease—meat does. Meat raises bad cholesterol and clogs your arteries. Meat provokes a state of inflammation—an immune system response that, when it becomes chronic, underlines virtually every one of our chronic disorders, including heart disease. Meat provokes heart disease in many other ways as well.

MYTH: A diet high in carbohydrates leads to obesity.
FACT: Every large-scale study comes to the same conclusion—vegans (who eat no animal protein) weigh less than vegetarians (who eat some animal protein), and vegetarians (with their eggs and dairy products) weigh less than meat eaters (with their red meat, chicken, and fish). There is another category, "pesco-vegetarians," who eat only fish and plant-based foods. Predictably, they weigh more than vegetarians and less than meat eaters.
Carbs are not behind the obesity epidemic—meat and calorie excess is. Meat disrupts your intestinal bacteria, which leads to weight

gain. Most meat contains antibiotics, which lead to weight gain. Meat creates acidosis and inflammation, which lead to weight gain. And that's just the tip of the iceberg—we'll explore the full story of protein and weight loss in Chapter 12 the chapter on obesity.

MYTH: Meat is only a health risk from animals raised on "factory farms."
FACT: True, factory farming multiplies the problem, contaminating your meat, milk, or eggs with bacteria, viruses, antibiotics, and industrial chemicals. But archaeological studies, which analyze the bones of our ancient ancestors who never ate a single factory farmed animal, have found higher rates of cancer among those who ate more meat. And contemporary studies point to the same conclusion: Meat—even grass-fed, clean-raised, organic meat—is a carcinogen; that is, it contributes to the formation of cancer. Dairy products and eggs may also be carcinogens.

MYTH: Many cultures, past and present, have eaten a high-protein diet and thrived.
FACT: Through the history of our time on Earth, no culture that has thrived on a high-protein diet. Some cultures have eaten such a diet. But when they do, they do not thrive. Without a single exception, they survive while suffering higher rates of disease, disability, degeneration, and premature death.

Why I Wrote This Book

As a weight-loss surgeon who runs a large surgical and medical weight-loss clinic in Houston, I am on the front lines of the battle against obesity. I witness daily the negative impact of the so-called experts' ill-designed diet plans as patients come to my office in dire need of help, having tried all the famous high-protein diet plans multiple times. I have treated thousands of people for obesity and obesity-related disorders, and I have learned what works and what doesn't.

What doesn't work is massive amounts of animal protein. What does work is a plant-based diet—not necessarily vegan, but featuring far smaller amounts of animal foods—with the vast majority of calories coming from fresh, whole fruits and vegetables, along with nuts, seeds, beans, and grains.

In other words, the exact opposite of the diets my obese patients follow before they come to see me. Their diet logs are a veritable animal graveyard. Eggs and bacon for breakfast, a sandwich with a few slices of meat for lunch, some jerky for a snack, and chicken for dinner. The amazing thing to me, now that I've recovered from proteinaholism, is that despite the evidence of their own bodies, my patients continue to believe the same old myths: protein is good, and more protein is better. If I ask them why they think they're not losing weight—why, in fact, their weight is going up—they never blame the jerky, the chicken, or, God forbid, the bacon. Instead they look ashamed and mutter, "Carbs."

"What carbs?" I'll say, looking at day after day without a single apple or a salad—since of course, fresh fruits and vegetables are carbs.

"Oh, I had some pizza on Tuesday," they might say, looking sheepish and unhappy. Or, "There were those fries on Wednesday." Or maybe even, "At Sunday brunch, I couldn't stop myself. I had a donut."

What's wrong with blaming carbs for their inability to lose weight? First, the vast majority of calories from pizza, fries, and donuts come from fat rather than carbohydrates. Second, in focusing on these supposedly evil carbs, my patients let animal protein and saturated fats off the hook. When I tell them to eat more fresh fruits and vegetables, it's not that they actually object. They're just so focused on getting more and more protein into their diets that they don't have room for plant-based foods.

So I had to ask myself, why? Why did my patients cling so desperately to this notion that eggs and bacon and fish and chicken were such healthy foods, disregarding the watermelon and apples and kale and oatmeal that had become my own weight-loss staples?

In our world of Google and Wikipedia, we no longer have to worry about not having information. We have tons of it. Our challenge is to know what to do with that information and differentiate wrong from right. In the realm of nutrition, the anecdotal stories of miraculous cures and unbelievable weight loss have catapulted to the forefront. Meanwhile, science has been ignored or, worse yet, manipulated. The result is a belief in certain dietary practices that in reality are making us sick and fat.

There are some thoughtful experts writing books appealing to the public to stop thinking of foods as macronutrients but rather as whole foods. They are asking readers not to think in terms of how much protein to eat but rather to concentrate on eating whole natural foods. As Michael Pollan, author of the bestselling *The Omnivore's Dilemma,* so eloquently puts it, "Eat food. Not too much. Mostly plants." The problem with this appeal to real food is that the public is so wedded to the concept of protein that whole foods have to be carefully examined for their protein content. Worse yet, the public believes that protein means animal protein. People either do not know that plant protein exists or, if they do, believe it is inferior.

And what do people mean when they say they are going to have "a protein" for dinner? What are beans, or avocados? They have protein, carbs, and fat. People give lip service to fruits and vegetables. We all agree that fruits and vegetables are good for us, though for reasons that drive me crazy, we add a disclaimer to fruits that they are only good "in moderation." But while we might believe these whole foods are good, we do not believe that veggies or fruit are nearly as important as "protein." In fact, we have developed a food calculus whereby we now compare one food to another. So we may nod our heads when experts argue that you should eat whole foods like a carrot or an apple, but in the back of our mind we are still questioning the protein content of the apple. Given this calculus we would rather eat a chicken breast or a protein shake. This incorrect emphasis on protein results in the fact that we only eat about 5 to 7 percent of our calories from fruits and vegetables!

We should be talking more about whole foods. The reductionist practice of breaking foods down to their component parts has really confused the situation. However, during the writing of this book I must be a reductionist. I cannot argue that the emphasis on protein is harmful if I do not roll up my sleeves and immerse myself into the world of reductionist nutrition. I need to take on protein mano a mano. Otherwise, no matter how much I tell you to eat an apple, you will always reach for the beef jerky, now available absolutely everywhere. More important, I also have to show you that there is a dramatic difference between the physiologic effects of plant versus animal protein.

I began to realize that for me and many of my patients, the transition to a plant-based diet required a huge reversal of everything we believed, much as Copernicus had asked the people of his time to give up the notion that the sun moved around the earth and to accept, instead, that the earth revolves around the sun.

After all, the protein obsession is one that just about every physician promotes. Ten thousand diet books proclaim it (actually, an Amazon search for "low-carb books" just yielded 9,710 results, so please forgive the slight exaggeration). The Atkins industry and its spin-offs (*South Beach, The Zone, Protein Power,* etc.) trumpet it. The Paleo movement argues for it. A whole legion of fitness and lifestyle bloggers insists on it. And the cattle, pork, chicken, dairy, and egg industries fund our protein obsession to the tune of billions of dollars per year, paying for TV ads, commissioning biased studies, lobbying and threatening government officials, and creating the illusion that one of our most dangerous addictions is totally normal and safe.

A Labor of Love—and Penitence

I'll be honest with you: I didn't particularly want to write this book. As the head of a burgeoning weight-loss clinic and bariatric surgical practice, I have more patients than I can handle. I'm the very involved father of two young girls. I love spending time with my wife. Since my discovery of the plant-based lifestyle, I've taken to competing in marathons and triathlons (you'll see—once you regain your health and vitality, the sky's the limit!). Between my practice, my family, and my hobbies, I've got more than enough on my plate.

So I didn't want to devote years of late nights, early mornings, and weekends to this book—but I had to. For three reasons.

First, and most pressing, I just couldn't stand seeing one more patient come into my office, clutching her diet log, explaining to me that her past week's weight gain was somehow due to eating "not enough protein," even though she'd had eggs for breakfast, salmon for lunch, and chicken for dinner, consuming two or even three times the amount of protein in the already too-high RDAs.

Second, although painful for me to admit, I wrote a book that's been part of the problem. In 2008, I published *The Expert's Guide to Weight-Loss Surgery.* It did very well. It earned 4.5 out of 5 stars on Amazon.com. And it reached a lot of people desperate to lose weight and regain their lives. Every chapter in that book was meticulously researched, based on the best evidence available at the time. Except for—you guessed it—the one on nutrition. Without a second thought, I breezily recommended the

Zone diet, complete with its ratio of 30 percent protein and 30 percent fat to 40 percent carbohydrates. (Nobody in the weight-loss community batted an eye, of course; I was only promoting what everyone else believed.) I couldn't put that genie back in the bottle, but I could unleash an even more powerful and effective genie to help people regain their physiques and their health. You're holding it in your hands.

And third, I couldn't take one more day of looking at our shameful U.S. health statistics, in which more people are overweight than not—66 percent—and in which a full third of the population is obese. I couldn't stand being a physician in a country that spends more on health care than any other nation in the world—and yet has the worst health statistics of any developed country. Our national obsession with protein is literally killing us: sapping our vitality, undermining our health, shortening our life span. I consider the current situation nothing short of criminal.

But it doesn't have to be that way. The solution can be right there in your shopping cart, in your refrigerator, and on your plate—as soon as you understand how animal protein affects you and how to make a healthier choice. The solution can be in your doctor's office, too, as the medical profession becomes better educated about nutrition and as more physicians begin giving their patients better advice. And the solution can be in our national policy, if we're able to stand up to the billion-dollar budgets of the food industry lobbyists and their buddies at the USDA, and if we're able to see past the ads proclaiming the health benefits of meat, milk, and eggs.

As a bariatric surgeon and recovering proteinaholic, I consider myself a fighter on the front line. Switching from hamburger and steaks to hummus and kale has enabled me to drop weight and turn into an Ironman competitor, stronger, faster, and healthier than I've ever been in my life. My irritable bowel syndrome cleared up. My cholesterol levels dropped to normal. My blood sugars are exemplary. My inflammation readings are excellent. A plant-based diet has been the gateway to a whole new life of health and vigor—and it's done the same for my patients.

As a weight-loss surgeon, I see the heaviest people in the country, the ones for whom standard diet and exercise simply have not worked. When these people switch from overconsumption of animal protein to a healthy, plant-based diet, they experience the same things as me. Their pounds come off, this time for good. Their cholesterol levels drop. The blood sugars stabilize. Good-bye heart disease, hypertension, and diabetes. Hello, energy, stamina, and a healthy weight. Their biggest problem shifts from having the energy to get up in the morning and face another day of pain, fatigue, and embarrassment to deciding how to spend their newfound zest for life. What they will do with their "one wild and precious life," as poet Mary Oliver puts it.

Decide for Yourself

If you're feeling skeptical as you read these words, I understand. My 2008 self would have been screaming BS! right about now. You and I and everyone have been programmed to regard protein as the perfect nutrient, the more the better. We're sold compelling narratives (Paleo especially tells a great story about returning to our noble caveman roots and becoming "real" men and women once again). We're intimidated by our doctors and other health authorities, not realizing that they have, if best, a layperson's understanding of nutrition.

To switch to a plant-based diet, you have to make the journey that I made: from thinking that animal protein is the healthiest possible food to becoming aware of its many dangers. You need to see through the way the media, the food industry, and the medical establishment have sold you a bill of goods, convincing you—falsely—that animal protein should be the foundation of a healthy diet, and the more of it, the better. You need to understand the scientific debates over the effects of animal protein and to cut through the noise: the confusing, often dispiriting information culture in which you can find "evidence" to support just about any conclusion, so that you no longer know what to believe.

The mental part of this journey consists of two phases.

First, you need to know the research: What have scientists actually discovered? The entire body of nutrition research is huge and varied, and you can always find a study that contradicts everything else—or seems to. That doesn't mean that "we don't know anything" or "nothing is certain." If you can find one hundred massive studies following thousands of people over many years that say one thing, and a single study covering only a few people for a few months saying the opposite, it's pretty easy to decide which evidence to believe. So in this book, I'll lay out that evidence and let you judge it for yourself.

Second, to cut through the noise, it helps to understand why the media gets it so wrong. The way scientific studies are reported, it's easy to become confused. Once you understand a few basic concepts about how to sift through the welter of information and settle on a few key facts, a lot of that "information anxiety" will disappear. Yes, it's confusing for all of us—even for me, and I'm an M.D. who lives and breathes medical research and practice full-time. But there is a way to break through the confusion—to sort for yourself between the solid news and the hype—and once you learn how to do it, you will know the extraordinary relief of being able to come to your own conclusions.

That's what I want this book to achieve: to enable you finally to feel confident that you know which foods are healthy choices. Then you can decide for yourself.

In these pages I'm going to take you on the journey I took myself, pointing out the overwhelming and consistent evidence for the dangers of animal protein and the virtues of whole fruits, vegetables, and other plant foods.

I'll take you to a Siberian yurt and a Kyrgyz hut—showing you two cultures that live side by side on the steppes of Russia, one eating meat, one eating plants. Guess which one is healthier? I'll give you a tour of Dr. Dean Ornish's remarkable experiment, where he put men with prostate cancer on a plant-based diet and taught them how to reduce their life stress, and then compared their cancer's progression with that of people who kept on eating meat.

I'll show you how the cancer cells in a petri dish start multiplying at an explosive rate as soon as you add IGF1—a hormone that increases with increased animal protein consumption—and how those same cancer cells begin to shrink as soon as you add the blood of people who've been eating a plant-based diet. I'll also give you the benefit of my many years of studying and applying it in a clinical setting.

Then, if you're interested, you can use the meal plan and recipes in Chapter 17 to help you make the healthy changes that I have made—the same healthy changes that have helped hundreds of my patients.

I don't expect you to take my word for any of this. We've all been exposed to far too many "diet gurus," miraculous fat-shedding foods, flip-flopping media reports, and confusing debates to put our faith in anyone's opinions anymore. Many people just tune it all out, shaking their heads and figuring, *Might as well eat whatever I want; everything's going to kill me anyway.*

If you can relate to that remark or have thought it yourself, I don't blame you. And I don't want to make things worse by becoming just one more confusing opinion. Luckily, faith is not a required ingredient on your plant-based journey. Aside from all its other benefits, one of the best things about the plant-based diet is how quickly it creates meaningful and obvious improvement. So you can let your body convince you, so I don't have to.

Sound good? Then let's get started. The first stop on our journey is one of my finest public moments, when I was celebrated for my work as a committed professional proteinaholic. The reality of my situation, as you'll see, was quite different . . .

This book has a companion website, Proteinaholic.com, that's designed to help people transition to a healthy diet and lifestyle. With recipes, cooking tips, inspiring stories, research updates, and coaching support, there's something for everyone.

You can start by downloading the free Proteinaholic Recovery Plan, including additional recipes, links to videos, and a simple step-by-step formula for improving your diet.

See you there!

CHAPTER 2

My Road to Ruin

I stood in front of my bedroom mirror and didn't much like what I saw. My heavy cheeks. My doughy physique. My big belly. I was only thirty-five, but already I looked like an old man. The flesh on my face sagged. My eyes were ringed with deep, dark circles. My face appeared tired, discouraged, as though I could barely drag myself out of bed in the morning. I was a physician—a specialist in weight loss—and yet I didn't look trim, or fit, or even very healthy. I looked the way I felt—frail.

I didn't understand. I ate what I considered a normal, if not explicitly "healthy" diet—what every physician I knew considered a healthy diet. Eggs and bacon every morning. For lunch, a double cheeseburger or maybe a turkey sandwich—layers of meat piled high between the bread. For dinner, steak or barbecue or spaghetti and meatballs. Lots of protein. Lots and lots of protein.

I had told my patients to eat this way, and they did. In fact, some of them—the overachievers—ate more protein than I recommended. I also insisted that they exercise, but they never seemed to do that. Neither did I, mainly because I was too tired and run-down to get myself moving.

Now, however, the *Houston Chronicle* was about to call my bluff. An editor had just asked me to be the cover story for the newspaper's health magazine. I guess they figured that a surgeon who specializes in weight loss should know about being healthy. When the editor asked me what I did to stay fit, I panicked and told them that I ran stairs at Rice University stadium. What I meant was, *In the past, I ran stairs once in a while.*

"Run stairs?" the editor said. "Great idea. Let's set up a photo shoot!"

Yikes! I had walked right into that one. So I bought myself a brand-new running outfit, showed up at the photo shoot, and believe it or not, I ran those stairs. I ran them hard, too, my adrenaline fueling every step. Each time I heard the camera click, it motivated me to keep running. Until—and it didn't take long—my legs were trembling so hard I could barely stand, and my breakfast, the usual eggs and bacon, was threatening to come up.

"You know, guys," I finally managed to drawl, "I've really got to get back to the hospital now."

"Sure," the photographer said. "Just one more—the cover shot."

They posed me, one leg up on the next step, head high, chest out, a fierce warrior's grin upon my face. When I look at that picture today, I have to laugh, because it could really make you believe I was a healthy guy at the peak of my physical fitness. They snapped the shot, I shook their hands . . . and then I speed-walked, as casually I could, straight to the nearest bathroom. I lunged for the first toilet I could reach and promptly threw up every gram of protein in my throbbing, aching stomach.

I had fooled the guys from the *Chronicle,* but I felt like a complete hypocrite. Not only did I feel lousy all the time, my labs made it clear that I was well on my way to the same chronic diseases that my patients were suffering: hypertension, heart disease, and diabetes. Who was I to tell them what to do when I obviously didn't have a good solution myself? Sure, I could keep doing weight-loss surgeries and just approach the job as a technician, but that felt woefully inadequate. I didn't want to just help people lose weight. I wanted to help my patients get healthy.

I began to question everything I had been taught about the human body. In medical school, we were given the idea that disease is pretty much inevitable. Humans just seemed to be destined to get some kind of chronic disorder—heart disease, diabetes, cancer, maybe Alzheimer's. Not much you could do to prevent it—basically, all you could do was medicate it. If your medications had side effects, you treated those with still more medications.

Of course, surgery was always an option. When I had entered medical school, there wasn't much talk about bariatric surgery, but now I was a specialist in the field. I didn't think twice about how crazy this was—why putting bands around patients' stomachs or performing a gastric bypass was the first thing we did, rather than a last resort. Worse, a disturbing number of patients were coming back a year or two later, having regained much of the weight they'd lost. Well, I had rationalized, maybe another, better surgery would be discovered soon. They had just started talking about putting a band around a bypass. Perhaps that would lock in the weight loss more permanently.

I had come to view the human body as a kind of expensive, unreliable car—something that was always breaking down and needing to be repaired. I was totally focused on treating disease—prevention hadn't really entered my mind as a possibility.

That's how my patients felt, too. When I had to tell someone that he had a serious condition—diabetes, say, or heart disease—I was often met with a look of resignation. *I knew something like this would happen sooner or later,* that look said. *I don't even expect to be healthy—it's just a matter of when I get the bad news.*

Now, still aching from my heroic and hypocritical run, I began to wonder how we had all come to accept such a bleak prognosis. How could the human body be so fragile? Why couldn't we count on staying strong and vital throughout our lives? Were we really all doomed to skyrocketing blood sugars, clogged arteries, and the kind of obesity that has made us the fattest nation on earth? There had to be another way.

So that day I said to myself, *Enough*. No more of this medicine that focused only on "sick care" while completely ignoring health care. No more telling my patients to do something that we were all too exhausted and unwell to do. I would pick up the ball that Western medicine had dropped. I would go on a mission: a quest to discover the foods that would keep us strong, vital, and healthy.

In pursuit of my quest, I would search the world and comb through the scientific literature, looking for the secret to better health. I would study the cultures that don't suffer from the typical Western diseases—obesity, heart disease, diabetes, cancer—and figure out what they were doing right, starting with the foods they ate each day. Obviously, they knew something we didn't. It was time to find out what.

I wanted to find another way to eat, but I didn't want another diet. Zone, Atkins, Paleo—most of my patients had been on all those and then some, and it hadn't done anybody a damn bit of good. Oh, sure, maybe some people lost a few pounds the first month—maybe they even lost twenty or thirty pounds the first six months. Within a year, though, they were right back at my door, all the weight regained plus a few pounds extra. Even my surgical patients were starting to regain their weight—that definitely wasn't supposed to happen.

So, no more diets. No more counting calories, resisting temptation, obsessing about food. Instead, I wanted to learn how to eat for health, to follow the wisdom of Hippocrates, the founder of Western medicine. "Let food be thy medicine and medicine be thy food," Hippocrates had said three thousand years ago. It was time I started listening.

The vow I made that bleak afternoon led me on the journey of research and practice that has inspired this book. It led me to the healthy plant-based diet—loaded with fresh whole fruits, vegetables, nuts, seeds, beans, and grains—that has melted away my excess weight, replacing fat with muscle and lethargy with energy. I now have so much extra energy that I have to run marathons and train for Ironman triathlons just to use it up! I'm never hungry. I'm never sick. My labs are perfect.

More important, my patients are flourishing. Some of my patients who agree to go on a plant-based diet don't even end up needing weight-loss surgery—they find themselves losing weight almost without effort. They are seldom hungry, even though they never count calories and don't restrict what they eat. They, too, have excellent labs and boatloads of energy. And those patients who choose surgery and then eat plant-based food also well exceed expectations in maintaining their weight and regaining their health.

In the rest of this book, I'll share with you the results of my quest, culminating in the chapter with a meal plan and recipes that can help you switch to a plant-based diet should you choose to do so. But first, I'd like to tell you the rest of my story, because I've come to believe that this story is not mine alone. America has become a nation of proteinaholics. And while struggling to free ourselves from our protein obsession, many of us have learned lessons very similar to mine.

"I want to help people"

Some kids play catch with their dads. I went on rounds with mine. Is it any wonder that I wanted to be a doctor from the moment I can remember wanting to be anything?

My friends still rib me about an incident that took place in high school. I was on the football team—in those days, I could run stairs!—and as the victim of a spectacular tackle by the opposing linebacker I was knocked out cold. As I started to come to, groggy and confused, the first words out of my mouth were, "Can I still be a doctor?"

I've thought a lot recently about why I was so passionate about medicine. It definitely goes back to my dad. Not that I wanted to be exactly like him, but I wanted to have, like he did, a job with a purpose. Unlike the fathers of most of my friends, he didn't just go into work and clock in for the paycheck. He went off each day on a mission, and he didn't punch out promptly at 5 P.M., either. He was always going in to the hospital to check on a patient or calling the hospital to get the latest numbers on a post-op. Clearly, his job meant something, and for as long as I can remember, that appealed to me. I guess you could say that his work seemed less like a job and more like a life's passion, and that appealed to me, too.

So off I went to medical school, where I plunged into a challenging curriculum of cellular biology, organic chemistry, and pathophysiology. One thing was missing, though I didn't realize it at the time: nutrition. Want to guess how many hours my fellow med students and I spent studying the ways that food affects the human body? A grand total of one. And if you're thinking I spent those sixty minutes learning about which foods keep us healthy and which foods make us sick, you'd be way off base. That single hour of nutrition was all about how to administer an IV formula to a patient so sick he couldn't eat on his own. As for what kinds of foods might be good for the rest of us humans? Not a single word.

I'll never forget how excited I was on the day I finally got my M.D. Although the administering of the Hippocratic Oath has become more of a routine exercise than a solemn ritual, the words stuck with me: "First, do no harm." That oath would come back to haunt me when I realized just how much harm I and my colleagues were doing to our patients—just how badly our "protein, protein, and more protein" advice was setting them up for obesity, hypertension, heart disease, diabetes, and cancer. But then, what could you expect of people who hadn't learned a single thing about nutrition?

My Life in Diets

I don't want you to think I was a complete stranger to diets. Even though as a child I ate the usual junk food—the processed sugar cereals and the sweets—I cut back on that stuff as I hit my twenties. Prevailing wisdom was that sugar and processed carbs were the obviously harmful parts of the American diet, and so, like every other dieter I knew, I tried to resist their temptation. Good thing I felt entitled to eat all the protein I wanted. After all, wasn't protein a weight-loss food?

By the time I got to residency, I had already put on quite a few pounds. Yet I never questioned whether that was due to my low-carb, high-protein diet. Luckily, we lived in scrubs, perhaps one of the most forgiving uniforms ever designed. Good thing, too, because the most convenient food available came from the Wendy's Hamburger restaurant, located right there in the hospital. It seems ironic to me now, if not downright sinister, that my hospital was leading the country in treating the diseases caused by fast-food diets and yet welcomed a Wendy's onto its ground floor. Every day, you could see a long line of people waiting patiently to get their bacon cheeseburgers before going in to see their cardiologists.

At the time, however, the irony was lost on me. All I knew is that I was working hard and I needed some good, hearty food to keep me going. Of course, I gained even more weight, and I was far from the only one. You hear about the freshman fifteen, but for us residents, it was more like the intern thirty. Like I said, thank heavens for scrubs.

So we all began to diet—but not for our health. We knew better than anybody the associations between obesity, cholesterol, heart disease, and stroke. But all we cared about was the day when we would leave the hospital corridors to go on a date, or maybe even to the beach. Our scrubs wouldn't save us then—so bring on Dr. Atkins!

Yup, Atkins. Why not, when there was a Wendy's right there? ("Hold the bun, please!") Besides, Atkins was the big fad at the time and we all had at least one friend who had raved about the instant weight loss and the unlimited supplies of bacon. (We didn't hear about the headaches, constipation, nausea, and bad breath; we just experienced those symptoms for—and kept them to—ourselves.)

Not one single resident picked out a diet based on health. None of us weighed the evidence—we didn't even look at it, despite having ready access to all the medical databases and the habit of reading studies. When it came to dieting, we didn't know any more than the most uninformed of our patients.

Not surprisingly, I loved being on Atkins—at least at first. I had eggs and bacon in the morning, hamburger without the bun for lunch, and roast beef or steak for dinner. My mealtimes became a glorious meat extravaganza! Why shouldn't I love it?—it was pretty much how I had been eating all of my life. For the first week, I was in hog heaven.

Then I started to get sick. Sure, I saved a few hours by never having to go to the bathroom more than once a week, but I paid a big price in personal comfort. I couldn't take it and fell off the Atkins wagon in less than a month.

Many of my friends lasted longer. Some even lost substantial amounts of weight—for about six months. Sooner or later, though, they all regained their lost weight and then some.

Practicing Surgery

My ignorance of diet continued as I began my surgical practice. I ate as I always had eaten and never connected food to disease—despite taking long medical histories of my patients, I never once asked what they ate.

Had I only been more aware, the links between food, lifestyle, and illness were everywhere. Most days I removed one, two, or even three gallbladders, often from patients with the typical profile of "fat, female, and forty." (That's the medical profession's phrase, not mine.) Did I ever connect the word *fat* with the need for gallbladder surgery? No, I did not. I removed the gallbladder and pronounced the patient cured.

I also performed many operations for diverticulitis, in which patients develop an outpouching of colon tissue. I did know that diverticulitis is a direct result of insufficient fiber. When you don't get enough fiber, you can't poop properly. The fecal matter collects in your colon, and you aren't able to push it out without a lot of straining. The resulting pressure on the colon walls can cause them to break down, to balloon out, and even, sometimes, to pop.

Diverticulitis is one of the few diseases where conventional doctors do offer a dietary solution. The average American consumes less than 15 grams of fiber each day, so I followed the "standard of care" and told my patients to shoot for 25 to 30 grams—what you'd get if you eat a bowl of bran with some berries for breakfast, a whole-wheat pita sandwich for lunch, an apple with some almonds for a snack, and some whole-wheat pasta with veggies and beans for dinner. Not a high bar, but it might have been the moon as far as my patients were concerned.

To each diverticulitis patient I handed a printed sheet listing high-fiber foods: fresh fruits, raw or lightly cooked vegetables, beans, seeds, nuts, and grains. Invariably, the patient would stuff the paper in her purse or maybe even leave it in my office. *Diet, really?* their blank stares seemed to say. *Just give me some meds and get me into surgery so I can get back to my regular life.*

To my disgrace, I didn't mind. I never actually believed my patients would increase their fiber. I am not sure I really believed it would make a difference. After all, as a surgeon, the primary relationship seemed between me and the disease. The patient was basically a bystander.

I was also doing a lot of cancer surgery, especially breast cancer. Of course, now I know how big a difference diet can make to this particular disease (see Chapter 13), but at the time I thought cancer was simply the result of bad luck. The good luck came in the form of my sharp knife and keen surgeon's eye, along with a few strong poisons.

Meanwhile, in response to the burgeoning obesity epidemic, a brand-new field had begun to emerge: weight-loss surgery. With the confidence—perhaps even the arrogance—of surgeons, we were certain that while diets had failed to stem the skyrocketing rates of obesity, surgery would succeed.

Enter the Bariatric Miracle

I'll tell you the truth, I was skeptical at first. I did not really believe that surgery could fix obesity.

Despite my growing waistline, I also harbored a bit of prejudice against the obese. At the time I had no understanding of the genetics of obesity or the hormones that control hunger. Like most people, I believed that overweight people lacked willpower. Now I think it's very sad that obesity has become one of the last bastions of acceptable discrimination while millions of Americans are suffering. When this obesity results from our national obsession with protein—as it all too often does—the situation is even sadder. And when that obsession with protein is supported—even promoted—by physicians, well, then, the situation is downright tragic.

But ten years ago I didn't know any of that, and, when my department chair asked me to enter this exciting new field, I agreed. In those early days, the concept was to cut the stomach into a small pouch and then join it to the intestine.

The reasoning behind this procedure is actually pretty interesting. Our bodies evolved in times of frequent famines, punctuated by an occasional feast. For weeks at a time, our ancestors grubbed along on whatever berries, grasses, or bark they could scrounge from a hostile environment. Then, every so often, they would encounter a bountiful harvest or conclude a successful hunt and have access to an abundance of calories.

In response, we evolved large stomachs that could stretch to accommodate that excess food. As agriculture developed, those same large stomachs filled up during harvest feasts, as our ancestors desperately tried to store body fat against the winter. (I realize the Paleo movement has told quite a different story about those early days, which we'll examine in Chapter 7.)

If you're not faced with starvation, however, you're likely confronting the opposite problem: obesity. With a fast-food restaurant on every corner, you're never very far away from your next meal. Even in the dead of winter, you're likely to get your three meals a day and then some. That stretchy stomach becomes a detriment when facing a 24/7 all-you-can-eat buffet.

To make matters worse, we evolved hormonal mechanisms that support a ravenous hunger and that cause us to crave sweet tastes. Of course, back when our ancestors evolved, "sweet" meant "fruit," or in case of a rare bonanza, honey. Now the closest many of us come to fruit is fruit-flavored Skittles, or the raspberry jelly inside our midmorning Krispy Kreme.

Enter the gastric bypass. By creating a smaller stomach, the surgery keeps us from the kind of overeating that our ancestors did occasionally but that we do on a regular basis. The surgery also bypasses the portions of the intestinal tract that produce our "hunger" hormones. Finally, by creating a direct passage for food to go into the intestine, the surgery creates intolerance to sugar and alters our sugar cravings.

I began doing gastric bypass at my hospital in early 2002 and immediately loved it. For a surgeon, this turns out to be a truly gratifying operation. It involves developing technical skills, which surgeons value, and it results in the immediate gratification we seek: take a problem, do some cutting, and the problem is visibly and immediately fixed. Again, the patient is simply a bystander. Their only job is to lie down on my OR table and let me do the rest.

Best of all, gastric bypass works extremely well. Patients on average lose 75 percent of their excess weight. The surgery has an 85 percent success in curing diabetes, and significant success in reducing high blood pressure, high cholesterol, and sleep apnea. I wasn't just listening to the statistics. I was watching the faces of my patients as, for the first time in their lives, they actually began to lose weight.

Those first few months of this surgical miracle, I felt as though I was starring in my own version of that movie *Awakenings*—in which Robin Williams plays doctor Oliver Sachs, a neurologist who brings a catatonic patient, played by Robert De Niro, back to life. As De Niro awakens, he is filled with wonder at being able to live again.

My patients had some of that same wonder. Most of them had been obese for their entire lives. They had done Atkins or a similar diet a dozen times—losing weight, gaining it back, losing it again, gaining it back. They never lost enough. And it always returned.

After my surgeries, though, they could finally succeed. For the first time in their lives, they didn't feel oversized, excessive, burdened by pounds and pounds of extra fat. For the first time in their lives, they felt normal.

I don't know if you've ever experienced losing a great deal of weight, but I can tell you that it's not just a cosmetic thing. You can move in a whole new way. Your body stops being your enemy. You feel lighter and freer. You can stroll down the street, walk up a hill, and even climb stairs without having to pause for breath. For the first time in a long time—maybe the first time since childhood—you feel comfortable in your own skin.

I would sit in my office for the follow-up visits, seeing one person after another come bounding through my door, showing off their new clothes, their new curves, their new stores of energy. Each time someone gave me a big hug and told me that I had changed their lives, I felt like an absolute hero, especially when I checked their labs and saw that they had finally escaped dangers of heart disease, diabetes, and stroke. I couldn't help thinking—and it wasn't just the God complex talking—*Wow, I really did save this person's life.*

The Honeymoon Ends

Bariatric surgery, as I mentioned, required everything from me and almost nothing from the patient. I sent them home with a prescription for some postoperative vitamins, a follow-up appointment, and a recommendation to eat a lot of protein. (I cringe to recall it, but we actually told them to eat their protein first.) What I didn't know then, but came to realize over time, was that the surgery didn't touch the root cause of obesity: the patient's terrible diet. And since that cause remained, not helped in the least by my pro-protein advice, some of my patients eventually started to gain back the weight.

Just as Oliver Sachs saw his patients slip back into their comas, I watched some of my own patients slide back into obesity. Three or four years after the surgery, I'd see them in my office, desperation in their eyes. *I've started to gain weight again,* they'd say. There were no sadder words.

It wasn't that the surgery hadn't worked. It actually works too well. For the first year following bariatric surgery, you can lose lots of weight even if you don't change your eating habits all that much. From double cheeseburgers to single cheeseburgers. From four eggs and six slices of bacon to two eggs and one slice of bacon. From a half chicken to a quarter chicken; from two pieces of fried fish to one. My patients were still eating lots of protein, dutifully following my advice.

Most people are forced to cut calories when their stomachs become so much smaller, so they do lose some weight. But that doesn't mean they are healthy. Bariatric surgeons know this now. We actually speak of a honeymoon phase—that first year or two when the weight just falls off regardless. Two or three years later, though, a sizable minority of my patients were back in for weight gain and/or nutritional deficiency. Some had fallen completely off the wagon and were not even trying to keep their weight in check. Some of them were trying very hard in the only way they knew how—cutting carbs and loading up on protein. It breaks my heart that I didn't know enough to tell them that it was protein that had helped to make them fat in the first place, and protein that was going to bring back the fat.

Meanwhile, the medical world agrees: Why bother with diet when you've got a dramatically effective surgery at your disposal? Conventional medicine now views weight-loss surgery as the only effective cure for obesity. But with more than 15 million U.S. residents who qualify for this procedure—or roughly 80,000 patients per qualified weight-loss surgeon—that's a heck of a lot of surgery. When you consider that the full surgery costs $25,000, or $18,000 for a bariatric sleeve, you can see the potential economic burden on the health-care system: a current backlog of up to $375 billion worth of surgery, with no end in sight.

And think about the larger implication: a medical system that sits idly by and waits for overweight people to become obese so they become candidates for this expensive surgery, rather than proactively teaching them to change their weight, their health, and their fate through better food choices.

Few things can kill the "God complex" more effectively than a patient desperately seeking guidance when you have nothing to offer. My knee-jerk instinct was to consider more surgery. Maybe we could make the stomach even smaller. But the research told me that surgery to reduce the stomach further would not work and was too dangerous to consider.

What if I went back in and changed the intestinal plumbing, creating a situation where food was not absorbed? Well, if food isn't absorbed in your intestines, it has to come out some way, and the resulting diarrhea can be rather bothersome. Also, if you aren't absorbing your food, you are also failing to absorb your nutrients. Vitamin deficiencies after malabsorption surgeries can be severe and debilitating.

Finally, in despair, I decided that the solution was exercise. I began telling all my patients to hire a trainer and begin slugging it out at the gym. Never mind that I was too run-down and exhausted to follow this advice myself. And so, as it turned out, were they.

Physician, Heal Thyself

So there I was in my thirties: happily married, working at one of Houston's premier hospitals, successful, well respected—and overweight. By this time, I was a full-out proteinaholic. I literally cannot remember eating a single vegetable, though I suppose I must have. I know I never ate a single meal without meat, though I was pretty fond of milk, eggs, and cheese, too. Whether it was breakfast bacon, barbecued chicken, deep-fried catfish, or a big, thick sizzling steak, my meals consisted of meat, meat, meat, and more meat.

I came by my condition honestly. I'd grown up eating this way, and just about everyone in my Texas world ate that way, too. All the experts I knew urged me to be a carnivore. Whenever I wanted to build muscle—something I never actually managed to do until I became a vegan—any trainer I hired pushed the protein solution as enthusiastically as if he was getting a commission on every bite of steak. One trainer even urged me to eat six chicken breasts each day. Six? When I later read about a massive European study associating chicken with obesity and lymphoma, I had to close my eyes and shudder.

Now here's the thing that, as a present-day vegan, really makes me laugh: although everyone is always asking me whether a plant-based diet is really healthy, nobody ever asked me the same question about eating meat. Nobody ever said, "Hey, Garth, are you getting in your RDA of six servings of fruits and vegetables?" Nobody said, "You know, Garth, the USDA recommends that we consume 35 grams of fiber each day, and since there's no fiber in animal foods, you better step up those beans, grains, and veggies." Nobody ever said, "My God, Garth, your omega-6 to omega-3 fat ratios are supposed to be 1 to 1, but yours is all the way up to 15 to 1! Quick, eat less animal fat (which is rich in omega-6s). Nope. Not a word about the well-documented associations between serum cholesterol and dietary saturated fat (which every piece of meat, chicken, and fish is loaded with, as are eggs and dairy products). Not a peep about the importance of antioxidants, flavonoids, vitamins, and minerals—the micronutrients that promote optimal function of just about every part of our bodies, and which you can only get enough of by eating loads of fruits, vegetables, grains, and beans. Eat cheeseburgers every day and nobody bats an eye, but order a salad for lunch and you'd think you'd just turned into one of those starving children featured on the 11 o'clock news.

I didn't ask myself, either, if my protein-heavy diet—and my avoidance of fruits and vegetables—might be responsible for my constant exhaustion and ever-increasing weight. Then, I had a series of experiences that served as my "hitting bottom"—getting to the point where I was finally ready to take responsibility for my own life.

Hitting Bottom

Wow, I thought, *this eye exam sure is taking longer than usual.* Although I wasn't nervous, I should have been, as my optometrist tried to tell me. When she backed away from her scope and looked at me with concern, I didn't even understand that she was worried. When she told me what she had found, it made no sense, to the point where her words didn't even register.

So she told me again—carefully, because she could see it wasn't getting through—that the small vessels of my eyes were filled with cholesterol.

The second time I heard her. Cholesterol? In my eyes? Wait a minute. I was no cardiologist, but even I knew that this type of excess cholesterol is rarely seen in a man my age. It's rarely ever seen in anybody. Usually you have to be well over fifty—or even older—with decades of exposure to high-fat foods.

Well, as much meat, eggs, and dairy as I consumed, I guess I had been overachieving. But disturbing as this news was, I was still a surgeon, secure in the bastions of Western medicine, and so I knew how to solve this problem: I would simply take a pill.

Sadly, this response was all too typical for me and my colleagues. We'd become so accustomed to disease that we were never very surprised by it. Coming out of medical school, I had the overwhelming feeling that we were dealt lemons for bodies—like poorly made cars that were bound to break. So although I wasn't thrilled with the diagnosis, high cholesterol seemed like such a fact of life that I hardly even considered it a disease.

Sure, there was the risk of heart disease, stroke, and a bunch of other dangers. But I could always rely on those magical meds.

It so happened that my wife was pregnant with our first child at the time, and I needed labs and a physical for a life insurance policy. Otherwise, I might not even have gotten myself checked out. But the labs confirmed what the optometrist had found, and then some. My cholesterol was through the roof. My liver function tests were also elevated, indicating that I now had fat growing in my liver. Throw in high blood pressure and elevated triglycerides, and it soon became clear I was fairly sick. Would I even live to see my child grow up? Rush through that life insurance policy!

I might have had a "God complex," but I was not completely blind. I knew quite well that meds can help but do not cure. Once you start taking a statin—the most common drug used to lower cholesterol—you are on it for life. Not for a year or two, not even for ten years. Forever.

It's not like you just pop the pill and go on about your day. Statins and similar medications have lists of complications that are a mile long. When I had to go over them with my patients, I could see the panic rising. After all, statins affect the heart, blood pressure, kidneys, bowels, and nervous system. They set us up for diabetes. They can cause brain fog so severe that some people have been misdiagnosed as having Alzheimer's. If you didn't need them to keep from stroking out, you might even think they violated the Hippocratic Oath.

Worse still, once you've been on meds for a while, many of them just stop working. I had quite a few patients who, in just three or four years, had bounced from one med to another to another to another, each with its own set of side effects and complications.

So when I left my doctor's office following all that lab work, I was pretty shaken up.

"Take this statin for cholesterol and this med for triglycerides," my doctor had told me, almost cheerfully running through the standard treatment. "And let's add a beta-blocker for blood pressure, but if you get dizzy or feel ill we will change to another. Now remember, if you get severe leg pains, let me know."

No big deal, right? Except I had just turned thirty-six and was now on three medications for life.

This wasn't even my first visit to the doctor that year. For the past decade, I'd been suffering from severe cramps and irritable bowel syndrome (IBS)—a condition that can truly spoil your life. Not to get too graphic about it, but every time I left the house, I had to know where the nearest bathroom was. I can remember sporting events, parties, and even dates ruined by me having to run for dear life. I'm kind of surprised that I made it through my wedding.

Yet conventional medicine is so inured to debilitating chronic conditions that none of my physicians seemed even slightly concerned, especially since my colonoscopy and endoscopy results showed "nothing to worry about." In other words, I had no tumor, no infection, and no structural issue—just an ongoing, chronic, and very painful malfunction of a basic part of my anatomy. "Irritable bowel is pretty common," my physician had said. He'd prescribed some pills, which hadn't helped.

IBS for the rest of my life? And now high cholesterol and fatty liver? I was getting somewhat depressed, although not actually alarmed, because in my view, everybody was dealing with this kind of thing in one way or another. Every one of my patients had either constipation or diarrhea. Some lucky patients had both, not to mention high blood pressure and skyrocketing cholesterol, too. I just assumed this was part of the fragile human condition.

Then came that fateful run up the stairs of Rice Stadium. I don't know why that got to me when I had somehow managed to brush off the scary lab work, the overweight, the fatigue, the IBS, and my patients' relapse rate. But that afternoon I looked at myself in the mirror and said no more. I didn't know then that proteinaholism was at the root of all my problems. But I was about to find out.

The Medical View of Disease

Before I could discover the truth about protein, and more generally about the awesome power of a plant-based diet to improve human health, I had to unlearn a whole array of invisible assumptions I'd picked up along with my medical training. The first is that disease just happens, usually without cause.

It seems strange to me now that in my entire medical career, I had never even wondered whether disease was necessary. I just assumed it was inevitable and focused on how to treat it. The patient, as I mentioned, wasn't enlisted as part of the battle—just me versus the disease.

This was the way all of us were trained—the way virtually every conventional physician in the United States is still trained. We spend thousands of hours studying disease but never even stop to consider why disease appears in the first place. For logical causation, we substituted what I can describe only as superstition: Cancer isn't the result of a systemic disequilibrium—it's an invasive monster. Heart disease isn't the logical outcome of excess fat and chronic inflammation—it's genetic bad luck. Diabetes isn't the product of a diet that consistently raises your blood sugars—it's just what happens to some people.

We view each disease as a lone villain—indeed, each condition is normally treated by its own separate doctor. If you have both heart disease and diabetes, you get two different specialists, each of whom prescribes a separate battery of meds and procedures. Most often, the two doctors don't even communicate with each other.

Worse yet was the fact that the patient was a side note in this battle. Patients were identified by their problem. The "colon cancer" in room 200 is ready for surgery. My fight was with the disease itself. This mind-set created a very aggressive notion of medicine. I must attack disease head on with surgery or medicine. Let's not get touchy-feely about the situation. There is a disease and it must be destroyed.

I have heard people accuse doctors of prescribing meds because drug companies bribe us, or because we make money by doing so. Surgeons are likewise accused of getting out the knife so that the patient will get out her wallet.

Sure, there are some bad apples in medicine. But the vast majority of doctors I know prescribe medications and surgeries because we've been taught that's the most effective way to combat disease. And after all our training and specialization, it feels unprofessional to say, "Eat better," instead of "Take 20 milligrams of Lipitor and schedule your open-heart surgery for next week."

Moreover, our patients are trained to demand quick fixes that require no effort on their part. They want us to take actions that feel dramatic and effective. Nobody wants to be told that they've caused their own problems by dining on steak or breakfasting on bacon. They want their problem treated—and in a way that they recognize. Most patients get very offended if you refuse to write them a prescription, especially if you suggest that they themselves are "at fault" (not what I say or mean, but sometimes what the patient hears) by not eating better or exercising more.

My Quest

I went along with the program because I really didn't know better—but I was beginning to feel like a hypocrite. I remember that as a medical student, I once attended a conference about lung cancer. While passionately presenting the latest treatments for this debilitating disease, one of the doctors actually held a cigarette! I watched, disgusted, as he pontificated about cancer between puffs. But me, with my paunch and my weak legs, telling my patients to eat healthy and go to the gym—was I really any better?

But now, sick and tired of this dysfunctional approach to weight loss and disgusted with my own role in it, I began my quest for a better way. So here I was staring myself down in the mirror. Overweight and suffering, I felt terrible, and my labs suggested I was sick and destined to the same chronic diseases my patients were suffering.

I also began getting a vision of a scene from *Star Trek IV,* where Doctor McCoy travels back in time to present-day Earth and is shocked at our health-care system. He is horrified by the barbaric nature of surgery, and if you think about it, he has a point.

All of a sudden everything I had been taught seemed wrong. How could the human body be so fragile? How could we be destined to disease? Was there some knowledge I was not taught in medical school that could help me address these diseases both personally and professionally? I vaguely recalled that there were countries where heart disease, cancer, diabetes, and obesity weren't nearly as prevalent as in the United States. Was it possible that they had something to teach us?

I vowed that I would go on a mission. My quest was to discover the perfect diet. I would search the world and search the scientific literature. I wanted to pick up where medicine dropped the ball. To do this I would study the cultures that don't suffer the typical Western diseases, and then decipher what they eat on a daily basis.

Equally important, I wanted to learn how I could change my own behavior. I didn't want to spend the rest of my life on drugs, getting sicker and fatter with each passing year. I didn't want to go on another diet, another short-term heroic sprint of willpower that would leave me more depleted and dejected than before. I wanted to truly change my life and come up with a protocol that could help change the lives of my patients.

Are you suffering like I was before I discovered the truth about protein? You can share your story and hear from others who have gone on to make remarkable recoveries at Proteinaholic.com.

CHAPTER 3

My Quest for the Ideal Human Diet

I sat in bed, the book propped open on my lap, my head spinning. This couldn't be true. And yet . . . it explained everything.

The volume was *The Blue Zones,* the first stop in my reeducation as a patient and a doctor. It looked at the longest-lived people in the world and described their lifestyles: how they ate, drank, exercised, worked, and socialized. The author, Dan Buettner, called these centers of longevity and health "blue zones." The overriding theme was that these blue zones had several traits in common, one being the reliance on a predominately plant-based diet.

Perhaps not surprisingly, this challenge to medical orthodoxy did not come from a doctor or even a research scientist. Buettner explored the world and wrote about it for *National Geographic* magazine. In 2005, he published a cover story about the longest-lived peoples in the world, which he then turned into the 2008 bestseller, *The Blue Zones.*

The book described a large body of research, as well as a series of National Geographic expeditions, that sought to answer the question: What do groups of people who live long, healthy lives do differently from the rest of us?

The question echoed one that had been growing in my own mind as I faced, day after day, a parade of increasingly sick patients, as well as my own growing health problems.

I was a highly trained surgeon, which arguably made me an expert on health and disease. I had skills and procedures and tools that could fight human frailty, but I never questioned whether that frailty, disease, and suffering was inevitable or in fact avoidable.

My quest began at precisely the moment I looked around the hospital at all the failing bodies and asked myself, *Does this have to be our destiny?*

I began by looking at epidemiology, the branch of medicine that studies the distribution and causes of disease and health. I wanted to broaden my perspective from that of the surgeon who simply sees a parade of diseased tissue and misbehaving organs completely cut off from the rest of life. I wanted to know, not just how to deal with disease and obesity, but if anyone had figured out how to avoid those conditions in the first place.

Epidemiological Research

Growing up in Texas, USA, it never occurred to me that America wasn't number one in everything. As the greatest country in the world, it stood to reason that we had the greatest health care, and the healthiest people. Then I read a sobering fact in a journal article: the United States spends significantly more on health care, per capita, than any other country (in fact, twice as much as our nearest competitor, Japan), but residents of about fifty other countries live longer than we do. I'm no Warren Buffett, but that didn't strike me as a particularly impressive return on investment.

I knew that other countries didn't have better technology, or more highly skilled practitioners, or more advanced clinical protocols. The answer had to lie somewhere else. That's when I cracked open *Blue Zones,* which was subtitled "9 Lessons for Living Longer from the People Who've Lived the Longest." The book profiled five "longevity hotspots" around the world, where the average life expectancy is much higher than the U.S. average, where older people remain vigorous and active and engaged, and where residents are up to ten times more likely than Americans, on average, to live to one hundred and beyond.

In bed that night, I began reading Chapter 3, "The Blue Zone in Okinawa." Along with the Seventh-day Adventists of Loma Linda, California, the Okinawans are the most rigorously studied of the Blue Zone populations. Good records and lots of verifiable data mean that the Okinawan experiment is much more science than story.

The subhead of the Okinawa chapter stopped me in my tracks: "Sunshine, Spirituality, and Sweet Potatoes." Sunshine, I could accept. Being active outdoors, gardening, walking—all that made sense, especially to me, with my life so busy I hardly had any time or energy for outdoor recreation or relaxation. Sure, long walks in the sunshine could definitely improve health, if you were lucky enough to have the energy and find the time.

Spirituality, likewise. I think the quest for meaning is a vital part of our development and aging.

But sweet potatoes? Come on—those are carbs. They'll make you fat and give you diabetes. Surely the Okinawans treated sweet potatoes as a condiment, a little color on the plate next to the meat that gave these folks their vitality. As it turned out, my prediction couldn't have been more wrong. The average Okinawan in 1950 was getting a whopping 69 percent of total calories from the purple sweet potato they call "imo," making it the number one staple food on the island. Before World War II, according to Buettner, the standard Okinawan greeting was not "Hello," but "Are you getting enough imo?"

All that sweet potato was not only providing a ton of carbs, it was also crowding out what I then believed to be the most important part of the human diet: protein. According to a 2007 study published in the *Annals of the New York Academy of Sciences,* protein provided only 7 percent of the calories in the Okinawan diet (Willcox, Willcox, et al. 2007, 2009; Sho 2001). That was unheard of—significantly below the U.S. recommended daily allowance, which was already scandalously low, in my opinion. Ten percent was the minimum required to prevent protein deficiency, not to thrive. And yet here was one of the longest-lived, most vigorous populations in the world, eating in direct contradiction to my unquestioning faith in protein. They lived well into their eighties and beyond, free of cancer, diabetes, heart disease, and Alzheimer's. They remained active, engaged, and vigorous. They had the life I wanted—the life my patients wanted.

The other Blue Zones also featured a predominantly plant-based diet. None of them were fully vegan or vegetarian, but meat and dairy and eggs were luxuries enjoyed regularly only by the wealthy, and just on festivals and special occasions by everyone else. The Sardinian peasants who enjoyed long, active lives ate lunches consisting of mostly bread, radishes, onions, fennel, and vegetable minestrone "to which the richest add some pasta." Most families ate meat once a week or less.

So here I was, giving my patients and readers the exact opposite advice, based on an unquestioned belief in the primacy of protein. My patients and I were getting sicker and fatter, while the Okinawans and Sardinians and the other Blue Zone populations were slim, active, and healthy into their eighties, nineties, and hundreds.

At that point I made a crucial decision: from now on, I would use science, rather than "common knowledge," to guide my recommendations. By itself, the Blue Zone data didn't constitute proof; I saw it more like a finger pointing in the direction of the truth. But it provided a useful litmus test: I would only promote a diet to my patients if there was a healthy population already eating that way. I had encountered data suggesting that plant-based diets contribute to human longevity. To maintain my protein-rich advice, I would have to find some equally compelling and well-documented examples of populations thriving on high-protein diets. How hard could that be?

As it turned out, impossible. The same basic dietary pattern—a minimally plant-based diet low in protein and fat and high in carbohydrates—featured in the Blue Zones also held sway in every other long-lived population on the planet. Every single one. In fact, it was hard to find traditional societies (those with a track record worth paying attention to, like hundreds or even thousands of years of success) that incorporated more than a little meat into their diets. The exceptions like the Inuit and the Maasai, much touted by the promoters of the high-protein Paleo myth, actually have dismal health and life expectancy (more on this later). Geography has even provided us with natural controlled experiments in which genetically homogeneous populations are separated into two areas, one eating more meat and the other eating more plants. In every case, the plant eaters live considerably longer, largely free of the diseases that plague their meat-eating relations.

The more I looked, the more I found. Previously unbeknownst to me, a number of researchers worldwide had compiled mountains of evidence correlating animal protein to various diseases that plague Western cultures. The EPIC trials, the giant Nurses' Health Study, the Adventist Health Study, and other long-term research all showed similar findings despite looking at dissimilar populations. Over and over, I kept finding evidence that animal protein was correlated with illness.

There is so much literature on the health effects of a plant-based diet, we can now list with confidence specific conditions and diseases that respond as well or better to nutritional improvement than any medical treatment: high blood pressure, obesity, diabetes, heart disease, stroke, irritable bowel syndrome, macular degeneration, cataracts, cancer, erectile dysfunction, rheumatoid arthritis, ulcerative colitis, diverticulitis, depression, dementia, gallstones, gout, and metabolic disease. And if you follow the literature, you can find new associations and causal links reported on a weekly basis.

Flash-forward: In January 2015, I presented at a conference organized by the Texas Association of Bariatric Surgery. I asked the audience if they had heard of the EPIC studies. No hands went up. The Adventist Health Study? Nada. The Nurses' Health Study out of Harvard? Nope. The Health Professionals Follow-up Study, also Harvard? More blank stares.

My point isn't how ignorant my colleagues are. Seven years ago I was in the same leaky boat. I knew what I knew, and what I knew was entirely based on the questions I was trained to ask. And the central question in American medicine is, "What do I do for this disease?"

What got me to jump out of that leaky boat and swim to the shore of nutritional sanity was simply a different question. Anyone who asks that question, "How can we become healthier?," ends up more or less where I've landed, if they aren't blinded by pride or money.

Evidence-Based Medicine

As I noted, the Blue Zone data and information from other population research was highly disturbing to my worldview and practice, but not enough by itself to change my recommendations. To practice true evidence-based medicine, I needed to see Western medical doctors treating their patients and improving their health outcomes with a low-protein diet.

Joel Fuhrman's book *Eat to Live* provided my first glimpse into a nutrition-based approach to treating and preventing disease through a plant-based diet. A doctor with a large and successful family practice in New Jersey, Fuhrman prescribes dietary excellence—what he calls "nutritarianism"—as a first treatment for most of the ailments of which his patients complain. Unlike almost all other GPs, he doesn't "manage" his patients' health woes with pharmaceutical drugs. Rather, he shows them how to eliminate most of their symptoms by addressing the root causes— principally, the standard American diet.

I've since discovered dozens, if not hundreds of other doctors who practice medicine this way. Several of them were featured in the popular and hugely important 2011 documentary *Forks Over Knives*. I'm now proud to include myself among their number. But "hundreds" is still a shamefully small percentage of the physicians in this country, most of whom still believe that our proteinaholic diet has nothing to do with our multiple epidemics of chronic disease and obesity.

One problem is that doctors in private practice can talk all they want about their patients' improved outcomes, but their accounts are dismissed as "anecdotal" by the research community. Luckily, several of the doctors promoting healthy diets have managed to put together clinical trials and get them published. As I pored over the results achieved by the patients of clinicians who treated patients with a plant-based diet, I became more and more convinced that the evidence sides entirely with those of us who prescribe from the "farmacy" rather than the pharmacy.

Opposing Research

There was still a part of my proteinaholic brain that wasn't willing to concede defeat just yet. *What about all the other studies?* it demanded. *What about all the research showing that eating meat, drinking milk, and consuming large numbers of eggs is good for us?* I had to resolve that contradiction before I could start sharing a whole new gospel of nutrition with my patients. I didn't want to jump from one belief system to another; I wanted to examine all the evidence and, at long last, make up my own mind.

There are many, many studies that purport to show that large quantities of protein—and animal protein, specifically—are good for us. Since they contradict the evidence of the Blue Zones and other population studies, how can they coexist with that research?

I discovered that all the pro-protein studies have a couple of things in common. First, they're all really short. As in, they follow their subjects for days or weeks—seldom longer than a year. Do you know anyone who went on a high-protein shake diet and lost a staggering amount of weight in the first three months? If so, how were they doing at the end of a year? Almost no one can sustain that diet for longer than a couple of months. If your study cutoff point is twelve weeks, then you can trumpet the amazing weight-loss potential of the shake. If you follow your subjects for a couple of years, you have to paint a very different picture.

Second, these studies focus on what are called "biomarkers" rather than meaningful health outcomes. Examples of biomarkers include systolic blood pressure, level of LDL cholesterol, and PSA (prostate specific antigen). Doctors pay a great deal of attention to these biomarkers because they are believed to be "markers" of health: high blood pressure is correlated with heart disease, for example.

It's easy to understand why biomarkers are used as study outcomes. First, they can change much more rapidly than health, which makes them conducive to short studies. They are often inexpensive and convenient to measure. They are "objective," unlike things like "quality of life" and "vitality."

There are many problems with using biomarkers. First, they may not predict what we think they predict. Second, even if high cholesterol predicts cardiovascular disease, that doesn't mean that lowering cholesterol artificially, as in the case of statin drugs, affects the incidence of strokes or heart attacks. It may be that the biomarker level itself is a symptom, rather than cause, of the disease it supposedly predicts. Worst, if you're on a fishing expedition to show that a big glass of milk can "do a body good," there are an almost infinite number of biomarkers you can look at until you find a couple that do respond positively to milk protein.

A third commonality to most of the pro-protein studies: they suffer from small sample sizes, sometimes looking at just a few people utterly unrepresentative of the general population. Others extrapolate findings from animal research, or even experiments carried out in test tubes. Let's say that you had a penny, and you wanted to prove it was "loaded" (that is, tossing it wouldn't give you an equal number of heads and tails). If you tossed it ten thousand times, and it was an honest penny, you'd expect to see roughly five thousand heads and five thousand tails.

Suppose it was an honest penny, but you wanted to claim that it favored heads. All you'd have to do is perform one thousand different trials, in which the penny was flipped ten times each. Then simply publish all the trials in which heads appear more than tails, and ignore the rest.

Does research really happen this way, or am I just unbelievably cynical?

Consider that most of the pro-protein studies are funded by the very industries that stand to benefit the most from the findings. The Dairy Council, Egg Board, Beef Council, and other industry groups (and front groups claiming impartiality) support many of the research scientists who produce a steady stream of pro-protein research. Additionally, there's a well-known (in academia) phenomenon known as "publication bias." It means that certain types of findings are much more likely to get published than others. "Interesting" findings—and by that I mean findings that give people good news about their favorite bad habits—are much more likely to find the light of day in a scientific journal than studies that confirm a boring fact like "you should eat more vegetables."

Bigger Issues

I started reading about a plant-based diet out of concern for my own health. That concern quickly grew to include the well-being of my patients. And before I knew it, my motivation expanded twice more, to include concern for our environment and the welfare of the animals I had been mindlessly consuming for so long. The catalyst was a book by John Robbins, onetime heir to the Baskin-Robbins ice cream fortune who renounced his inheritance when he discovered the harmful effects of animal product consumption at every level. In his epic *The Food Revolution* (an update to his earlier, groundbreaking *Diet for a New America*), Robbins lays out as clearly and forcefully as possible the environmental damage done to our planet by animal agriculture.

He also opened my eyes to the fact that the steak on my plate had come from a living creature that had been born, raised, fed, and slaughtered with unbelievable cruelty, and that milk came from cows hooked up to milking machines, housed in crowded conditions in their own feces, never seeing the light of day or tasting grass, and fed a steady diet of hormones to increase production and antibiotics to keep them from dying of disease.

I also read Jonathan Safran Foer's *Eating Animals*, an open and hard-hitting answer to the author's sincere question, *If I really knew the realities of animal agriculture, could I still eat meat?* At the book's conclusion, Foer couldn't. And now, no longer, could I.

Had the science not shown a clear-cut benefit to reducing animal protein, I may have still pursued a vegan diet due to all I had learned about the ethics of animal agriculture and its effect on our environment. However, I would have never recommended it to my patients. I take pride in practicing evidence-based medicine. Turns out the science shows that what is good for our bodies is also good for our environment—and obviously for the animals we eat.

My Personal Transition

I would love to tell you that once I was armed with all this information about the health, environmental, and ethical problems with my protein-aholism, I woke up one day, decided to give up all animal products, and never looked back. Unfortunately (or rather fortunately for the hundreds of patients I've been able to counsel more effectively thanks to my experiences), it didn't work out that way.

I did start with a bang. As my wife was in the hospital giving birth to our first child, I vowed, *Things are going to change.* I wanted to be there for birthdays, lost teeth, first crushes, graduations, a wedding, grandchildren. My cholesterol-filled eyes welled with tears at the thought that I was eating my way to an early grave.

That day I ate my first-ever (to my memory) meatless meal. I remember it to this day—steamed vegetables and rice.

I didn't like it.

I hated vegetables. I didn't know how to cook. I didn't know anyone who ate this way.

My frame of reference around food was meat. So I ate the vegetarian equivalent: veggie burgers. I ate them at every meal. For every meal. They were okay—not meat, but bearable. And they certainly weren't making me feel a whole lot better. After a month of this, I had my cholesterol checked again. It had dropped somewhat.

For some reason, at that point I went back to eating meat for a while. The addiction was still strong, obviously. I wasn't feeling amazing. My numbers hadn't shifted so dramatically. But during this time I was really getting into the ethical and environmental impact of meat eating. Honestly, if I had eliminated meat only for personal reasons, that wouldn't have been enough for me. It was the videos of cows being slaughtered, the in-my-face reality of where that flesh came from, that brought me back for try after try.

Eventually, I was able to eliminate meat once and for all. Except for fish, because, well, I still felt like I needed some animal protein. (It's amazing how many contradictory beliefs one human being can hold!) That went well for a while, but my reading kept pulling me more and more in the direction of my values. Fish were also living creatures, large-scale fishing was an environmental disaster perhaps even worse than livestock farming, and farmed fish meat was just about as harmful to my health as any other kind. There's nothing good in fish that we can't get from plants, minus the sky-high mercury levels that appeared on my blood tests during my pescetarian phase.

I finally understood the great Czech-German writer Franz Kafka's decision to become a vegan. Looking through the glass at an aquarium, he is reported to have told the fish, "Now I can at last look at you in peace. I don't eat you anymore."

Dairy was the last thing to go. If I was a proteinaholic, it turned out that I was a double-cheese-aholic. There's a good biological explanation: chemicals in cheese called casomorphins actually mimic the effects of the real morphine in our brains and bodies.

In addition, cheese is everywhere. In salads. In vegetable main dishes. In sauces. Eliminating dairy forced me to take a hard look at myself, and at the values I now called my own. I started asking myself, *With all I know about the dairy industry, what am I doing consuming dairy?* Finally, I let it go. It got much easier over time, to the point where going dairy-free is completely effortless.

My wonderful wife, who supported me every step of the way, began cooking true plant-based meals as she recovered from childbirth. To be fair, she was only too happy to get me onto a different health track, as she had witnessed my gradual decline. What new mother wouldn't have been a little worried to be married to a thirty-seven-year-old "obesity expert" with high cholesterol, hypertension, and a growing belly? Without her support and guidance this would have been much harder.

A good cook, she relished the challenge of exploring the vast world of vegetables and whole grains that now made up my diet. My research, and my decision to act on it, spurred her to explore a whole new world of food. Think about it—how many different kinds of meat are there? Just a few. But there are thousands of different varieties of fruits and vegetables, nuts and seeds, beans and legumes, herbs and spices. You could literally spend your whole life coming up with new dishes and combinations of flavors and textures that had never been tried before. When you consider that just twelve plants and five animals compose about 75 percent of the world's food, and that there are approximately 300,000 known edible plant species (150 of which are in common use around the world), you can see that there's a lot of as yet unexplored culinary landscape for plant-based eaters.

Flash-forward: These days, when I go out to eat with friends at nice restaurants, I always ask the waiter if the chef can prepare a meal to my requirements. Invariably, I end up with the best-looking and best-tasting meal. Often the chefs personally present the dishes, so full of pride are they at their beautiful creations.

In addition to my wife's growing culinary skills, we found a delivery service in Houston that provided prepared plant-based meals, and I steadily progressed from veggie burgers to a more varied diet.

Slowly, I began exploring the world of plant-based eating. I discovered beans. I tried different vegetables. If I didn't like them the first time, I tried them again. And again. One day I found that I actually enjoyed the taste of kale. When I felt a meat craving, I replayed the slaughter videos in my mind. Eventually I was able to reprogram my taste buds to enjoy and look forward to eating produce, and to produce a disgust reaction at the thought of eating meat.

While I don't necessarily recommend this strategy to anyone trying to get animal products out of their diet, I will say that it worked considerably better than allowing myself occasional "treats" of animal products. No matter the diet, the concept of the "Cheat Day" is a disempowering and dangerous one. People who eat strictly for six days a week and then binge on their favorite "forbidden foods" on day seven spend the entire week fantasizing about that cheeseburger. Whatever you do, don't elevate the food you're trying to eliminate to mythic status in your mind. In Chapters 16 and 17, you'll get concrete suggestions for making the transition.

"Where Do You Get Your Protein?"

It's funny: when I ate meat, no one ever asked about my nutrition or my health. As I turned to a more plant-based diet, people began freaking out. On a daily basis, I started hearing the question that all vegetarians and vegans must face from their friends, family, coworkers, and even casual acquaintances: "Where do you get your protein?"

As I began eating more plants and fewer animals, people began to treat me like I was some sort of freak. They considered such a move to be ill advised. I would surely wither away. My health would fail and I would languish. Of course, this is rather odd coming from a group of people who, for the most part, were overweight, and far from thriving on their high-protein diets.

The irony of asking someone who follows a plant-based diet how they will keep healthy without the vital nutrients found in animals is lost on most of the meat-eating world. In my office, I check labs on everybody who comes to see me for weight loss. Let me tell you, meat eaters have extremely poor nutritional labs. They are predictably deficient in vitamin D, folate, thiamine, vitamin A, and even B_{12}.

What about my vegetarian patients? I cannot really answer that, because I don't have many. Vegetarians don't, for the most part, end up in a weight-loss clinic. In over ten years, I can think of just one who came to see me, a woman hooked on vegan cookies and cupcakes. Despite her penchant for baked goods, her lipids were stellar and she did not show any vitamin deficiencies. Even more impressive, she had no heart disease or diabetes.

People universally thought my diet was "extreme." I could understand where they were coming from, since I had held the same opinion just a few months earlier. But when I discovered the work of pioneering surgeon Caldwell Esselstyn, M.D., who was able to reverse heart disease in patients who had been told to go home and get their affairs in order by the medical establishment, I tended to agree with his assessment:

"Some people think the 'plant-based, whole foods diet' is extreme. Half a million people a year will have their chests opened up and a vein taken from their leg and sewn onto their coronary artery. Some people would call that extreme."

Many friends and colleagues pity me for my refusal to partake in what they consider to be gourmet food. They think I am missing out on the "finer" things in life. Even when I convince them that my diet is helping me live a long, happy life, this doesn't change their assessment that I am giving up too much. Most people reply that they would rather be unhealthy and die young, so long as they can live now. The inference being, of course, that I am missing out on life. They believe I am struggling to be healthy just so that I can eke out a few more years in the end, hooked up to tubes and monitors in the old age home, watching reruns of *Big Medicine* on TLC.

At least people do admire what they assume to be amazing willpower on my part. As they see it, I am struggling every day to avoid foods I crave and stomaching foods that taste terrible in order to reach some far-off goal. To many, I have some sort of yogic power over the senses. I understand this viewpoint, as it's based on the assumption that I share their cravings for the typical American food and lifestyle. After all, who doesn't love a big, juicy steak? The truth, that it is not at all hard for me to turn down a steak, or a chicken, or a donut, never crosses their minds.

It does not take superhuman willpower for me to decline a double cheeseburger, because I find cheeseburgers repulsive. My friends watch a fast-food commercial and crave the cheeseburger, thinking how great it tastes. I look at a picture of a cheeseburger and think how ugly it looks, so bland and colorless. I also picture the greasy stove where the meat was cooked, all black and oily. I picture some teenage kid listlessly flipping the frozen meat without any care for its preparation. I picture the slaughter-house where that meat actually came from. I imagine the horrible life and death of the cow itself, not to mention all the chemicals and antibiotics it was fed before its flesh was mixed with "pink slime" to become ground meat. I then picture that slime building up in my vessels and invading the cells that make up my body. Finally, and maybe most important, I picture how I would feel after eating that burger. Following a possible moment of initial enjoyment, I would begin to feel bloated and disgusted. I would get indigestion and experience fatigue. I can even picture the fat forming on my organs and slowing me down, sapping my vigor and will to live.

Offer me an avocado and kale salad, on the other hand, and just watch Pavlov's response kick in. The beauty of all the colors in a great salad really gets my juices flowing. I marvel at the care and preparation of the salad, and I picture the love that went into growing the vegetables on the organic farm. Most of all I can feel the salad, as corny as it may sound, nurturing my body. I feel myself grow stronger with each bite.

So it is no great feat for me to pass up the meat. Nor is it some Spartan chore to eat vegetables. I am just like everyone else. I seek things that make me feel good and avoid things that I just don't like. The difference is simple yet profound: unlike most people, I have trained myself to be more attuned to what is really good for me and what is not, and thereby changed my tastes. Rather than feeling deprived, I am privileged to have discovered and mastered a new and rewarding lifestyle. I don't live this way to be healthier when I am old or to live longer. I have adopted this new lifestyle because it makes me feel vibrant right now. As William Temple wrote, "Health is the soul that animates all the enjoyments of life." No truer words have been spoken. My quest for the right way to eat has truly set me free from all my old desires.

Getting Better All the Time

As I hit my plant-based stride, I began noticing how much better I felt. I had never, even as a child, experienced that kind of energy before. I had always thought it was normal to want to lie down after eating. The kind of fatigue and crappy feeling that had accompanied my meat-heavy meals had completed disappeared. Now I had excess energy to burn. I literally had to start exercising to keep from driving myself (and probably everyone else) crazy. Instead of forcing myself to sprint the stairs to avoid looking like a fool for the *Houston Chronicle,* I started training for long-distance races because I couldn't help myself.

More dramatically, my irritable bowel disease symptoms vanished. If you haven't suffered personally from this affliction, you can't begin to imagine how its absence improved my life. I could go out and enjoy myself without constantly plotting the shortest route to the nearest bathroom. When you've gone without it for so long, good health actually feels like its own sensation, rather than the absence of pain or discomfort or fatigue. My body was practically singing in appreciation of its newfound potential for movement and joy.

The changes cascaded into continuous improvement. I found that the more salads I ate, the more dark green and raw vegetables I added to my diet, the better I felt. My tastes continued to change to support the new way of eating. I fell in love with the rainbow of colors available on a plant-based diet, and with the accompanying crazy variety of tastes. No longer forcing myself to feel disgust when I thought of meat, I began to pity my dining companions for the blandness of their meat-filled plates. I couldn't wait to jump up and fill my plate at the salad bar for lunch.

On the true plant-based diet, my cholesterol plummeted, as did my blood pressure. The food played a direct role, and also allowed me to begin my life as an athlete, which did further wonders for my health.

My foray into competitive races after a lifetime of not being an athlete of any kind was inspired by some of my bariatric patients. After a lifetime of lying on the couch, they got up after the surgery and totally reinvented themselves as they lost weight. Some of them actually started running marathons, which made me think that perhaps I could someday do the same. I remember wondering, *How do these people find the courage to get up and run?* I looked for, and found, a source of inspiration in myself as I got stronger and healthier, day by day. My mantra became, "*Impossible* is a dare." Having spent my life in a rut, I wasn't going to allow myself to stay there.

A friend of mine ran triathlons and introduced me to that world. I set a daunting goal for myself as I prepared for my first one in 2009: train by running twenty miles per month. I competed in, and finished, a triathlon and a few marathons, and then asked myself what would become a recurring question: *What else can I do that I never thought I could do before?*

The answer came at once: complete an Ironman, a grueling event consisting of a 2.4-mile swim, 112-mile bike ride, and 26.2-mile run consecutively in a single day. "Despite"—I now know it was because of—my lack of animal protein, I was able to do it in a very respectable time. My goals have expanded, now that I'm in the eighth year following my initial recovery from proteinaholism. Now I'm no longer satisfied to merely finish the races. I'm looking to turn in competitive times, like the 3-hour, 25-minute marathon I'm itching to run to qualify for the Boston Marathon. I want to start finishing in the top ten in my age bracket, so I can become an even stronger voice and role model for the health and overall benefits of the plant-based lifestyle. I want to reach all the struggling athletes who have hit what looks like a nonnegotiable plateau, working out like mad and taking the trainer's advice to eat six chicken breasts a day for endurance and strength.

My personal growth preceded and supported my professional transformation into a very different kind of doctor. I'll talk about that in Part III. Before that, however, I want to unpack the evidence that I gathered during my quest for nutritional sanity. It took me months of intense research to arrive at these conclusions; in the next few chapters I'll share that journey in some detail. My goal is to equip you to make your own decision, rather than just take my word for it.

Ready to find out how protein achieved its vaunted place in our nutritional mythology, and why we're all so confused about nutrition? Let's explore the protein problem . . .

Have I qualified for the Boston Marathon yet? Follow my progress, and share your own, at Proteinaholic.com.

PART TWO

How We Became Proteinaholics

CHAPTER 4

The History of Protein

I grew up with an unchallenged belief in the nutritional supremacy of protein. It was sown in childhood, reinforced by society, and echoed by my medical mentors and peers. It was such an obvious fact, I had no reason to question it for almost four decades. Once I discovered that this was a story, not an incontrovertible fact, I became angry—and also curious. I wanted to know how I, and so many others, had been duped. Who crowned protein king, and why? Why hadn't science deposed the false sovereign? What financial and political interests kept that king in power? What I've found out is instructive, and also not a little bit disturbing. Let's take a walk back in time to before proteinaholism was the norm, to see how we got here.

When Only the Rich Ate Meat

For those of us who have grown up since the 1950s, it's hard to believe how much less animal protein people used to consume. Many immigrants to this country were still eating their own national diets, which, out of economic necessity, were primarily plant based. The Irish survived on oatmeal, bread, and potatoes. The Italians lived on pasta, beans, bread, and tomatoes, as well as colorful salads and creatively prepared vegetables. The

Eastern Europeans relied on borscht and similar vegetable soups, as well as on sauerkraut, potatoes, dumplings, and bread. The Chinese diet was all rice, soy, and vegetables, and, in some cases, bread. Later generations of Asian, African, and Latin American immigrants had similar plant-based diets.

In all these communities, meat was a luxury—something used in tiny amounts to flavor a soup, stuff a dumpling, add heft to a sauce. Once a week, there might be a festive meal based around a roast or a chicken, but even then, portions would be far, far smaller than we are used to today. Meat was such a costly way to store calories, it was reserved for special occasions and emergencies.

For today's immigrants, the same holds true. Even countries that eat meat frequently do so in significantly smaller portions than in the standard American diet. A Senegalese stew, for example, might have two or three small chunks of meat per person, served in a sauce of onions and other vegetables, all on a large helping of rice. A traditional Chinese stir fry—as opposed to what you get in a U.S. restaurant—is primarily vegetables and spices served over rice, with perhaps a few small chunks of beef, chicken, or tofu thrown in. In traditional cultures, meat is almost always a condiment—rarely the star of the meal.

Whatever the national diet, the rich ate far more animal protein in the form of meat, poultry, fish, eggs, and dairy products. And everywhere we look, the rich tended to weigh more. As you'll see later in this book, that's not an accident—the protein was making them fat. However, before obesity exploded into an epidemic, being portly—or even massively fat—was considered almost praiseworthy, as clear evidence of prosperity. Look at the photographs of some of our largest U.S. presidents: Millard Fillmore, Grover Cleveland, William Howard Taft. No one worried about those men's health or whispered that they needed to muster up some more willpower. They were admired, not ridiculed, for their girth.

If we want to understand how protein became king, we have to understand the context. In an environment of scarcity, it's almost impossible to become overweight. So it didn't matter that animal protein made you fatter: when you're trying not to starve to death, a little excess body fat is a good thing. Likewise, when life expectancies are short, you tend to worry less about the long-term consequences of a food—the way it might someday contribute to diabetes, or heart disease, or cancer. Who can think that far ahead, when the long, cold winter is now?

It was in a context of short, hungry lives that European scientists first began to study protein in the late seventeenth century. Toward the end of the seventeenth century and beginning of the eighteenth century, scientists began to study the makeup of the human body. During that study of the body, a Dutch chemist named Gerardus Mulder first discovered the chemical structure of protein. The word *protein* came from the Greek "proteos," meaning "of prime importance."

Scientists in those centuries got one thing right: they understand that "human meat"—our muscles, organs, and skin—is composed primarily of protein. But they leapt to an erroneous conclusion that plagues us to this day: that because we are protein, we need to eat protein. Hence the concept of "prime importance" began to refer to its place in our diets, rather than in our physical structures.

Of course, we do need to consume protein. We just don't need nearly as much of it as those scientists believed. And, we know now, we don't need to source our protein from animals—we can get all we need from plants (in fact, just like many animals do!).

Can you see how our scientific introduction to protein led us astray? For most of human history, we survived just fine on a plant-based diet, and that is how the longest-lived, healthiest people on the planet are eating to this day. But when scientists started trying to figure out what we should eat, they based it not on demonstrable outcomes but rather on a false analogy.

Early Plant-Based Advocates

Despite the growing reputation of protein as the "ultimate food" (whether you could afford it or not), some people did stand up for plant-based diets. The nineteenth-century American minister Sylvester Graham, of Graham cracker fame, was a staunch supporter of vegetarianism. He cited biblical verses like Genesis 1:29–30: "Behold, I have given you every plant yielding seed that is on the surface of all the earth, and every tree which has fruit yielding seed; it shall be food for you; and to every beast of the earth and to every bird of the sky and to every thing that moves on the earth which has life, I have given every green plant for food."

Like many reformers of his time, Graham advocated a number of other causes, including temperance and sexual abstinence. As a minister, he thought sex was sinful and believed that our lustful urges were fueled by a diet rich in meat, cheese, and butter. Stick to simple, plant-based fare, and, Graham preached, your ungodly urges would subside to manageable levels. Not exactly the best advertising for a plant-based diet, I have to say! It's no wonder his ideas didn't catch on.

It's too bad they didn't, because Graham was years ahead of his time. He advocated not just a vegetarian diet, but one that focused on clean, pure, whole foods. His "Graham bread" was made from unsifted flour and prepared without chemical additives, such as the alum and chlorine then used by commercial bakers. (Yes, they had preservatives and additives back then, too!) As I just mentioned, Graham's bread is the ancestor of today's "Graham cracker," so next time someone breaks out the S'mores at a campfire, feel free to imagine Sylvester turning in his grave.

Graham's views might have been unpopular, but they were opposed by powerful interests. The butchers and commercial bakers of Boston were so worried about his stance against meat and preservatives that they threatened to riot when Graham was scheduled to speak in their city.

My favorite argument of Graham's, which has lost no validity over the years, is that orangutans and gorillas clearly prove that you don't need meat or dairy products to remain strong. As a fit and healthy "Ironman" vegan, I heartily agree! (We'll fully debunk the "vegans are weak" myth in Chapter 16.)

Despite Graham's thunderous sermons and evidence-based arguments, animal foods only grew in popularity. Over the nineteenth and twentieth centuries, a number of factors have combined to create a halo effect around meat:

- Meat promotes excess weight and the creation of body fat, a useful quality in times of scarcity.

- Our bodies are themselves "meat."

- Only the rich could afford meat.

And thus was meat crowned king! The poor, who envied the wealthy, could not afford carriages and mansions and servants, but they could emulate the rich by putting their extra coins into the minor extravagance of fish or beef. And in an America obsessed with rags-to-riches opportunity tales and operating under the Protestant idea that worldly wealth was a divine thumbs-up on the state of one's soul, almost everyone wanted to fortify their bodies and celebrate their successes with the stuff of life itself, animal protein.

At the risk of sounding obvious, there are several important differences between these early days and our own.

First, no matter what the scientists recommended, only a few people could afford to eat much animal protein of any kind: meat, fish, dairy, or eggs. It's not like today, when one Atkins or Paleo bestseller sends hundreds of thousands of people to the butcher counter on a daily basis.

And second, with a few exceptions, even the frequent meat eaters consumed far, far smaller amounts of animal protein than you'd find in today's American diet. Even in the 1950s, when meat was becoming the star of most American meals, portions were smaller than they are now. So even though meat was our monarch, it still held a tenuous hold on our stomachs, if not our appetites.

Science Marches On

Scientists continued to study protein throughout the nineteenth and early twentieth centuries. However, their experiments didn't always meet today's standards, and the researchers didn't always draw logical conclusions from their data.

For example, the German physiologist Dr. Carl von Voit studied the diets of late-nineteenth-century laborers and found that they ate about 118 grams of protein per day. Von Voit then made a couple of classic errors. He confused description with prescription, and he extrapolated from heavy laborers to the population at large. He assumed that the workers ate what their bodies needed, so therefore 118 grams of protein must be the optimal daily amount for everyone.

Of course, we can imagine lots of reasons why a group of people—especially an impoverished group of laborers—would eat a less-than-ideal diet. We don't know what other foods they had access to, for example, or what other foods they had the facilities to store or cook. But von Voit concluded from his data that 118 grams of protein should be our daily target.

Von Voit's 118 grams quickly became the floor, not the ceiling of recommended daily protein intake. By the time Yale chemist Russell Henry

Chittenden began studying the question in a more scientific matter, the medical consensus advocated a whopping 130 grams of protein per day. Chittenden, a rare voice of sanity at the time, pointed out that excess protein breaks into potentially toxic nitrogen components. Chittenden's experiments on himself, athletes, and military men proved that even people with active lifestyle could thrive on less than half that number. His recommendation: just 62 daily grams. His conclusions had little impact, drowned out as they were by the medical love affair with ever-increasing amounts of protein, and the fact that no one was dying of obesity or other diseases of overconsumption at that time.

Why did these nineteenth-century and early-twentieth-century physicians advocate such copious amounts of protein? After all, even in the nineteenth and twentieth centuries, researchers using the best scientific tools available at the time demonstrated clearly that a low-protein, plant-based diet was the healthiest way to live.

The answer I've come up with has to do with the difference between chronic and infectious diseases. It's going to take a moment to get to the connection here, so bear with me.

A chronic disease results from a kind of disequilibrium in the system, most often caused by diet, toxic burden, lack of exercise, poor sleep, and/or stress. Chronic diseases take years to develop, and once you have one, you're permanently—chronically—sick unless you are able to make a huge systemic change. Chronic diseases—obesity, heart disease, diabetes, cancer, and the like—are the real health challenges of our time. That's why I'm so concerned with protein, because of the way it promotes chronic disease.

But I can only have that concern because, in the developed world, we have largely eliminated (at least temporarily) the threat of deadly infectious diseases. This major advance in infectious disease control occurred beginning in the 1950s, partly because of the widespread use of antibiotics (invented in the 1940s) and partly because of the improvements in water, sewage, health codes, and other public health improvements.

Before that, the disease environment was completely different. Many poor and working-class people were malnourished and subject to unhygienic living and working conditions in both cities and rural areas. They were highly susceptible to any bacterium or virus that crossed their path. In cities where people lived in close quarters, sharing the same dirty water and poor sanitation, an infectious disease would ravage a neighborhood with frightening speed. Influenza, tuberculosis, typhoid, polio, dysentery, measles, mumps, scarlet fever, and sexually transmitted infections regularly tore through the population, and if you were a physician in that era, treating those outbreaks was your main concern.

To a pre-1950s physician, animal meat must have seemed like a godsend. It helped people put on some body fat so they could withstand hunger. That extra body fat might also make the difference between resisting or succumbing to the ravages of disease—you don't want to be underweight when you come down with a major infection. With food so scarce and hard labor so common, obesity simply wasn't a concern for the vast majority of the population. And given that the average U.S. life expectancy at the turn of the century was only forty-six, if there were long-term negative consequences to excess protein consumption, few people would live long enough to suffer from them.

The problem is that Western medicine is still practiced as though we live in that bygone era. While it was possible to fortify some malnourished people against infectious disease by feeding them meat, the diseases themselves were still going to have their way. The only way to fight them effectively was through the tools of public health—sanitation, vaccination, education. In contrast, an individual can all but eliminate the risk of most chronic diseases through healthy diet and lifestyle. My medical colleagues still put their faith in pills and surgeries, the tools that were developed for—and triumphed against—infectious disease and traumatic injury. The diet they recommend corresponds to this outdated worldview as well. And they give lip service, at best, to the notion that the chronic diseases that disable and kill most Americans are almost entirely preventable by a very different diet, one in which protein is no longer "of prime importance."

The Evidence Mounts

Despite their cheery assurances of the salvational effects of high-protein diets, the medical establishment could not completely ignore the negative consequences of these diets. On September 24, 1907, a front-page headline in the *New York Times* proclaimed, "Cancer Increasing Among Meat Eaters." The article reported on a seven-year study linking meat consumption with a higher risk of cancer and suggested that part of the problem was the way immigrants were switching from their traditional plant-based diets to meat-rich fare once they began to establish themselves in America. The lead researcher was quoted as saying, "There cannot be the slightest question that the great increase in cancer among the foreign-born over the prevalence of that disease in their native countries is due to the increased consumption of animal foods."

In other words, the evidence that was later compiled in the Blue Zones explorations was obvious, even back in 1907. Scientists could already tell that immigrants' health declined when they began to prosper in America, against all expectations. And even back then, some scientists believed that animal protein was at the heart of the problem.

Ignoring the 1907 study, the U.S. government championed the concept that meat should be the star of every meal. In an insane conflict of interest, the U.S. Department of Agriculture (USDA) was charged in 1865 with both promoting the economic welfare of farmers and ranchers, and determining and promoting nutritional recommendations to the public. The political influence and money of the meat, dairy, and egg industries tipped the balance of USDA policy firmly to the "meat on every plate at every meal" side, public health be damned. The USDA maintained this position from 1913 to 1979 (Nestle 1999).

Despite the warnings of populists like Graham and scientists like Chittenden, U.S. meat consumption continued to grow, tracked closely by increasing rates of cancer, heart disease, and obesity. USDA figures show that meat eating rose from 124 pounds per person per year in 1909 to 201.5 pounds in 2004, an increase in less than five generations of an astounding 63 percent. The rise in milk, cheese, and yogurt consumption has been even greater.

Then, in the late 1950s, came that medical watershed I have already described: for the first time in human history, our biggest threats came not from infectious diseases and malnutrition, but rather from chronic disease and rising obesity.

I don't want to overdramatize the change; many people around the planet were still at much greater risk of infection and starvation than of chronic diseases of affluence. Most of the inhabitants of Africa, Asia, Latin America, and even much of Europe were still living hand to mouth, lacking clean water and good sewage, making them prey to the diseases that result from poor nutrition and frequent infection. Many Americans, especially those in rural areas or living in urban poverty, were likewise more concerned with infection and starvation. And many people across the planet simply didn't have access to the antibiotics, vaccines, and other medications that could thwart the power of infectious disease.

But many Americans did have access to those medications, and they were now living off the fat of the land—literally. The supply of food—especially meat—was going up, while the cost was going down. People were eating more animal protein and rapidly gaining weight. And with more and more Americans eating like royalty, more and more of them were suffering the afflictions heretofore reserved for royalty: obesity, gout, heart disease, stroke, diabetes, and cancer.

The McGovern Fiasco

The U.S. Senate formed its first Select Committee on Nutrition and Human Needs in 1969, on the heels of well-publicized accounts of malnutrition and starvation here in the United States. The committee was tasked with solving the problem of hunger, ignoring nutrition-based problems like heart disease and obesity. With South Dakota senator George McGovern as its chair, the committee began to address the problem. Over the years, it accomplished quite a bit. It pushed for expansion of the food stamp program, subsidized school lunches, and other antipoverty measures.

In addition to the battle against hunger, some experts were testifying about a diametrically opposed issue: overconsumption. Committee members were learning that heart disease had just become our nation's number one killer (a distinction it still holds today). When the committee convened a White House Conference on food, nutrition, and health, they listened with interest to the evidence linking the U.S. diet, rich in meat, saturated fat, and sugar, with the problem of heart disease.

The presiding spirit of the conference was Ancel Keys. A prolific scientist who held two Ph.D.s, Keys had spent the better part of his life looking at the relationship between heart disease and food, primarily by comparing the diets of different societies. In 1956, he had presented research at the World Health Organization (WHO) drawing attention to the impressive longevity and very low rates of heart disease enjoyed by countries that bordered the Mediterranean. (Yes, that was the beginning of the "Mediterranean diet" craze that continues—in grossly caricatured form—to this day.)

What happened in Crete had especially piqued Keys's interest. In the 1950s, the Rockefeller Foundation had gone to Crete to "modernize" the country. What they found were hardy, vibrant people who were far healthier than typical Americans. At the time, Cretans got more than 60 percent of their calories from plants. Meat consumption was extremely low, at about 7 percent of total caloric consumption. The typical Mediterranean diet contained lots of pastas, fresh breads, beans, tomatoes, soups, with loads of fresh vegetables at every meal, and lots of fruit for dessert. Cretans ate meat and fish at most twice a week, rather than three times a day.

U.S. figures at the time were just about the opposite. We got only 7 percent of our calories from fruits and veggies, and upwards of 48 percent from animal products.

Keys had already begun to wonder whether diet was playing a part in the rising rate of heart attacks among middle-aged American men. When he discovered the Cretan or "Mediterranean" diet, he was inspired to begin the Six Countries Study, one of the largest studies ever conducted on diet and its relationship to heart disease. His initial finding: the more fat in the diet, the more heart disease.

Keys had published his preliminary findings on the correlation between fat and heart disease in a 1953 paper, which attracted controversy. Keys looked at six countries' (Japan, Italy, England/Wales, Australia, Canada, and the United States) fat consumption and 1948-49 rates of degenerative heart disease. In a simple yet compelling-looking graph, he made the case that dietary fat was highly correlated with heart disease. He presented his findings at a 1955 World Health Organization conference, where both his conclusions and methodology were subject to a few critics.

Among the doubters were Berkeley statistician Jacob Yerushalmy and New York state commissioner of health Herman Hilleboe. In 1957, they published a "methodologic note" in the *New York Journal of Medicine* claiming that Keys had cherry-picked his data and slanted his conclusions based on the countries that would give him the results he wanted. They published a twenty-two-country study that they claimed gave a more accurate portrait—one that questioned a significant correlation between dietary fat and heart disease, but included a surprise: the dietary factor most closely associated with heart disease mortality was—wait for it—animal protein.

Keys, ever the scientist, rebuked his detractors efficiently. He pointed out why he chose those particular six countries, namely because they were the only countries with reliable data. He did, however, seem to change

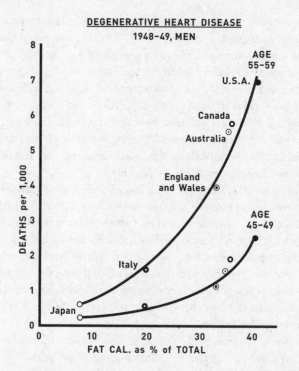

DEGENERATIVE HEART DISEASE
1948-49, MEN

his view a bit. He stopped blaming fat in general for heart disease—but he became even more concerned about saturated fat, a type of fat found almost exclusively in animal products. The later Seven Countries Study attempted to look specifically, in a prospective manner, at the effect saturated fat had on health.

Keys compared sixteen cohorts of men in seven countries: Finland, Greece, Italy, Japan, the Netherlands, the United States, and Yugoslavia. Nearly 13,000 people were interviewed about their diet and were then followed for several decades: a simply stunning large-scale, long-term epidemiological study. Keys chose these seven countries for their distinctly different diets and also because they kept excellent records. Additionally, he required that the countries had not changed their diets significantly due to the recently ended World War II. While these filters may seem trivial, it's important to understand their logic, since many subsequent studies have ignored them and reached quite different conclusions.

Choosing countries with vastly different dietary patterns ensures that the differences will be large enough to matter. If, for example, you wanted to prove that smoking was unrelated to lung cancer, you might compare a group of 4-pack-a-day smokers with a group of 3.5-pack-a-day smokers. At those levels, it would be hard to discern a dose-response relationship. By selecting widely varied dietary patterns, Keys was essentially comparing 4-pack-a-day smokers to 10-pack-a-day smokers and nonsmokers. With differences that big, you could trust the real effects to show up clearly.

Clean and comprehensive record-keeping is crucial, so the researcher and the public can have faith in the data. In the absence of reliable facts, all sorts of erroneous interpretations are possible.

Finally, countries that had experienced war-caused famines were excluded from Keys's study to keep the correlations accurate. Yerushalmy and Hilleboe had discovered several outliers in their analysis of 22 countries: Denmark, Norway, the Netherlands, and Sweden all had low rates of heart disease while consuming a high-fat diet. But all these countries had endured severe rationing of fat-rich animal foods during the 1940s. Were their low rates of heart disease related to current high-fat consumption, or to their prior relative abstinence? There was no way to tell, so Keys eliminated them from his analysis.

The Seven Countries Study, published first in 1961 and continuing to this day, provided strong evidence that as saturated fat increased, so did heart disease. I need to point out that saturated fat is closely associated with animal-based foods, which makes it a near-perfect proxy for animal protein.

Keys eventually moved to the southern coast of Italy, where he lived to the ripe old age of one hundred, a one-man testimonial to the power of his diet. I like to picture him growing old in his beloved village of Pioppi, sitting down to a big plate of pasta primavera after a vigorous walk on the beach.

Meanwhile, the McGovern Committee was preparing its own critique of animal protein and saturated fat. Inspired by Keys's Seven Countries Study, the committee members held a well-publicized series of hearings that resulted in their 1977 recommendations, grandly titled "The Dietary Goals for the United States" (Select Committee on Nutrition and Human Needs 1977).

These recommendations basically followed Keys's approach: less than 30 percent of calories from fat, less than 10 percent of calories from saturated fat, and less than 300 milligrams of cholesterol per day. The only way to achieve those goals is to eat less meat and dairy, because cholesterol comes only from animal products, and most of our fat and saturated fat come from animal products as well. Leaving no ambiguity, the committee also recommended that Americans eat less meat and dairy while consuming more fruits, vegetables, and grains.

Who knows what would have happened if these recommendations had been widely publicized and accepted. But when the report was released, all hell broke loose. The sugar lobby complained, "People like sweet things, and the McGovern Committee apparently believes people should be deprived of what they like!" The head of the National Livestock and Meat Board exclaimed, "Guided by my conscience, I am certain that actions of the animal industry to ensure Americans are properly fed with abundant meat and other animal foods is an honorable and morally correct diet course." The egg and dairy industries were equally enraged. One lobbyist even argued that trying to increase longevity was wrong—because if people were living longer, that would spike the cost of health care!

The idealistic McGovern paid a heavy political price for his nutritional activism. South Dakota is a cattle industry state, and when he ran for reelection in the 1980 Senate race, McGovern didn't have a chance.

The food industry growers and manufacturers didn't wait till 1980, however, to defend their pocketbooks. They called upon Senator Bob Dole of Kansas (another big meat-producing state). Dole actually got the committee to alter the report. In a reinterpretation worthy of George Orwell's *1984*, the report went from telling people to eat less meat to eat *more* lean meat, like chicken and fish.

It's not like there wasn't support for the original recommendation. The American Society of Clinical Nutrition convened an unbiased committee to review the McGovern recommendations and found them completely valid. The American Dietetic Association and the American Heart Association likewise applauded the committee's initial recommendations based on their own in-depth review of the evidence. The howls of outrage from the scientific community were to no avail, however. The food industry found and hired scientists willing to challenge the findings, and the committee was disbanded.

One part of the report did survive: the suggestion to reduce saturated fat. Unfortunately, most people didn't know what that meant, and they certainly weren't aware that every kind of animal product includes this type of fat—even lean meats. The only way to reduce your intake of saturated fat is to cut back your consumption of animal protein.

But thanks to Senator Dole and the meat industry, that wasn't the message the U.S. government ended up promoting, and it wasn't the one the media reported, either. Instead of switching to a healthier diet—less animal protein, more fruits, and more vegetables—we had simply declared war on fat.

From Real Food to Macronutrients

I'm fascinated by the concept of unintended consequences. We try to accomplish something, and the blowback from our efforts ends up sabotaging our goals in ways we didn't foresee. In this case, the McGovern Committee had wanted to help us avoid heart disease. Instead, the major effect—a highly problematic one—was to change the way we talk about food. And that change in language has contributed to our galloping epidemic of heart disease and other killers.

Before the committee, nutritionists, doctors, and policymakers spoke of whole foods: fruits, vegetables, grains, nuts, meats, fish, butter, eggs. After the committee publicized its guidelines, we stopped talking about food and instead referred to the macronutrient components of food: fats, carbohydrates, and of course, protein.

Ask your doctor what you should be eating in the course of a day, and she probably won't use words like *fruits and vegetables, rice and beans,* and *olive oil.* She won't even recommend *Lots of meat, chicken, and fish.* Instead, she'll probably say, *You want to get a nice, healthy balance of protein, fats, and carbohydrates.* She's talking about what are called macronutrients—she's no longer talking about food.

After the McGovern Committee, published dietary recommendations switched from whole foods to macronutrients, and so did dietitians, trainers, and doctors. Eventually, the public followed suit. As we chose foods that we believed contained less fat, we began eating more processed carbs, low-fat and skim milk, and leaner cuts of meat. Then, when eating fat-free cookies, candy, skinless chicken breasts, and half-and-half in our coffee didn't improve our weight, people began questioning their "low-fat diet" and started to demonize carbs.

"Carbs" in general weren't the problem, of course. The problem was that people were eating processed, refined carbs instead of fresh whole fruits and vegetables, beans, and whole grains. After all, green leafy vegetables are carbs, and so are broccoli, cucumbers, red peppers, and onions, and those are some of the healthiest foods on earth. But because of our focus on macronutrients, we aren't really thinking about those specific foods. We say "carbs"—and think starch.

Even to think about starchy carbs as a separate category distorts the picture. There's a world of difference between a bowl of steel-cut oatmeal and a sugar-sweetened cereal made from refined flour; between some boiled garbanzos or black beans and a fried corn chip or potato chip.

Moreover, some "carbs" are mainly fats. Muffins, for example, are anywhere from 40 to 50 percent fat by calories, yet they are unfairly lumped in as a carb. Ditto McDonald's french fries—over 43 percent of their calories come from the oil in which they are fried.

Some diet gurus even began to demonize fruit, conflating the natural sugars that occur in fruit with dead, processed, white sugar. This despite the fact that fresh, whole fruit is one of the healthiest foods there is, full of fiber, vitamins, and phytochemicals. If there is one food that could be said to be created specifically for human consumption, it would be fruit. Sweet and colorful, fruit is the plant's way of getting humans and other fruit eaters to spread its genes. Peaches, plums, and pears certainly didn't deserve the blame for our mounting obesity epidemic. I've never seen a single person who became overweight from eating too much fruit; Chapter 12 lays out the scientific reasons for that.

Meanwhile, the food industry jumped on the "low-fat" bandwagon, not with genuinely healthy low-fat foods, but with marketing campaigns that promoted highly refined, heavily processed white flour products loaded with white sugar, dyed with artificial colors, and preserved with dangerous chemicals as low-fat health foods. No one in their right mind could look at a 100-calorie pack of diet Chips Ahoy and think *That's just what my body needs to be fit and healthy.* That assessment, of course, tells you nothing about the value of brown rice, black beans, fresh kale, or a dish of fresh berries.

The real irony was the way people paired those unhealthy low-fat products with high-fat animal protein, as if the indulgence of fatty main dishes could be balanced out by a miserly dessert. My patients consume ever-increasing amounts of saturated fat in the form of chicken breasts, T-bone steaks, and eggs . . . and compensate with low-fat Oreos for dessert.

Can you see the problem with the argument repeated ad nauseum by advocates of low-carb diets: "We tried low-fat diets, starting in the 1970s, and they only made us fatter." Not really—we never stopped eating fat! Here's what really happened, based on data from the USDA's Economic Reserve:

Year	1970	2008
Total Average Calories	2057	2674
Calories from Meat, Eggs, Nuts	463	483
Calories from Oils	403	616

Does it look like America went on a low-fat diet from 1970 to 2008? To me it looks like more fat—along with more of almost everything else. The one type of food we didn't eat more of is the only one we should have—fresh, whole fruits and vegetables.

Since we were getting sicker and fatter over those four decades, two schools of thought presented two completely different dietary solutions: low fat and low carb. As they bickered, protein's halo grew brighter and shinier. Nobody, it seemed, had a bad word to say about protein, our "prime" nutrient. More and more, our food choices centered on animal protein. And our current nutritional paradigm, proteinaholism, was born.

What did you believe about protein before picking up this book? Share your "protein indoctrination" at Proteinaholic.com.

CHAPTER 5

Protein Usurps the Nutritional Throne

If we stop and take a snapshot of the moment we live in and looked at the culture as a whole—books, movies, magazines, TV and social media, grocery stores, and pharmacies—the picture would tell us that Americans believe three things about nutrition:

Belief 1: Protein is the most important nutrient.

Belief 2: The only place to get protein is from animals.

Belief 3: Our health problems largely result from not adhering to Belief 1.

We saw in the last chapter how these beliefs originated and spread. We see here how these beliefs are keeping us from adopting healthy diets, even in the face of overwhelming evidence. Even if you know nothing about nutrition, consider this protein paradox: some of us consume protein shakes and skinless chicken breasts in order to *lose* weight, while at the same time bodybuilders and gym rats chug protein shakes and gorge on chicken breasts in order to *gain* weight.

What accounts for the persistence of the protein myth? Here's an old joke.

Harold believes that he's dead. His doctor tries to convince him otherwise. He points out that Harold is walking and talking. Harold shrugs, believing that dead men can walk and talk. The doctor mentions that Harold is breathing, and he has a pulse. Harold remains unswayed by this evidence as well. Finally, the doctor asks Harold whether dead men bleed.

"Of course not," Harold replies. "Everyone knows that dead men don't bleed." The doctor pricks Harold's finger with a pin and they both watch the blood begin to flow. "Well, I'll be!" Harold exclaims. "Dead men do bleed."

Cognitive Dissonance

The joke provides an example of a psychological phenomenon called "cognitive dissonance." This occurs when someone has such a strong prior belief that the person filters out or reinterprets all evidence contradicting the belief. There's no way to convince Harold that he's not dead. Indeed, recent research suggests that presenting people with proof that their beliefs are incorrect doesn't change their minds. Instead, it actually reinforces their erroneous beliefs, as they work hard to defend them against fact and logic.

What I've discovered, through my work as a plant-based doctor counseling patients on diet, is that our society's belief in the primacy of protein is, if you'll pardon the pun, a sacred cow. Despite decades of evidence, from observation to epidemiological studies to large dietary surveys to clinical trials, the presupposition that protein is good, and more is better, is still firmly implanted in our minds.

As I mentioned, I wrote this book partly so I could stop having the same conversation with my weight-loss patients.* The one where they nod and assent to all my dietary advice, only to return for the next visit having complied with almost none of it. Here's an example, a paraphrased (and mercifully shortened) version of a conversation I recently had with one of my patients, a forty-two-year-old woman.

> **PATIENT:** *I am really frustrated, Doc. I have tried so hard to lose weight. I have done all the usual diets. I try so hard to make sure I am getting enough protein. I go regularly to my trainer.*

---

* I should mention that the thousands of patients I see for medical and surgical weight loss fall into one of two categories: the junk food junkie, or the "I am trying hard to lose weight by eating lots of protein" dieter. There are some variations, but believe me, people in each category eat pretty similar diets.

ME: *When you say you have done all the usual diets, what specific diets are you referring to?*

PATIENT: *You know, the usual. I did Quick Weight Loss a few times. I have tried Atkins many times and I have tried Paleo. I have been able to lose weight but I keep putting it back on..*

ME: *Well, take me through a typical day eating.*

PATIENT: *Breakfast I do eggs, or egg whites, or just yogurt. I usually add a protein shake. Lunch is another shake if I'm busy, or I pick up a Subway cold cut sandwich. Dinner is always chicken or fish with some vegetables. I really try and avoid junk food. Sometimes I get sweet cravings and have chocolate. I know I'm getting too many carbs, but sometimes I just crave them.*

ME: *Can you elaborate on "getting too many carbs"? (I know, I sound like a psychologist.)*

PATIENT: *Well, from time to time I'll eat a candy bar or crackers or chips. Sometimes I can't resist a doughnut. I know it is my downfall, so I limit it to once a day, if even. I do love pizza.*

ME: *Do you eat fruit?*

PATIENT: *Some. But like I said, I try to limit my carbs.*

ME: *What if I told you that carbs are not your problem? Your diet is actually low in carbs. What if I told you that you are eating far too much protein?*

PATIENT: *(With look of shock and indignation) Well, that would be the opposite of everything I have ever read. All I ever hear is "Eat more protein."*

ME: *And how is that working for you?*

PATIENT: *(Getting more annoyed) Well, I know this isn't working, but I think it's because I eat too many carbs. I even had pizza the other night.*

ME: *(Using her diet log with calculated percentage of calories from different nutrients) You are actually getting a low percentage of calories from carbs, only about 40 percent. Roughly 20 to 30 percent of your* calories are coming from protein, and 30 to 40 percent from fats. You're making a mistake when you think of things like doughnuts and pizza as carbs. In fact, they have more fat calories than carb calories.

As I read your diet questionnaire, I see you eat lots of chicken. Meanwhile, there's very little fiber consumption. Your diet is similar to most Americans'. Did you know that, while we are the most overweight country in the world, Europe is catching up? They have therefore started a large study to find out what foods are causing weight gain. They followed close to 350,000 people for eight years and found that meat consumption, especially chicken, was significantly associated with weight gain (Vergnaud, Norat, et al. 2010). In fact, in a subset of this large prospective study, researchers looked at vegetarians versus meat eaters and concluded that the higher the protein intake and the lower the fiber intake, the higher the weight (Spencer, Appleby, et al. 2003).

PATIENT: Well, this can't be. How can chicken make you fat?

ME: Well, it is a complex science (which I will explain to readers in detail in Part III). But, remember that meat is calorie dense, meaning that a small volume contains a lot of calories, so we tend to overeat just to feel full. Also understand that chickens in the 1950s used to run around eating natural grain and went to slaughter after upwards of six months. Now they go to slaughter as soon as six weeks and are far heavier due to artificial selection and an unnatural diet designed to produce fat birds in record time.

Modern chickens are cooped up in dirty cages, lacking room even to turn around. In order to keep them alive under those conditions, their food is dosed on a regular basis with antibiotics. So you are eating a fatter chicken pumped full of antibiotics that can mess with your natural bowel flora that can affect your weight; and it is filled with toxins that can cause inflammation in your body. On top of this mess rides the illusion that chicken is a healthy choice, so it is overconsumed.

PATIENT: Well, my family doctor told me I need more protein.

ME: (Getting a little snarky) And how much nutrition training has your doctor received?

PATIENT: Well, it's not just him. That is all I ever read or hear about on the Internet and on TV.

ME: *And how is all this diet information you refer to working for our country? We eat more protein than any other country in the world (except Iceland) and we are the most overweight, have some of the highest cancer rates, highest diabetes rates, highest heart disease rates, and the lowest longevity. The RDA recommends we eat 45 to 55 grams of protein a day, but you are doubling that, at least. As you can see, my waiting room is full—and every one of those people has been on some kind of high-protein diet.*

PATIENT: *(persistent) But isn't it our sugar consumption? Didn't the low-fat diets fail?*

ME: *We never actually ate low fat. Yes, sugar has risen and our total daily calories have risen, and that is in fact bad. But the rise in sugar was due to a "low-fat" diet ideology that arose in response to an already failing high-protein diet plan. Because we started hearing that fat was the culprit, Americans turned to "fat-free" junk foods like Snackwells that were loaded with sugar. And to add insult to injury, we didn't reduce our fat consumption. We just added sugar. Instead of going on a supposedly low-fat, high-processed-carb diet, we should have switched to a high-fruit-and-veggie, high-starch, low-protein diet.*

PATIENT: *You have to be kidding me. A high-starch diet?!*

ME: *If we are among the unhealthiest people in the developed world, shouldn't we look at the healthiest people? Cultures like those found in Okinawa and Sardinia, where people live much longer and healthier lives than we do, actually eat very low-protein, very high-carb diets. Okinawans eat lots of rice and lots of yams and very little meat. They get about 80 percent of their calories from carbs. They eat far less protein than you do, and far more carbs, and yet they are far healthier. And it is not their genes. If they move to the USA, or shift to a Western diet, they become as overweight and sick as we are.*

PATIENT: *(Blank, disbelieving stare)*

And so it goes, with patient after patient. Eventually, I do get through to many of them, usually when their desire to lose weight and to live overwhelms their previously held beliefs. The recovery community calls this "hitting bottom," and as a recovering proteinaholic myself, I'm honored to be there to guide them to a better, saner, and much more joyful existence.

I work at the most intense and volatile part of the addiction cycle, where the proteinaholism can crumble in the face of ill health and the real threat of future suffering. Before people get to that point, their unquestioning belief in the value of animal foods doesn't reach consciousness until they are confronted by a person who doesn't eat any.

Market Exploitation

In our capitalist society, businesses exist primarily to make money. And one of the best ways to make money is to sell people what they're already addicted to. Given our culture's worship of protein, it was only a matter of time before someone figured out how to make a fortune from the mass delusion. In so doing, Robert Atkins and the companies he started have given proteinaholism a modern twist (the "low carb" concept) that still captures the public imagination and dominates much of scientific discussion. It's to his story that I turn next in my exploration.

Do you still have proteinaholic voices in your head? Share your doubts and "yeah buts" at Proteinaholic.com.

CHAPTER 6

To Atkins and Beyond

The ascendence of protein from necessary macronutrient to the "stuff of life itself," the one nutrient that was so good for you, the more the better, created a fertile environment for anyone trying to get rich promoting a high-protein diet. Dr. Robert Atkins, a cardiologist, has been the most famous and influential proponent of such a diet. He was not the first, getting the idea after discovering the work of Dr. Alfred W. Pennington, who in the 1940s got 20 obese DuPont employees to lose an average 22 pounds in 14 weeks on a calorically unrestricted low-carb diet. This concept of lowering carbs goes all the way back to the mid-nineteenth century when William Banting, a well-known, and obese, undertaker at the time, changed his diet based on the recommendation of his doctor and lost weight; he wrote and published *Letter on Corpulence* describing his experience with the low-carb diet.

In 1961, Dr. Hermann Taller published a book, *Calories Don't Count,* that promoted a low-carb diet. It sold two million copies, despite the fact that Dr. Taller was charged with fraud by the FDA, for using the book to push sales of his proprietary safflower pills.

In 1967, the year Dr. Taller was found guilty by a jury, fined, and sentenced to two years in prison (suspended), Dr. Irwin Stillman published another high-protein and high-fat diet book, *The Doctors' Quick Weight Loss.* His approach was quite severe, as he forbade fruits and vegetables. Dr. Stillman died of a heart attack, while his most famous patient, Karen Carpenter, followed his advice on her way to dying of heart failure, a complication of the anorexia nervosa that made her such a compliant diet patient.

Atkins took up the mantle of this failed and dangerous medical fringe and did something none of his predecessors had been able to accomplish: make the low-carb diet respectable and popular. The most important tool at his disposal was his entertaining and genial personality. Before he chose a career in medicine, he had considered becoming a comedian. Atkins was able to recycle this old idea of a low-carb/high-protein diet and turn it into gold. He appeared as a guest on the *Tonight Show* with Johnny Carson, published an abbreviated version of his diet in *Vogue* magazine, and quickly became the darling of many other media outlets. His message resonated with everyone whose inner child still smarted at being told to "eat their vegetables." All of a sudden, a funny, kindly, and authoritative doctor was telling us that our worst vices were actually our best friends. What wasn't to love?

The book he published in 1972, *Dr. Atkins' Diet Revolution,* was a huge success, quickly selling millions of copies. The book lauded foods like pork rinds, meat, and cheese, while demonizing bananas, whole-wheat bread, and potatoes. His argument was that carbs, including fruit, cause a rise in insulin, and insulin is like poison to the system. Problem is that Atkins, and all the current low-carb evangelists, miss one gigantic, important scientific fact: protein, as well as carbs, causes insulin to rise!

One in-depth study of insulin response to different kinds of food gave a group of volunteers equal calorie servings of thirty-eight different foods, then measured their insulin response through drawing blood. If Atkins was right, then the highest-carbohydrate foods would cause the biggest spike in insulin. Instead, the researchers found that protein-rich foods elicit a disproportionately higher insulin response than would be expected given the sugar content. In other words, while a protein meal might not raise blood sugar, it substantially increases insulin, the evil hormone we are supposed to be avoiding by eating a high-protein diet (Holt, Miller, et al. 1997). This study alone should alert open-minded low-carb adherents to the intellectual bankruptcy of the movement.

Ultimately, most people don't care about the science. As long as something sounds good (and by that I mean it justifies a desired behavior and/or supports an existing belief), we usually don't pay too much attention to the details. The real question people had about the Atkins diet was much simpler: Will it help me lose weight?

In fact, you can lose weight with Atkins, and you probably will. A very large study called the A to Z Trial was published in the prestigious *Journal of the American Medical Association (JAMA)* in 2007. In this trial, people were randomized to either the Atkins diet, the Zone diet, the Ornish diet (vegan), or the LEARN diet. Each group had to read the book associated with the diet and then attend a weekly class (Gardner, Kiazand, et al. 2007). The Atkins group jumped off to an early lead with weight loss, and the multimillion-dollar Atkins corporation, understandably excited, embarked on a frenzy of advertising and public relations to announce their victory.

There are several reasons for the dramatic weight loss. Once you understand these details, you might not be so enthusiastic about it. After all, one way to lose ten pounds quickly and permanently is to cut off your head. The fine points matter here.

First, much of the weight loss comes from water. To understand how this works, recall from high school biology that sugar from carbs is the fuel every cell in our body needs for energy. We have such a desperate and immediate need for this sugar that our bodies include redundant storage systems in case we miss a meal or two. We store excess carbs as glycogen in the liver and in our muscles as emergency fuel source. On the Atkins diet you are not consuming carbs, so your body has to mobilize the glycogen to get sugar to fuel your cells. The glycogen is stored with water, so as you mobilize your glycogen you also lose water weight.

Second, the Atkins diet has two effects that can dramatically reduce our desire to eat, thus lowering caloric intake. One of these is nausea, nature's way of telling us that we're eating badly. As the body goes into starvation from not receiving its primary fuel and reverts to emergency fuel sources, it initiates an inefficient process of extracting fuel directly from fat cells. This process produces chemicals called ketones. One side effect of ketone production is nausea, which can make you eat less. An additional side effect of ketones is the stimulation of even more diuresis (water loss). The second way the Atkins diet reduces our caloric intake is through the painful lack of variety. People get so uninspired and bored, they unconsciously reduce the amount of food they eat.

Atkins claimed that the weight loss had to do with some magical breakdown of fat. Defying a fundamental law of physics, he argued that calories don't count. He claimed that by eating his diet you would magically burn more calories than you consume. This intriguing assertion was put to the test in 2004 by a BBC show called *Horizon,* in collaboration with researchers at University of Kansas. They put identical twins on different diets. One followed a low-fat diet and the other followed an Atkins diet. They then put the twins in a special sealed chamber and measured calorie expenditure. It was the same. The brother on the Atkins diet was not magically burning more calories.

A more rigorous trial was conducted on 12 men. Each participant was given a diet either high in pork protein, soy protein, or carbs. They then went into a special chamber that measured their energy expenditure. Then they would switch diets and repeat the process. In the end, the high-protein diets had a very slight 2 percent increase in basal metabolic rate, hardly enough to cause any substantial weight loss (Mikkelsen, Toubro, et al. 2000).

Indeed, many scientific articles have shown that in the end, a calorie is a calorie. A large study looking at many papers that had been written on Atkins and high-protein/low-carb diets showed that weight loss is simply a result of decreased calories. There is no magic behind decreasing just carbs. Sadly and predictably, long-term weight loss on these diets is rare (Bravata, Sanders, et al. 2003).

One researcher placed 35 obese women on diets consisting of exactly 1,200 calories per day, but varied the percentage of fat from 10 percent to 40 percent. There was absolutely no difference in weight loss over a 12-week period (Powell, Tucker, et al. 1994). Another study took a similar approach, keeping calories the same but varying the participants' carbohydrate content from 25 percent to 75 percent. Again, no difference in weight loss. They did show that the higher protein group had higher nitrogen breakdown components, which can cause future health problems (Alford, Blankenship, et al. 1990).

Mark Haub, a professor of nutrition at Kansas State, best displayed the importance of calorie in versus calorie out by performing an extreme self-experiment and posting the results on his Facebook page. Haub went on an 1,800-calorie "junk food" diet for 10 weeks. Two-thirds of his meals were junk food. He ate every three hours and consumed mainly Twinkies, Little Debby Snack Cakes, Doritos, and Oreos, careful always to stay under 1,800 calories. He did eat some veggies and took a multivitamin. After 10 weeks, he had lost 27 pounds and reduced his body fat from 33 percent to 24 percent. His bad cholesterol dropped by 20 percent and his triglycerides dropped by 34 percent. Obviously, these beneficial changes were all from simply eating less.

This is not to say that Haub's experiment proves that cookies and corn chips constitute a healthy diet. Please don't run to the convenience store brandishing this book and telling everyone the "good news" about Frito-Lay and Nabisco junk foods! Had Haub remained on this diet for life, he would soon have been suffering health issues due to the lack of nutrients and antioxidants. Interestingly, as soon as he added meat back to his diet, his cholesterol and weight increased.

So back to the A to Z diet study. The significant water loss due to diuresis and the decreased calorie consumption caused by nausea did result in initial weight loss. Over time, however, the Atkins group began to gain back weight so that, at one year, the difference in weight loss between groups was not significant. The Atkins group lost about four to five pounds more after one year than the Ornish ("low-fat vegan") group.

Still, five pounds is five pounds, right? Maybe Atkins didn't achieve spectacular results, but it still kicked Ornish's butt, right?

Not so fast. When I read the published study, it turned out that the media had conveniently omitted a fairly significant fact: the Ornish group was not actually eating anything resembling a true Ornish diet! Ornish, whom we will discuss in Chapter 11 for his work on heart disease, recommends a diet with less than 10 percent of calories from fat. In this study, the people on the Ornish diet reduced their fat intake only from 35 percent to 30 percent. A truly healthy vegan diet should give a great boost in fiber to over 35 grams per day, but the Ornish group increased only from 16 to 19 grams. Finally, you would expect that a vegan diet would decrease protein consumption (at least you would if you were surrounded by the chorus of "Where do you get your protein?" that accompanies plant-based eaters wherever they go), but in this study the so-called Ornish group actually increased its protein intake. In other words, these people were not remotely compliant with the diet. In fact, the only thing that really determined how well someone did in this study was how well they followed the particular diet they were given. It had nothing to do with the macronutrient breakdown, as was suggested by the authors (Alhassan, Kim, et al. 2008). In the end, those who ate less lost weight. Earth-shattering, I know.

Atkins has been put to the test like this before with the same results (Dansinger, Gleason, et al. 2005). In fact, a review of 15 controlled trials with high-protein diets show short-term weight loss in 7 of them, with the weight returning at about the one-year mark. The authors of this review do point out that low-fat protein, such as found with plant protein, may be different and beneficial (Hu 2005).

The weight regain we eventually see should be expected. As we've seen, the body uses carbs as its preferred and natural source of energy. Deprive someone of carbs, and eventually willpower and resolve cannot override the body's desperate need for them. The carbs cravings will hit, and hit hard. Ask anyone who's been on Atkins for a while: a slice of Pepperidge Farm white bread starts to look and smell like manna from heaven.

Ketosis, the body's switch to fat metabolism as an emergency fuel, causes its own unpleasant and ultimately harmful side effects. In their fantastic and comprehensive review of popular diets, nutrition professor Marjorie Freedman, Ph.D., and her colleagues point out that the Atkins diet is not only disadvantageous for weight loss, it's actually accompanied by the kinds of side effects you usually find on the flip side of magazine ads for pharmaceutical drugs: constipation, bad breath, headache, nausea, and fatigue, among others. With those kinds of side effects is it any wonder that virtually nobody can stick to the diet? Freedman, after an amazing review of the science behind popular diets, including Atkins, concludes that the best evidence for weight loss comes from a diet high in fruits, vegetables, and grains and low in fat (Freedman, King, et al. 2001).

Atkins capitalized on the almost universally held worship of protein and relied on our willingness to rationalize what we want to believe. We have grown up eating meat. Wanting to be consistent and avoid cognitive dissonance at almost any cost, we naturally want to believe that meat is good for us, even in the face of overwhelming evidence to the contrary. Atkins obliged by giving us scientific nonsense, like carbs increase insulin production and protein supercharges our metabolism, and we buy into it. Millions of people bought his books and other similar titles, while we have continued, predictably, to grow sicker and more obese with each passing year.

The Atkins empire lost steam in the 1980s, as more and more irritable, constipated, and nauseated former adherents literally became sick and tired of the boring diet and its consequences. Alas, we are quick to forget. By the turn of the millennium, we were ready for another dose of low-carb nonsense. In 1992, Atkins returned in a big way with *Dr. Atkins' New Diet Revolution*. Backed by a hefty advertising budget, the new book (essentially a rehash of the first one) achieved the unfortunate distinction of bestselling diet book ever, and again spent time as number one on the New York Times Bestseller list. Sadly, it was not listed in the fiction category to which it was most suited.

The country suffered collective amnesia about the constipation, bad breath, nausea, and weight rebound and returned to the pork rind, cheese, and butter trough yet again. Atkins made millions from this mass protein binge. This time, his empire even found a way to make money from the side effects, by selling supplements to counter the most unpleasant effects of his recommendations. His diet was "perfect," but people required all kinds of vitamins to offset the fact that the food they were told to eat lacked what their body needed to survive. When his patients got gout thanks to his high-animal-protein diet, he put them on meds. The fact that people were getting sick never seemed to make him rethink his dietary strategy. Like his protein-worshipping public, he too wanted to believe in the unbelievable. In our case, we relished our freedom from calorie counting and low-fat "cardboard" foods. In his case, his denial of the evidence was making him millions.

Did Atkins save our health with his recycled book? Obviously not. We continued to get sick and overweight. Millions tried the diet, and millions eventually failed. Atkins did succeed in making the diet respectable, and pervasive in our culture and our individual psyches. People would lose weight in the beginning, and that experience was so monumental and profound that they were unable to revise their opinions when the weight returned and their health decayed.

Before I see patients in my office, they fill out a diet history. The Atkins section is almost universally checked. When I ask directly, people rarely remember the side effects at first. They think the diet worked, but they failed the diet because they had to eat a carb, not realizing that the carb craving is their body screaming for the fuel it needs. Rather than attributing this catastrophe to an unsustainable and dangerous diet, Atkins's adherents from then until now blame themselves for their lack of willpower: "I know I shouldn't, but sometimes I eat the bun along with the hamburger. I just can't help myself."

Atkins opened a Pandora's box of low-carb nonsense from which we are far from recovering. From Atkins sprung all sorts of diets, including Quick Weight Loss, the Scarsdale diet, Medifast, the Zone diet, the South Beach diet, the Sugar Busters diet, and many more. Their differences are superficial, and they cite insulin dumps from excess carbs as our biggest enemy. They refuse to acknowledge the science showing they are actually promoting excess insulin release, and none admit the long-term health consequences of their high-protein diets.

Atkins's Death from Heart Disease

Atkins actually suffered a cardiac arrest in 2002. Can you imagine how devastating it was to the now huge Atkins corporation? Its seventy-one-year-old evangelist of health had a heart attack, despite his adherence to his own heart-healthy diet of bacon, scrambled eggs, chicken, and cheddar cheese. The company's public relations team acted quickly, explaining that the good doctor suffered from a viral cardiomyopathy (disease of the heart) completely unrelated to diet. A year later, Atkins passed away in a hospital. The story was that he slipped in the snow, hit his head, and went into a coma.

It is possible to get a viral cardiomyopathy and die from an arrhythmia. The arrhythmia may have caused his heart to stop, but records from his private doctor showed that he did have cardiac occlusive disease (obstruction of coronary arteries), which is definitely diet related, and known to be caused by high-fat, high-protein, animal foods.

Then, a damning blow. A physician in Nebraska requested the medical examiner's report, and by mistake, they sent it to him, even though he was not caring for Atkins. The report showed that Atkins did have plaque in the vessels in his heart, which caused his heart attack. It also showed that at time of death he weighed 258 pounds, which makes him obese at a height of six feet. The Atkins PR machine countered that he weighed 195 when he suffered his accident, that the additional 63 pounds was caused by fluid retention while in the ICU. While the general public might swallow a statement like that without question, those of us who work in hospitals raise our eyebrows. If Atkins's problem had been an isolated head injury, the last thing physicians would do is let him swell like that. Second, while I have seen people swell from ICU stays, 60 pounds is just too much to be credible.

The story is a sad one. The release of his medical documents is certainly not ethical, and the fact that his widow had to defend him publicly while mourning him is unfortunate. My point, however, is that we have to learn from our mistakes or we are bound to repeat them. Atkins was seventy-two at his death, which may be old in this country, but young compared to populations that consume heart-healthy diets. In photos and videos, Atkins clearly looks overweight, but since two-thirds of the country is overweight, we just think he looks normal. He was never what you'd call a picture of health. If you look at online debates between the high-protein experts versus the plant-based experts, you can visually see the difference. Speakers like John McDougall, Neal Barnard, Joel Fuhrman, Caldwell Esselstyn, and T. Colin Campbell are all svelte. Drs. Esselstyn and Campbell, both in their eighties, are completely healthy, and they radiate health in their demeanor and levels of activity. Of course, appearances are not everything. There do exist healthy-appearing meat eaters and very unhealthy-appearing vegans, but you can't help but be impressed by the health of the leading experts who promote and follow a plant-based diet.

The Weston A. Price Foundation

One of the most vociferous critics of plant-based diets was a man named Stephen Byrnes. He was a naturopath and founding board member of the Weston A. Price Foundation (WAPF). WAPF is one of the strangest organizations I have ever seen. They spew torrents of pseudoscientific mumbo jumbo that are simply baffling in their lack of resemblance to actual facts. It is as if they are inventing ideas and advocating the worst possible recommendations to the public. And they do it with such confidence that people, even smart people, are taken in. Authentic scientists always doubt hypotheses; meaning, we're open to evidence that calls into question our assumptions. WAPF leaders use scientific words, but the similarity to actual science ends there. No matter what evidence is shown to the contrary, they are completely confident in their beliefs and find ways to rationalize their crazy views. How crazy? They believe that we should be eating lots of butter and lard. (They often frame this advice by pointing out that margarines and other trans fats are worse, which is like arguing over whether you'd rather die by being shot by a revolver or a 9 mm.) Other favored WAPF foods include extracts from animal glands, bone broth, and animal organs, especially brains. And, they insist, we should avoid feeding our kids too many fruits and vegetables.

There is a mountain of scientific evidence to contradict everything they claim. The kernel of truth they've latched onto like the Holy Grail is the understanding that saturated fat is not the sole cause of heart disease, as was believed by some researchers and low-fat advocates in the 1970s and 1980s. There's an impossibly big leap between the statement that saturated fat may not be the prime reason for heart disease and the completely faulty conclusion that saturated fat is actually good for you.

Since I study the science of nutrition daily and have vast experience in this field, I have tried to point out to WAPF members and followers how they may be misreading, misunderstanding, and ignoring the science. The responses have been fascinating. Rather than engaging in honest scientific debate (by sharing their own evidence and explaining what may be wrong with mine), they prefer to lash out in mockery and childish insults. What little science they can muster is easily invalidated, which, rather than making them see the light, actually further fuels their antics. They don't stand behind scientific articles (which, to be fair, would be impossible for them), but rather attempt to prove their points by quoting one another's blogs.

I would dismiss them as a fringe group were it not for the fact that their ideas—and worse, their practices—have developed grassroots and web-based support. Like their cousins the Paleo advocates, whom we'll meet in the next chapter, WAPF insanity is wrapped in a story that makes people feel better. Like children throwing a tantrum, they shout profanities at the "food police" (whoever they are) and "politically correct" dietary guidelines. And their fantasy of feeding the world's population on grass-fed beef, free-range chicken, and pastured pork would require several dozen planet Earths, rather than the one we've been given.

Most real scientists are not blogging. Their voices are not heard. The Internet, monetized by advertising paying for page views, has developed an insatiable hunger for the controversial and the loud, and the Weston A. Price Foundation is both controversial and loud.

If WAPF beliefs are incompatible with scientific evidence, where do they come from? The group's namesake is Dr. Weston A. Price, a decent guy who would probably be horrified at the movement that's hijacked his name. Price was an American dentist who, in the 1930s, began to question why we develop cavities. In this I see him as a kindred spirit, a practitioner who questioned the prevailing protocol of treating symptoms and problems and sought to understand the root causes and prevent them in the first place.

His quest took him around the world, where he examined different cultures and their dental health. The list of cultures is long, varied, and impressive: " . . . the Swiss of Switzerland, the Gaelics in the Outer and Inner Hebrides, the Eskimos of Alaska, the Indians in the far North, West and Central Canada, Western United States and Florida, the Melanesians and Polynesians on eight archipelagos of the Southern Pacific, tribes in eastern and central Africa, the Aborigines of Australia, Malay tribes on islands north of Australia, the Maori of New Zealand and the ancient civilizations and their descendants in Peru both along the coast and in the Sierras, also in the Amazon Basin." His 1939 book, *Nutrition and Physical Degeneration,* has become the bible for WAPF members. By that I mean they all talk about it, though few, apparently, have actually read it.

I have read the book. It's pretty good, and certainly interesting. Price was a kind of "reverse missionary"; rather than imposing our "superior" beliefs on the primitive third world natives, he sought to bring their wisdom back to help us. The first thing he noticed was that they had better dentition than do "civilized" Westerners. Not only were cavities almost nonexistent, but they also had better jaw structure and straighter teeth. He also noted that if they moved to a "civilized" area, they would develop tooth decay.

Before we look at Price's conclusions about nutrition, understand that his research was purely observational. Rather than providing the "scientific proof" that WAPF acolytes claim, his wanderings and observations can provide questions for further research, but no answers. One contemporary review of his book *Nutrition and Physical Degeneration* hit the nail on the head: "his approach to the problem is more evangelical rather than scientific . . . This is a story of an observant, but not wholly unbiased, traveler who relates entertainingly what he discovered during various trips to primitive peoples" (JAMA, 1940). An example of this bias is his assumption that starchy foods cause tooth decay, despite direct evidence to the contrary. In Price's own words, "Another difficulty is the fact that many primitive races have their teeth smeared with starchy foods almost constantly and make no effort whatsoever to clean their teeth. In spite of this they have no tooth decay." The alternate explanation, that starchy foods are protective of dental health, seems obvious to the modern reader, but literally did not occur to Price.

Price did make many keen observations, but he did not engage in any kind of scientific evaluation. By today's standards, his work is curious, but not serious science. Modern-day researchers would replicate this study by making sure they had a random and reliable sample with enough people in each group. They would then attempt to remove any confounding factors (other things that could potentially influence the results but are not relevant to the question at hand), such as age, sex, mineral content of water, and so on. The teeth would be examined by a third party with no interest in results, and a multivariate regression analysis (fancy statistics) would be done to see what elements of the diet caused the dental deformities. For instance, Price found fewer problems with dental arches within the "uncivilized" cultures. Is this due to their diets, or might the main cause be the pacifiers and bottle feedings common to first world cultures?

Interestingly, Price was not antivegetarian, a fact that would surprise his so-called followers were they to take his work seriously. He called the Pathans, a North Indian tribe of lacto-ovo vegetarians (eating milk and eggs but no meat, along with wheat and vegetables) "the most perfect people in India." He was likewise enamored of the Gaelics, the Swiss, and the Neur tribe of Africa. All these tribes subsisted on grains and fish mainly. In his encounters with the Inuits, he notes that they ate large amounts of seafood but also consumed wild berries, nuts, flowers, and kelp.

Dr. Price wrote an enlightening letter to his nieces and nephews, detailing how they should eat to stay healthy, and how they should feed their children. Here's a direct quote: "The basic foods should be the entire grains such as whole wheat, rye or oats, whole wheat and rye breads, wheat and oat cereals, oat-cake, dairy products, including milk and cheese, which should be used liberally, and marine foods." He also advised his young family members to consume vegetables and especially lentils. There are no admonitions in this letter about eating lots of butter or eating tons of meat, although he may later have changed his views to incorporate more butter. It is therefore very difficult for me to understand how current foundation members extrapolate Price's observation to a philosophy that consists of eating as much fat as possible and avoiding grains and legumes like the plague.

The founding president of the WAPF, Sally Fallon, published an "interpretation" of Price's letter on the foundation's website in 2006 (see www.westonaprice.org/health-topics/abcs-of-nutrition/the-right-price/), which is a masterpiece of cherry-picking (although in this case, she passed up the cherries in favor of organ meats and butter). In prose worthy of

George Orwell's "Big Brother," she insists that Price's real recommendations were the opposite of those he himself penned:

" . . . as Price perceived so clearly, the only way for humans, with their
limited ability to take in food, to properly nourish themselves is to eat
mostly nutrient-dense foods; and the emerging science of biochemistry
confirmed the dietary habits of primitive peoples by revealing just which
foods best meet these requirements—all of them animal foods, and not
necessarily steak or chicken but seafood, and milk products and organ
meats from animals raised on mineral-rich soil. These were the very foods
valued so highly by the peoples Price studied."

Whatever you believe about Price's advice, it didn't seem to do him
much good: he passed away from a heart attack at age sixty-eight.

Back to Stephen Byrnes, one of the most vocal members of the foundation. Describing himself as a "recovering vegetarian," he is best known
for his scathing diatribe, "The Myths of Vegetarianism." Written with the
aggressive, blind zeal of the fresh convert trying to prove himself to his new
tribe, Byrnes appears to be deeply and personally offended by the thought
of someone eating only vegetables and avoiding animal products. His bio
attached to the piece reads, "Stephen is enjoying a healthy robust life on a
diet of butter, cream, eggs, whole milk, and offal." Soon after writing this
article, he died of a stroke at the age of forty-two (sources disagree on exact
age). Taking a page from the Atkins response to the untimely death of their
leader, the WAPF PR machine went into effect, but with less discipline.
Some wrote that he had AIDS. Some say he died because he did not take
the HIV medicine; others say he died because of the medication. Many
claimed it is common to get a stroke with AIDS, which is not true. The
WAPF website explains that Stephen had a stroke because he was under
stress and was an excitable person. In reality, a stroke at his age is very rare
and should not be exacerbated by having HIV. In the mystery surrounding
a cardiovascular death of a person just entering middle age, a high-fat diet
is always the prime suspect.

The deaths of a few people doesn't prove anything, of course. Maybe
Atkins did have a viral infection. Maybe Byrnes's stroke was inevitable,
and no diet in the world would have prevented it. I just find it odd that
these leaders of a dietary movement are dying from the diseases they claim
their diets prevent. Moreover, if they were so confident, why not allow an
autopsy to study the effects of the diet on the body?

One famous diet "guru," Nathan Pritikin, did just that. Pritikin was an inventor and businessman, not a doctor. In 1957, at the age of forty-two, he was diagnosed with heart disease and high cholesterol (and a few years later, with leukemia). Contemporary science taught that stress, not diet, was the primary cause of heart disease. Pritikin questioned this bit of dogma, based on his exposure to classified documents that showed a significant decrease in heart disease deaths in Europe during World War II.

Further research led him to conclude that diet was the source of disease. He found a California cardiologist, Lester Morrison, who had also seen the European wartime data. In the early 1950s, Morrison experimented by putting 50 of his sickest cardiac patients on a diet that mimicked the food-rationing diets (low in animal products, high in fiber) while allowing 50 others to maintain their high-protein American diets. The results, which he shared with Pritikin, were striking: by 1960, all the high-protein patients were dead, while 38 percent of the low-protein patients were still alive.

Pritikin decided a diet very high in fruits, vegetables, beans, and grains was the answer to his health problems. It was a wise decision: once he adopted this low-protein diet, his angina went away immediately and his cancer was held in remission. He went on to write several books and founded the Pritikin Centers for Longevity.

After twenty-seven years in remission, unfortunately, Pritikin's cancer returned. Chronic lymphocytic leukemia unfortunately is not curable, and it was impressive that he remained in remission for so long. He started on chemotherapy but was devastated by the swelling and pain brought on by the treatment. This made it impossible for him to run, which had been his favorite activity. He had enjoyed stellar health for so long, he became depressed when it at last abandoned him.

Pritikin elected to take his own life rather than suffer further illness or treatment, but before he did so he wanted to make a point to a skeptical medical community. He asked to be autopsied and his heart evaluated, with the results—whatever they were—published in *New England Journal of Medicine.*

The autopsy result was remarkable. His heart was free of any plaque and resembled that of a much younger man. His blood vessels were likewise pliable and free of disease (Hubbard, Inkeles, et al. 1985). Far different from the grim diagnosis he first received of a shortened, disabled life, Pritikin's autopsy teaches us that a plant-based diet can add vigorous and joyful years to our lives, even in the face of formidable health challenges.

The low-carb movement appeared to be on its last legs in 2004, with the bankruptcy of Atkins Nutritionals, and a growing public and professional recognition of the long-term bankruptcy of the whole diet. Then, a few men began telling us a story of our caveman past that has resurrected the low-carb diet in a new guise. In the next chapter, let's look at the truths and myths of the Paleo diet.

Do you have an Atkins diet story—either a personal one or from someone you know? Share it with the community at Proteinaholic.com.

CHAPTER 7

The Latest Flavor of Proteinaholism: Paleo

For hundreds of years, high-protein diets have come and gone, never actually resulting in any long-term benefits. Now many intelligent and environmentally conscious people have been seduced by Paleo, the "new and improved" Atkins diet for the twenty-first century. Perhaps in rebellion against cubicles and Lunchables, a substantial segment of educated people now believe that the cavemen had it right: the key to a long healthy life is to eat what the Neanderthal man consumed (never mind his probable life expectancy of thirty years). I'll be the first to admit, the image of muscular, lithe prehistoric men bringing down and subsequently feasting ravenously upon a woolly mammoth is an enticing, macho image. The problem is, it's a complete fantasy.

While underground versions of Paleo have been around for some time, the concept was popularized by the book *The Paleo Diet*, by Loren Cordain, Ph.D. In case you're wondering, that Ph.D. isn't in anthropology, something Cordain shares with most of the others writing authoritatively about the actual diets of Paleolithic humans. Without having to labor under the burden of actual scholarship, Cordain and the others are free to speculate about the makeup of the Paleo diet, generally identifying the foods each of them already enjoys. Cordain himself, like most of the Paleo faithful, is a big believer in meat. On his website, beef is listed as a superfood. Some Paleo advocates balk at this generalization, noting that the only meat ever eaten by cavemen was wild game, never farmed animals. As with most faith-based systems, ideas have evolved. Many Paleo supporters now claim grass-fed beef is the answer, as if a cow is in anyway similar to what a caveman may have hunted. In fact, the original notion of a Paleo diet has now morphed into a giant industry, consisting of a confusing mess of products. Paleo bread, cookies, and protein bars are all touted as functionally equivalent to what prehistoric man may have consumed, which of course is ridiculous. In reality there is simply no food that we eat today that is remotely similar to what they ate in prehistoric times.

Common to all Paleo diets is an emphasis on meat and protein. To be fair, they also recommend eating produce, although each sect offers a different set of forbidden fruits and other plant food. For example, most Paleo diets view legumes as the enemy, even though every population study that has investigated the claim has correlated high legume consumption with health and longevity. Wheat is strictly off the menu, since it allegedly makes us fat and stupid (see *Grain Brain* and *Wheat Belly* for particularly egregious examples of entertaining writing and bad science). When we get to the "What I Eat" portion of Chapter 16 , we'll see overwhelming evidence that wheat, whole grains, and legumes are actually very good for us.

The upside of Paleo from a dietary perspective (and it's not insignificant) is the elimination of most industrially processed foods, including sodas, donuts, cookies, white bread, and dairy. It's no wonder that so many people feel so much better during the honeymoon phase of the Paleo diet; they've just gotten thousands of calories of daily poison off their plates. There's also societal benefit brought about by the Paleo movement and its compelling story of returning to a noble human lifestyle: many people have begun thinking about their food in a critical way, no longer willing to unquestionably swallow industrial food. My hope, of course, is that they will continue to evolve and question their diet choices until their quest coincides with actual science, as opposed to wishful thinking.

Many Paleo leaders suggest that a balanced Paleo plate consists of two-thirds plants and one-third meat. If that sounds reasonable, consider how unlikely it would be for actual Paleo man to have such an abundant supply of meat to be able to eat it three times a day. In addition, that "balanced" plate actually isn't very balanced, as meat has a much higher caloric density than fruits and vegetables. Let's say your plate was filled with one-third Porterhouse steak, one-third baked sweet potato, and one-third raw kale.

First, we have to decide: How are we calculating the thirds? We can do it by weight, by volume, or by calories. Let's do it all three ways and see what the plate looks like.

First, by weight. Let's plate 100 grams of each of the three foods. There are roughly 282 calories in 100 grams of Porterhouse steak, 90 calories in 100 grams of baked sweet potato, and 49 calories in 100 grams of raw kale. So that plate would provide 69 percent of its calories from meat, and only 31 percent from plants. That plate doesn't really look like the typical Paleo meal. It's got far more plant food than animal food, and despite that still manages to deliver more than two-thirds of its calories from the meat.

When we divide the plate equally by volume, things get even more skewed calorically. Let's pile on a cup of each. One cup of porterhouse steak has 640 calories, while a cup of baked sweet potatoes provides 181 calories, and a cup of chopped raw kale has 33 calories. This plate now delivers fully 75 percent of its calories from meat. The vegetables hardly have a chance.

The fairest way to divide a plate in thirds, nutritionally speaking, is by the energy content of the food: in other words, calories. Let's create a 600-calorie meal, in which the steak, sweet potatoes, and kale all contribute equally. There would be 71 grams of Porterhouse steak, 222 grams of baked sweet potato, and a whopping 408 grams of kale.

Even that last plate, with the meat overshadowed by the vegetables, still consists of way too much protein. Essentially, despite the ban on processed food and dairy, the dietary pattern is identical to prior low-carb incarnations. That's why I consider Paleo the "new and improved Atkins." Dr. Atkins favored pork rinds while Paleo zealots turn up their noses at such swill, preferring a piece of beef jerky instead. The improvement in diet is actually very slight, and most patients I see who try Paleo are eating a meal plan almost identical to the Atkins diet.

To be fair there are some healthy Paleo advocates who are eating large portions of fruits and vegetables, and only consuming meat that they hunt themselves. Sadly, these true Paleo advocates are few and far between.

The Paleo "Evidence"

The core of Cordain's argument is that whatever prehistoric man ate must be what we are genetically engineered to eat. Anything that came later—like all the fruits of the agricultural revolution, including grains and legumes—is therefore off the menu.

This argument is very similar to that of Dr. von Voit (whom we met in Chapter 4), who said we need 118 grams of protein a day because that is what laborers eat. Since Cordain assumes that Paleo man ate lots of meat, it logically follows that meat must be what we are created to eat.

There are several obvious fallacies with this argument. First off, prehistoric man was an obligate consumer. He ate what was available because otherwise he starved. He made decisions on food based not on optimal health, but rather survival. Second, there's no such thing as "the" Paleo diet; patterns of eating varied tremendously from region to region and season to season. The idea that there existed one specific Paleo diet is pure fiction (Eaton and Konner 1985).

In addition, the idea that our genes are exactly the same as a caveman, and the idea that we could not have evolved to process legumes and grains, is obviously flawed. Marlene Zuk is an anthropologist who specializes in the diet of early man. She was quite taken aback by the erroneous statements made by Cordain when she first heard him talk. Her book, *Paleofantasy*, is an excellent look at how our genes have changed to allow us to thrive under a completely different food environment.

In fact, much of what Cordain and the Paleo movement believe about the origins of our diet are completely false, according to actual forensic anthropologists. Many of Cordain's erroneous notions were brought to life in a debate he had with T. Colin Campbell, a transcript of which was published in the *Journal of Nutrition and Athletic Excellence*. His claim that ancient man ate mainly meat and protein is based on an ethnographic atlas and the fact that we have found hunting tools. An ethnographic atlas is basically an observational study, like Dr. Price's book, from which no statistical inferences can be made. The atlas found a lot of animal bones and what appeared to be hunting implements. Therefore, according to Cordain, ancient man ate lots of meat. What's laughable about this, of course, is that bones and stones are precisely the sorts of material that might last long enough to be found by researchers tens of centuries later. The remnants of the nuts, seeds, berries, leaves, roots, and stems that composed the lion's share of the diet would have been long gone, and therefore unable to offer their evidence to the atlas makers.

Imagine cataloging high school cafeteria Dumpsters to discover the eating habits of American youth. You'd find more peas and corn than tater tots, which might lead to you conclude that peas and corn were a staple. And you might assume that pizza was not even part of the diet, based on the fact that so little was thrown out. If you waited three hundred thousand years to perform the survey, all you might find left would be a few soda cans, leading you to conclude that Mountain Dew was the staple of the American teenage diet in the twenty-first century. (Sadly, you'd be more accurate than the Paleo theorists have been about prehistoric humans.)

Ethnographic atlases can also be notoriously biased. In our cafeteria study, the high schools we choose to include and ignore will determine what we conclude. The Dumpsters in South Central L.A. will look markedly different from those in Greenwich, Connecticut, and neither will closely resemble Dumpsters in Houston or Bellingham, Washington. The atlas Cordain relies upon was heavily biased toward men. From a man's view, the hunt was very important and symbolic, but evidence exists that most of the Paleolithic diet was in fact plant based and gathered by the women (Milton 2000).

So if ethnographic atlases can't provide the answers, what other evidence is there? Studies presented in the *Proceedings of the National Academies of Science* used isotope analysis on fossil teeth of *Australopithecus* to show that ancient man was a heavy plant consumer. In 2008, *Australopithecus sediba,* a two-million-year-old hominid fossil from South America, was examined to determine diet. Food matter in the fossilized teeth revealed that the diet appeared to be mainly tree leaves, bark, and fruits. The diet was very similar to that of chimps, and this was in an open savanna habitat with plenty of animal food available (Henry, Brooks, et al. 2011; Henry, Ungar, et al. 2012; Schoeninger 2012). In fact, no matter what region of the world is studied, analysis of Neanderthal teeth proves that these humans ate mostly plants, including legumes. This is odd, because people who follow a Paleo diet avoid legumes since they believe they were "invented" as part of the agricultural movement, and furthermore we are not genetically capable of processing beans. With an astonishing unwillingness to face facts, Paleo advocates actually argue that beans are poisonous to humans, despite the overwhelming evidence linking bean consumption with human longevity. All long-lived cultures consume legumes, and studies have shown that legume consumption decreases heart disease and increases years of life (Menotti, Kromhout, et al. 1999; Kromhout, Bloemberg, et al. 2000; Darmadi-Blackberry, Wahlqvist, et al. 2004; Chang, Wahlqvist, et al. 2012). If that's the definition of a poison, then make mine a double!

In addition, the evidence shows that the shift to eating grains may have occurred far earlier than ten thousand years ago, the figure Cordain would have us believe. Tools for grinding grains and plants have been found in Italy, Russia, and the former Czechoslovakia, many of which have been carbon dated to over three hundred thousand years ago.

Nathaniel Dominy is a professor of anthropology who writes widely on the subject of diet and ancient man and is one of the foremost experts. He notes that plants made up the bulk of calories for primates and hunter-gatherer societies. The hunters may have received all the glory, but the bulk of the calories came from the women doing the gathering. More important, he has found that our genes may have evolved to eat starch, and that may have been the key to our evolution and brain development. Paleo pseudoexperts claim that meat allowed our brain development, which really is just odd given that we did not evolve a new gene to facilitate eating meat, nor was there a sudden surplus in available animal protein. Dr. Dominy has looked at genes and found that we differ from chimps mainly in the way we can process starch. Turns out, our ability to eat and process bulbs (onions) and tubers (potatoes) may have been the key for our brain development and our ascension from the chimps. These same findings were also presented in the comprehensively researched book *The World History of Food* (Cohen 2012).

I can understand thinking that Paleo men ate lots of meat based on unfounded but persistent cultural assumptions, but some Paleo claims simply defy what is known about contemporary human biology. For example, Cordain states that humans are designed to process the uric acid that comes from eating meat. He obviously has not treated any people with gout and/or uric acid kidney stones, which I see frequently in people who eat a lot of animal protein.

He also claims that fruit and veggies will cause N-nitroso compounds, which have been linked to colon cancer, to form in the gut. This is so wildly wrong, I'm rendered practically speechless. (Luckily, not for long!) Randomized control trials show that meat causes the formation of N-nitroso compounds and colon cancer (Hughes, Cross, et al. 2001). Nitrates found in vegetables would need heme iron, only found in animal protein, to convert to the N-nitroso compounds. Finally, he asks rhetorically why a cat doesn't get colon cancer, seeing that it eats meat. A cat doesn't get colon cancer because a cat is a carnivore. Its anatomy and physiology are completely different from a human's. That's about as logical as trying to prove that humans need to consume diesel fuel because Volkswagens thrive on the stuff.

If you look at comparative anatomy of humans and other animals, we are much more related to chimps than cats (or any other animal, for that matter). What do chimps eat? Plants, plants, and more plants, with an occasional insect chaser. Very rarely do they eat other monkeys, and only in times of food scarcity.

It's a common misconception that humans are carnivores. It's one of the first things people say to me when they want to argue with my food advice (after the obligatory protein rant). Are we carnivores? Feel your teeth. Look at your hands. Can you chase down an animal and rip its hide off with your bare hands and teeth? Do you look anything like a lion? We are omnivores; our intelligence and anatomical adaptation has allowed us to survive harsh situations by being able to eat anything, but that does not mean what we eat is the best thing for us! If we are to eat solely based on our anatomy, we would do best eating just fruit and lots of fiber (Eaton and Konner 1985).

Carnivores walk on all four limbs. They have large, sharp teeth. Their jaws are hinged, with no side-to-side motion. Got a dog? Just try moving Fido's mouth side to side. It is not possible. Their jaws and teeth are made for clasping and shearing, not for grinding and chewing like ours. A carnivore has acidic saliva and acidic urine, consequently dealing with the high acid intake of meat far better than we do. They also process cholesterol much more efficiently. Part of the reason cats and other carnivores don't get colon cancer is that, unlike us, they have very short intestinal tracts. They move food through in under four hours as opposed to our eighteen hours or more. A true carnivore can live on meat alone. We cannot. Alden Todd's harrowing book *Abandoned: The Story of the Greely Arctic Expedition 1881–1884* describes a phenomenon seen in men who had to survive exclusively on lean meat (in this case, it was their travel mates) known as "rabbit starvation." Eating a diet exclusively of meat would lead to skin diseases, stomach distention, and hair and teeth falling out.

We have small mouths, grinding teeth, and long intestinal tracts. We produce amylase in our saliva to break down starch. Unlike carnivores, we do not produce our own vitamin C, so we have to get it from plants. We, like other primates, can live exclusively on a plant-based diet. Compared to all the different species, the primates have the closest anatomy and thrive on a predominately fruit diet. If you think you cannot build muscle on bananas, I challenge you to pick a fight with an ape.

Cordain makes one claim that's echoed mindlessly and endlessly by those touting a high-protein diet: that we should eat like the Inuits. They eat a diet very high in fat and protein and yet don't get heart disease. The first time I heard about the Inuits was at the annual meeting of the American Society of Bariatric Physicians, an organization of physicians dedicated to helping their patients lose weight. The society has a decidedly high-protein, low-carb bent. They lean toward high-protein diets for the reason Atkins is so popular: adherents achieve short-term weight loss, and it is easy to get people to eat lots of meat. Patients who need to lose weight simply won't return to the doctor's office unless they see quick and dramatic results.

This particular meeting was sponsored by the Atkins corporation, a multimillion-dollar business venture that thrives on rampant public proteinaholism. We were given an Atkins diet book and treated to a lecture by Gary Taubes. Taubes is a journalist, not a scientist, yet he was the keynote speaker at this supposedly scientific meeting. He and another speaker described the Inuit diet loaded with blubber and devoid of fruits and veggies and suggested that they were amazingly free of Western illnesses. This fascinated me, so I decided to explore the story of the Inuit health paradox for myself. I discovered that Taubes's description bore little resemblance to the actual facts.

Inuit is a name referring to the original tribes of the Arctic, Canada, Greenland, and the United States, and their descendants. They are more popularly known by a term they find pejorative, "Eskimos." Because they live in a frigid climate, they lack access to produce and depend on large amounts of seafood. They eat blubber and consume lots of fat. Interestingly, when compared to Danish people living at a similar latitude, they have lower overall cholesterol and higher good cholesterol. That is because of their diet, however, not in spite of it. While they eat more total fat, they eat far less saturated fat (fewer than 9% of the calories) in their diet. By comparison, most Western diets consist of approximately 15 percent saturated fat.

The Inuit also consume far more polyunsaturated omega-3 fatty acid. When they do eat meat, it is caribou that have been grazing on grass, and therefore high in omega-3. Their total omega-3 intake is upwards of 14 grams, compared to 3 grams in Holland and a pitiful 0.2 grams in America. The rest of their traditional diet is plant based: wild berries, kelp, flowers and nuts when available (Feskens and Kromhout 1993).

That's the kernel of truth in Taubes's story. Unfortunately for the Inuit (and their Paleo imitators), the rest of the story isn't so rosy. Turns out the Inuit are not healthy at all. They suffer from many chronic diseases and live, on average, ten years less than statistically matched Canadians (Choinière 1992; Iburg, Brønnum-Hansen, et al. 2001). In fact, they have the worst longevity of all populations in North America.

There are many reasons for their short life expectancy: high rate of infections and TB, as well as a high suicide rate. While these may not be diet related (although more and more evidence suggests a strong connection between diet and the ability to fight of infection, and between diet and mood), Inuit also die of cancers of the GI tract and stroke, afflictions strongly correlated to diet (Paltoo and Chu 2004).

Autopsy studies show they have less heart disease, likely due to their high omega-3 and low omega-6 and low-saturated-fat diet, but they are by no means free of heart disease (McLaughlin, Middaugh, et al. 2005). And there's a possibility that autopsy statistics showing low heart disease are unreliable, based on really poor data collection (Bjerregaard, Young, et al. 2003; Bell, Mayer-Davis, et al. 1997). In fact, one of the likely reasons for their apparent low rates of heart disease and some cancers is their short life expectancy: Inuit eating their traditional diet simply don't live long enough to demonstrate heart disease and cancer. In fact, the Westernization of their diet—adding the very foods the Paleo movement vilifies—may actually be prolonging their lives. A recent review of the literature suggests that a diet high in seafood does not lead to less heart disease and may lead to worse health (Fodor, Helis, et al. 2014)!

The Paleo propaganda also lionizes the Maasai, a nomadic tribe inhabiting southern Kenya and northern Tanzania. The Paleo supporters point to the fact that the Maasai are cattle ranchers and eat lots of meat, including the organs, as well as copious amounts of blood. As in most traditional societies, nothing from the animal is wasted. And because of this meat-heavy diet, according to Cordain and others, the Maasai are healthy and do not suffer heart disease like we do.

The Maasai do not suffer heart attacks because, like the Inuits, they do not live long enough for their heart disease to progress sufficiently. They live only forty to fifty years, on average. The Maasai typically die from infectious disease, but an autopsy study of fifty Maasai revealed as much heart disease "as an elderly American man" (Mann, Spoerry, et al. 1972). The autopsy study does note that they seem to have large vessels to compensate for the plaques. This adaptation is likely thanks to their living at high altitude, as well as their nomadic lifestyle, requiring them to walk much farther on a daily basis than Westerners. They also live at subsistence, eating far less than we do, and are infected with parasites that keep them leaner. In short, these significant differences make a comparison between the Maasai and Western populations truly meaningless. And to top it off, they do not achieve anywhere near the level of health we want.

If we are going to look at how different, non-Westernized, native cultures eat, why not look at the diets of the Blue Zone cultures that I mentioned in Chapter 3? Blue Zones, as you'll recall, are regions of the world where people live significantly longer lives. The first study of a Blue Zone was in Sardinia (Poulain, Pes, et al. 2004). The study looked specifically at people living in the mountains of Sardinia and found them to be healthier than Sardinians in other parts of the island. There can be many reasons that the villagers in the mountains lived longer than surrounding areas, but a main one is their diet: predominately plant and starch based. Breads and pastas were common, wheat being one of their main staples prior to Westernization. Animal meats were saved for special occasions. They did eat some cheese, especially from goats grazing on natural grasses and therefore high in omega-3. Their protein intake was much lower than that in our Western culture.

Again, this is not a formal scientific study, but more like an ethnographic atlas. Nonetheless, much can be learned since these are modern cultures, rather than fossilized remains unearthed from ancient campsites. No matter which Blue Zone culture you look at, plants, especially starchy vegetables and legumes, make up the base of the diet. Legumes, frowned upon by Paleo believers, are a large part of every Blue Zone diet. Here's a question that Paleo promoters can't answer: If legumes are so poisonous, then why are people who eat them living such long lives?

The most widely talked about Blue Zone is the Japanese island of Okinawa. Unfortunately, their traditionally healthy diet is being invaded by Western culture, and their youth are decidedly less healthy. Fast-food restaurants are taking the country by storm. Nonetheless, we can learn a lot from the elder Okinawans.

The traditional Okinawan diet is light on fish, despite what you might expect from an island population. Remember that the majority of their calories (70–80%) comes from the purple yams they call "imo"(Sho 2001). Thus the Okinawan diet is mainly starch, with only 7 percent to 9 percent of calories coming from protein, and a paltry 4 percent of calories coming from animals. Starch is a dirty word in the United States, but Okinawans, unlike the Inuits and Maasai, live incredibly long healthy lives in large measure thanks to starch. They also eat lots of fruits and vegetables (Willcox, Willcox, et al. 2007, 2009). In fact, their daily diet is devoid of meat, and they traditionally eat pork only at festive occasions once or twice a month.

One of the most interesting Blue Zones is that of the Seventh-day Adventists in Loma Linda, California. Can you believe that in America, one of the unhealthiest countries in the civilized world, we have a Blue Zone? The religion is interesting in that it advocates a clean lifestyle on a physical, as well as spiritual, level. Seventh-day Adventists view the body as the temple of the soul and therefore worthy of good treatment. Smoking is frowned upon and exercise is celebrated. Adherents have varied views on meat consumption. Many Seventh-day Adventists believe that people should eat as the biblical Daniel did while in captivity. Daniel "avoided anything unclean" and therefore was a vegetarian. Many Adventists are vegetarian, and over 4 percent are completely vegan (no dairy, no meat, no fish).

From a research perspective, the Seventh-day Adventists of Loma Linda have been a godsend. The community has been open to being studied by researchers at Loma Linda University. They make a wonderful "natural experiment," as they practice similarly healthy livestyles but differ in how much animal food they consume. Some eat meat, some exclude land animals and consume just fish, others eschew all meat but have dairy, while a few eat solely plant-based food. One of the first research studies that focused on the Seventh-day Adventists was commissioned by the American Cancer Society and compared their nonsmoking population to a typical American community. This was one of the first studies showing that smoking greatly increases risk of lung cancer. Researchers noted with some interest that there was an anomaly in the data: lung cancer was not the only condition that visited the Adventists less than average

Americans: they also had lower incidence of many other cancers, as well as heart disease. In Part III, I will refer several times to the Adventist Health Studies, as many valid and reliable research articles have come from this population.

In *The Blue Zones,* Buettner shared quotes from an interview with one of the lead researchers of the Adventist Health Studies, Dr. Gary Fraser. Fraser concisely summarized years of research on the relationship between diet and disease in one sentence: "Not eating meat is clearly important because it seems to have an impact on heart disease and cancer." He also notes that body weight is closely correlated with health and points out that vegetarians in Loma Linda are sixteen pounds lighter than meat eaters, while vegans are a whopping thirty-two pounds lighter!

The unarguable fact is, no culture in human history has truly thrived on a high-protein, meat-based diet. To the contrary, anthropology of both past and present civilizations demonstrates that starches, grains, vegetables, beans, and fruit are the foods that have enabled humans to flourish. Whether you look at the Incas, the Aztecs, the Middle East, the Far East, or even Africa, you can see that agriculture and the cultivation of starch, not high-protein meat, underpins their growth and success.

Dr. Denis Burkitt, born in Ireland, was an English surgeon who served in the Royal Army Corp and therefore had the opportunity to travel widely through Kenya, Uganda, and Somalia. He found that the native people ate very high fiber and starch diets. He also noted that the high fiber resulted in bulky stools that were softer than the typical Englishman's bowel movement and less odorous. There's a scientific reason for this interesting observation: the sulfur that comes from amino acids in animal-based protein creates a strong and unpleasant odor. Burkitt also noted native Africans moved their bowels more frequently that did his own countrymen (Burkitt 1971). Here was a man obviously dedicated to his job, and definitely observant. I sometimes wonder what the Africans thought of this strange white man examining their excrement. His real interest, of course, was not simply the texture, size, or frequency of the African natives' bowel movements, but rather how that data might shed light on their practically nonexistent rates of bowel disease.

Burkitt, like me, was a general surgeon. Spend a night on call with a general surgeon and you'll see a nonstop parade of diverticulitis, appendicitis, gallbladder attacks, and colon cancer. Yet when he traveled to Africa he rarely saw these diseases. He knew the cause was not genetic, as he treated many Africans in England who had adopted a typical Western diet and consequently developed these ailments. His book, *Don't Forget Your Fibre,* shares his studies and stresses the importance of a high-fiber diet in preventing disease. Note that Burkitt did not advise eating more meat to get protein. As animal foods, including dairy and eggs, contain no fiber whatsoever (Burkitt 1981), they are among the foods that people seeking health should most avoid. And if the avoidance of painful and life-threatening diseases of the bowels isn't incentive enough, studies show that Africans on a traditional high-fiber diet also have extremely low rates of heart disease (Thomas, Davies, et al. 1960).

The more Burkitt studied, the more convinced he became that the answer to the vast majority of diseases of modern man was not more advanced surgical procedures or better drugs, but rather a complete change in our diet. He noticed, as I eventually did myself, that medicine was not curing diseases, but simply managing their symptoms, and, in best cases, slowing or halting their progression. Why, he wondered, did doctors not seek to achieve what would be a real boon for their patients: preventing disease in the first place? Imagine, he wrote, a cliff where people keep falling off and dying. Instead of erecting a warning sign at the top of the cliff telling people not to approach, modern medicine just places ambulances at the bottom (Burkitt 1991).

We can learn a lot from medical explorers, like Burkitt, who have studied how healthy and slim native peoples have lived. A 2002 article in the *American Journal of Cardiology* shared the observations of some "medical Marco Polos," doctors who visited non-Western civilizations and were struck by the utter lack of "Western" diseases among their populations. One example was the young physician Cornelis de Langen, who was sent by the Dutch government to teach internal medicine in Jakarta, Indonesia, in 1916 (Blackburn 2012). He noted that the Javanese ate largely vegetarian diets, including hefty portions of rice. They were thin, had very low cholesterol, and almost no heart disease, gall bladder disease, thrombosis, or embolisms. De Langen's understanding of the connection between diet and disease deepened when he looked at their Javanese counterparts who worked for the thriving tourist industry, especially the cruise ships. They were much more exposed to the typical Western diet and therefore had higher rates of obesity and were exhibiting the typical Western diseases. As you might now suspect, they ate more meat and consequently more protein.

To test his theory that the animal-rich Western diet was the culprit, de Langen conducted one of the first known experiments to manipulate cholesterol levels. He took five Javanese and, for six weeks, replaced their traditional starch-based vegetarian diet with one rich in meat, butter, and eggs. Their average cholesterol skyrocketed an average of 40 mg/dl in just a month and a half (Blackburn 2012).

There are many reports that compare genetically related (and even identical) groups that had developed different diets and cultures. One of my favorite studies looked at the Kyrgyz tribe, living mostly in Afghanistan and Turkey, but descended from nomadic plainsmen of Mongolia. Genetically they are closely related to the peasants of Siberia. Early-twentieth-century Kyrgyz follow a lifestyle that had not changed much in hundreds, perhaps even thousands of years. Their diet was very high in protein and fat. They ate mainly meat, all grass-fed and raised on the plains. Their milk was whole milk, fresh and unpasteurized. They consumed no processed foods at all. In short, veritable poster children for the Paleo diet!

So how was their health, living so close to the Paleo ideal? Alas, it was horrible. Despite their high levels of physical activity, they were obese, had very high cholesterol, and died young. Compared to their genetically similar Siberian counterparts, who thrived on potatoes and wheat and lived well into their seventies, the Kyrgyz were a supremely unhealthy society (Bjornsson 1942).

When you look at traditional Asian cultures, you typically observe people eating very high-starch, low-protein diets and enjoying long, healthy lives. General Tso's Chicken is not a traditional Asian dish, nor one that would have been affordable on a regular basis to any but a tiny elite upper class. The ordinary people enjoyed rice and veggies. Atherosclerosis, hypertension, and obesity are almost unheard of in traditional starch-based native cultures, but they are extremely common in areas of China and Africa where meat, eggs, and butter have been a key part of the diet (Khor 1997). Even modern-day people who live in the pasture lands of Xinjiang Province in China, and eat a diet high in meat, have high rates of the usual Western diseases, far higher than their genetic relatives eating a more plant-based diet in the rural parts of China.

In 1908, a researcher named William Roger Williams studied the health of the Argentinian gauchos, the original cowboys of South America. As you might expect, they subsisted on lots of beef. And not McDonald's quality either; this was grass fed, much purer than any Paleo adherent can buy today. Yet Williams noted that they had a high rate of cancer. He had also traveled in Egypt, where most inhabitants consumed a largely vegetarian diet with little meat, and where cancer was almost unheard of.

Speaking of Egypt, we know that pharaohs and other members of the political ruling classes sought immortality through embalming and entombment in giant pyramids. While the jury's out on that effort, modern science has been able to assess the heart health of some of these mummies through CAT scans. These studies show that heart disease, far from being a recent human affliction, actually goes way back in history, appearing wherever people ate large amounts of animal products. Mummies over four thousand years old showed evidence of clinically significant cardiovascular disease. Paleo advocates argue that this was due to agriculture, but CAT scans have also been done on fossils of humans who lived in preagricultural hunter-gatherer societies, and they too showed evidence of heart disease (Thompson, Allam, et al. 2013; Allam, Thompson et al. 2011).

It's no coincidence that the upper classes, the ones who could afford mummification, were the ones dying young from heart disease. The bodies of ancient Egyptian peasants and slaves, who ate wheat and grains, have not survived to be scanned, but I have little doubt what they would show. Modern-day Bedouin and Yemenite Jews live very similar lives to what we know about ancient Egyptian peasants. Careful analysis shows that they eat a very high-carbohydrate diet almost completely devoid of animal protein. The wheat and barley they grow themselves make up the majority of their diet. They are slim, have very low cholesterol, and despite (actually, because of) the very high-carbohydrate diet, have almost no diabetes (Groen, Balogh, et al. 1964)!

What would happen if their diet changed from a high-carbohydrate to a higher-protein diet? We may find some answers in a fascinating and unfortunate natural experiment that has played out in modern-day Tunisia. The traditional Tunisian diet has been high in grains and other carbohydrates, and low in protein. Then something alarming happened: from 1997 to 2009, the rate of death from heart disease in Tunisia increased 17 percent, which correlated with spikes in cholesterol, blood pressure, and weight. The obesity rate among Tunisian men increased by an almost unbelievable 74 percent during that twelve-year period. And during the same period, the smoking rate went down, and access to modern health care increased!

What happened that could possibly cause this rapid decline in health? Starting in 1997, Tunisia underwent rapid economic growth. With Tunisians' newfound wealth, they were able to afford different kinds of food. Their animal protein consumption increased from 14 percent to 27 percent of total protein. Meat and milk consumption doubled over a single decade. Most of that meat and milk went to Tunisian men, not women, which is why weight gain and heart disease rose more in men. Rural Tunisians, relatively unaffected by this growth, maintained their traditional diet. Eating three times the wheat of their wealthier countrymen, while consuming very little animal protein, they have far less heart disease, obesity, and diabetes! There are many other factors that are no doubt affecting the health of urban Tunisians, including a sedentary lifestyle and urban pollution, but there can be no doubt that the rapid rise of animal protein has caused a commensurate decline in the health of the modern-day urban Tunisian.

One of the most interesting populations to study is the Pima Indians of Arizona. The Pima lived for many years along the Gila and Salt Rivers of Arizona. These rivers were their source of life, irrigating their lands, drawing game to hunt, and supporting fish to catch. Despite the availability of animal foods, the Pima were mainly farmers. Their diet consisted of wheat, corn, squash, beans, fruit, along with some rabbit and fish. It is estimated that, like many of the Blue Zones, they ate 70 to 80 percent of their calories from carbs, 10 to 15 percent from protein, and 8 to 12 percent from fat.

So far that's a fairly normal tale. Healthy populations subsist mostly on plants. Nothing surprising, unless you're still in the thrall of low-carb propaganda. But here's where things get interesting.

In 1848, Arizona became part of the United States. With its statehood in 1912 came increased colonization. Settlements upstream from the Pima constructed dams that dried up the Gila and Salt Rivers. The Pima, deprived of their livelihood, were forced to become dependent on trading posts, and later on government subsidy. At first they starved, but by the turn of the century the government was providing them with sufficient flour and lard. After World War II, a modest economic boom in the area led to even greater Westernization. Today, the Pima eat about 35 percent carbs, 50 percent fat, and 12 to 18 percent protein! The total number of calories has also increased dramatically (Boyce and Swinburn 1993).

So how have these changes in diet affected their health? Before the turn of the century there were no cases of diabetes among the Pima, but now approximately half of adult Pimas are diabetic. They have among the highest rates of obesity in North America. Of course, their diet now has many processed carbs, but it is also loaded with animal fat and protein. Researchers have come from all over to study the Pima to attempt to understand the underlying disease process of diabetes. While their environmental situation is noted, most researchers focus on the genetics of the Pima that make them so susceptible to diabetes (Knowler, Saad, et al. 1993).

Sure, it's interesting that this group of people develop more diabetes than normal when fed the standard American diet. Certainly there are things we can learn from them. But do you know what's far more interesting to me? The fact that they have a genetic predisposition to diabetes but never had diabetes until they gave up their very high-carbohydrate/low-protein diet. Even possessed of a gene that makes them highly susceptible to diabetes, they did not develop diabetes. Rather than chasing genetic cures, wouldn't it be easier to fix our diets?

You may think I'm speculating wildly here. Perhaps the Pima would have developed diabetes anyway for some reason. Luckily, there exists another Mexican tribe, relatives of the Pima, who still eat a traditional diet. How is their health these days?

You may have heard of the Tarahumara Indians of Mexico. They were made famous in Christopher McDougall's book *Born to Run*, because they are among the world's best long-distance runners. More interesting to me is that they are very close genetic relatives to the Pima. That being the case, they are also genetically susceptible to diabetes. Yet despite their genetics, only 6.9 percent of their population suffer from diabetes (Schulz, Bennett, et al. 2006). They eat mainly pinole, a dish of roasted corn that is mashed and combined with water, spices, and sugar. They also eat lots of beans. Almost 100 percent of their daily 85 grams of protein come from veggies; almost none come from meat. Like their traditional Pima cousins, they consume 70 to 80 percent of their calories as carbs. Not only do they not have diabetes, they also have less heart disease, low cholesterol, no bone disease (despite not drinking milk), and can run faster and longer than many of the top runners in America. Put a Pima next to a Tarahumara and you would be shocked to realize they are genetically related (Cerqueira, Fry, et al. 1979; Ravussin, Valencia, et al. 1994)!

Stories like this abound throughout the world, everywhere we look. The Vanuatu, for example. It's an archipelago of islands in the South

Pacific. Like the Tarahumara and the Pima, the people on the different islands share a common genetic heritage, but live on islands experiencing varying degrees of economic development and Westernization. This makes for an excellent environment to study the effects of diet on a native and ancient culture. Studies show, unsurprisingly, that the more Westernized the island, the higher the rate of obesity and chronic disease. Specifically, researchers found that increased animal protein was a key factor in obesity. To be fair, processed carbs add extra calories and certainly play a part (remember, I'm definitely *not* advising you to start eating bagels and Wonder Bread in place of meat), but the increased consumption of animal protein, especially canned fish, is strongly correlated with weight gain (Dancause, Vilar, et al. 2013).

The point here is that ancient man never really ate a high-protein diet, and throughout history most societies have thrived on a lower-protein, very high-carb diet. In fact, we simply do not know of a culture that ate a predominately animal protein diet and thrived. The diseases of Western civilization can certainly be blamed, in part, on increasing calories and more processed carbs; however, through the next few chapters I will show you the science that demonstrates that dangerous amounts of animal protein are the real smoking gun.

For the latest research comparing paleo and plant-based diets, visit Proteinaholic.com.

PART THREE

Death and Disease
by Protein

CHAPTER 8

Research Truth and BS: How to Speak Science

In Chapter 3, I told you about my rapid transformation from sick, over-weight, and sluggish patient to healthy, lean, energetic triathlete. Had I been an accountant, a bricklayer, a rock musician, that would have been the end of the story. But I was a doctor, a surgeon—and a weight-loss surgeon at that. My old proteinaholic views on nutrition were public record, enshrined in Chapter 12 of my 2008 book, *The Expert's Guide to Weight-Loss Surgery*. Just to rub my nose in it, here's a sample passage advising patients what to eat once they begin recovering from the surgery:

"Strained cream soups and yogurt-based shakes and smoothies are good choices. A little cream of wheat with protein powder added or grits thinned with skim milk—even tuna and chicken salad that have been blended until there are no distinct pieces remaining—are also good options. Sugar-free pudding and gelatins are okay, too; add protein powder for added nutrition. Well-mashed scrambled eggs or egg substitute and puréed low-fat cottage cheese are also good protein sources."

Ugh.

A book is one thing, while television is a whole other level of exposure. In 2006, an old college buddy and I got together and were chatting about our careers. He, it turned out, had gotten into television. When he heard about my career in bariatric surgery, his Nielsen rating detectors started going off. "That would make a great reality show," he mused.

The following year, *Big Medicine* debuted on TLC. Here's the network's description of the show: "The father and son team of Drs. Robert and Garth Davis perform innovative bariatric surgeries at the Methodist Weight Management Center in Houston. The series chronicles the emotional transformations of obese people who have opted to undergo weight-loss surgery, capturing the process before and during the operation, through recovery and post-op care . . ."

Big Medicine ran for two seasons and established me and my dad as "celebrity" weight-loss surgeons. So by the time I discovered that my views on diet and nutrition were all wrong, I had a thriving practice based, in part, on those errors. I began to feel sheepish: How in the world was I going to start telling my patients the exact opposite of what I had been preaching for years?

And feelings of embarrassment aside, my recovery from proteinaholism begged a larger question: How should I be treating patients differently, based on everything I now know?

My transformation, while dramatic and extremely personal, was still anecdotal, a case study of one. Before I was going to change my practice model, I needed to dive into the nitty-gritty of clinical research. Not just the Blue Zone correlations, or the prospective population studies. I had to immerse myself in the totality of evidence, including biochemical laboratory research and controlled clinical trials, in order to treat my patients confidently with my newly adopted plant-based protocols.

And while I was known for my contributions to the weight-loss field, I was acutely aware that the real goal was improved health and freedom from disease, not simply a slim body still in failing health.

I wanted to see if a plant-based diet could treat obesity, sure. But to prescribe it enthusiastically, I wanted to see evidence that it could help diabetic and prediabetic patients. Patients with hypertension and other cardiovascular diseases. Patients facing the terrifying diagnosis of cancer. Patients suffering from any condition likely to shorten their life span.

The more I looked, the more conditions I found that could be prevented, arrested, reversed, and even cured with a protocol that included a plant-based diet. Diseases as varied and disabling as rheumatoid arthritis, ulcerative colitis, diverticulitis, and depression responded well to a plant-based intervention. In study after study, I found support for my decision to treat all my patients the way I had successfully treated myself.

So Parts III and IV of this book, for me, are a bit of redemption: a chance to right my prior book's mistakes, this time with evidence-based dietary recommendations. These sections will be absolutely full of science. Maybe too much for many people, but if I leave out too much, I will be accused of speculating. My use of plant-based diets for my patients is not an ideologic decision but rather an evidence-based practice.

Before we jump in, though, I want to make sure that I don't just add to your confusion by contradicting everything you've heard before. Prior to surveying the scientific evidence favoring a plant-based diet, let's look at how to evaluate scientific research. So the next time someone says, "But I heard that cholesterol levels don't matter," or "I saw an article that bone broth was really good for me," you'll be able to look at the data and decide for yourself if the sources are valid and trustworthy.

A Glut of Information and a Famine of Wisdom

People who know nothing about nutrition often offer the following statement as unassailable truth: "There's no such thing as a diet that's right for everyone." Where does this firm belief in "nutritional relativism" come from? It's common sense that people with food allergies and sensitivities should avoid foods that trigger them, but the science is clear and overwhelming that there is a fundamental dietary pattern that has been shown to be superior in every population where it's been studied.

A number of popular and misinformed nutritional "experts" promote a fantasy they call "bio-individuality," meaning that we're all different and need to eat based on our body's own inner wisdom. That's fine in theory, but in practice it usually means choosing the foods we crave over the ones that can heal us. Imagine telling a cocaine addict to listen to his body. He'd be bent over a mirror with a glass straw up his nose as soon as his current high started to fade.

But nutritional relativism is much bigger than that. It's largely been created by a tidal wave of conflicting information, much of it intentionally created expressly to sow confusion and doubt. Bloggers and social media outlets jump on any study that appears to support their worldview and create sensational headlines as "click bait" to increase page views and advertising revenue. The layperson, sincerely looking for guidance on how to eat healthy, is easily swept up in the rhetoric. Without the medical community guiding them, too many make decisions based on the writer's or speaker's eloquence and charisma, rather than an honest review of the science. In fact, the people actually doing the science are largely absent from social media and the popular press, leaving a vacuum that allows industry-funded charlatans to sell their nonsense.

Without a science-based rudder to steer the correct course, our eating patterns have changed dramatically. Fad diets—many of them plainly crazy and some alarmingly dangerous—are the norm. The diet supplement business is thriving. We spend $80 billion a year on diets and diet supplements, yet we have managed only to diet ourselves fatter. We've become obese and ill not just from consuming the wrong foods, but also the wrong information. The goal of this chapter is to help you become a smart consumer of information, so you can protect yourself and your loved ones from bad science and harmful food choices.

My Scientific Credentials

Although medicine didn't teach me about nutrition, it did make me an expert in experimental design. Med school, internship, and residency, and the process of becoming board certified, all trained me to read, understand, evaluate, and integrate complex scientific studies. After my "popular" introduction to the idea of a plant-based diet through books and websites, I began to devour the scientific literature with the same ravenous appetite I already had for research on bariatric surgery and other relevant medical topics. I started attending professional meetings for medical weight loss and treating patients without surgery. I used my ability to read scientific journals and my access to countless articles to examine the actual science of nutrition in depth.

I keep up with nutritional literature, poring through dozens of journals and analyzing many scientific articles each month to be sure I'm sharing the best and latest information with my patients and readers. And because I have a busy clinical practice, I get to see the results of that information in action. Native American leaders would often apply the following question to any new idea or philosophy: "Does it grow corn?" In other words, does the sparkly new idea or exciting concept actually work in the real world to benefit human beings? Since I see hundreds of patients each week, I quickly get real-world feedback on the truth and usefulness of scientific findings.

My ongoing research, as well as my successful clinical application of the plant-based diet, continue to confirm my initial conclusion: humans should be eating mostly plants, and limiting or eliminating animal products.

Once I saw the weight of evidence and applied it to help my patients lose weight and get healthier, I had to confront the question: Why is there still such heated debate on this issue? Our current understanding of nutrition reminds me of the 1946 R.J. Reynolds advertisement, "More doctors smoke Camels than any other cigarettes." We've known that cigarette smoking is a health disaster for at least the past fifty years. No present-day doctor would dare recommend smoking, and no citizen would believe that doctor if he or she did.

When it comes to nutrition, the evidence is even clearer than with nicotine. And the stakes are higher: far more people will suffer and perish from bad food than ever did from cigarettes. So I had to ask: What's wrong with how nutritional science is conducted, reported, and understood in our society? And given that truths are generally drowned out by half-truths and downright falsehoods, how can ordinary citizens figure out what's right and wrong?

The answers to these questions are of far more than theoretical value. When you can see behind the curtain, you'll know how to protect yourself from "information-borne illnesses." The goal of this chapter is to teach you how to "speak science." Specifically, I'll show you how to evaluate the research studies you hear about on TV and read about in blogs, magazines, newspapers, and on your Facebook feed. You don't need to become an "expert"; a little interest and effort can keep you from becoming a sucker for bad ideas.

Key Issues

Little Dots and Big Pictures

The single biggest problem with science and science reporting is reductionism, a mind-set that obsesses over tiny details at the expense of the big picture. Have you ever zoomed in on a digital photograph? When you make the picture big enough, the overall image is no longer apparent;

instead, you see individual dots, or pixels, each with a specific color. Even if the scene depicted is a blue sky, not every pixel will be blue. Some will be black, others white, still others red or brown or dark green or orange. The effect of the blending and melding of all the individual pixels generates the complete image.

I want you to hold on to that metaphor as we look at scientific research. Individual studies are the dots; the full breadth of research is the whole picture. Just as there are orange pixels contributing to the blue sky, there are studies whose findings appear to contradict the preponderance of evidence. Can you imagine someone insisting that, based on his discovery of an orange pixel, the entire sky in this photograph must therefore be orange? All it takes to disprove this absurd suggestion is to pan back out and view the big picture.

But in science, views of the big picture (what we call the "preponderance of evidence") are uncommon, and not greatly valued. It is very difficult to actually study the big picture. Instead, scientists tend to focus on a few, easily controlled variables. Most academics live in a "publish or perish" environment, where their jobs depend on them being able to get studies into the journals, so science tends to gravitate to the study of these easily controlled variables.

Studies differ in how much of the whole picture they can show. A decades-long population study, rigorously carried out, tells us much more than a lab study conducted over four days. And there's a massive trade-off, generally speaking, between how much a study can teach us, and how much it costs to run. All things equal, the shorter the study, the less it costs. So science tends to favor short and sweet studies that produce isolated pixels of data over long, comprehensive studies that can give us entire swaths of landscape. To extend the metaphor, a single snapshot of the sky gives us much less valuable information than a time-lapse video taken over an entire season.

The problem is not the small studies that produce the pixels. Our sky photo needs the orange pixels to give us a vivid picture of the blue sky. The problem, rather, is that we—scientists, journalists, policymakers, and the public alike—don't realize that there *is* a big picture. When the *New York Times* reports on the discovery of a new orange pixel, we need to see it in context of the big picture. Our society worships pixels and doesn't believe in photographs. Therefore we see a story about an orange pixel and start wondering what color the sky is.

Once we've lost our ability to tell the difference between reality and fantasy, all sorts of nefarious forces can sneak into our minds and public discourse to profit from that confusion. The point being: never take one isolated study as "proof". If you want to really research the science then you need to cast a wide net. It is vital to look at the big-picture studies, as well as the smaller studies looking at individual variables. You then should be able to put this all together. For instance, let's say there is a study that shows drinking milk increases a hormone that may increase risk of prostate cancer. That doesn't mean milk causes prostate cancer. But if there are several studies that confirm this change, and there is a controlled trial showing that men who drink milk have higher PSA, and there are long-term epidemiologic studies in several countries that show men who consume dairy have higher rates of prostate cancer, then you now have developed a much fuller picture.

Industry Influence

The food industry, one of the largest in the country, has a vested interest in keeping the public confused. Their marketing and PR departments have studied at the feet of the tobacco companies, whose private motto for decades was "Our product is doubt" (Freudenberg, 2014). If they sell a food product found to be harmful, they simply refer to the odd assortment of obscure articles that actually show the food to have some benefit, or even a study that shows one ingredient of their product to be good for you. Many scientists are on the payroll of food companies, hired to prostitute their professional credibility by publishing misleading articles and promoting bad science at industry meetings. The dairy industry actually held a meeting where they developed a goal to "neutralize" the science that dairy may be bad for the public.

Is meat good or bad for you? Who knows, right? We've all seen evidence for both sides. And if we don't really know, here's where we end up: we believe what we want to believe. So when the TV commercial featuring a juicy steak sizzling in a grill pan, we focus on what we've heard about life-giving protein and ignore the little voices warning of heart disease from saturated fat and cholesterol and the cancer-causing heterocyclic amines. And off we go to the steakhouse.

Because the food industry can afford a much bigger megaphone than the honest nutritional scientists toiling away in their offices and labs, we hear about many more orange pixels than there actually are in the big picture. After a while, it starts looking like the entire sky is tinged with orange, to our surprise and delight.

This probably isn't the first time you've heard about wealthy and powerful interests hiding or distorting facts to maintain their wealth and power. What we need to do to break their grip is examine, in some detail, exactly how they succeed in promoting a false and self-serving "orange pixel" agenda at the expense of true blue sky.

Funding Determines Outcome

While certain scientists have traded all their professional credibility for industry money, others believe themselves to be impartial and independent. Unfortunately, virtue doesn't keep the lights on in the lab or pay the stipends of graduate assistants. So even the most noble seekers of truth have to raise the money for their research somewhere. And evidence shows that researchers who accept corporate money find in favor of their benefactors' interests a curiously high percentage of the time. I know many scientists who insist that industry funding is essential in order to conduct studies, and I do think they believe it will not influence results.

However, there have been many studies over the years showing that big pharmaceutical companies can influence science in their favor. Recently, it has been found that big agribusiness is doing the same thing. A review was performed of 206 recent studies on the health effects of milk, juice, and soda. Of those studies, 111 declared financial ties to industry, receiving part or all of the funding for the study from the manufacturer of the beverage in question. (Keep in mind that these are only the *known* ties. Many other financial arrangements can be hidden.) The 111 industry-funded studies showed zero unfavorable findings. That's right, not a single one found evidence that the beverages in question were harmful. Let that sink in for a moment: no study that received funding showed anything bad about consuming soda, juice, or milk. Can you imagine anything more ridiculous? The 95 unbiased articles, on the other hand, found evidence of harm 37 percent of the time. This is a very significant difference, demonstrating clearly that science can be bought (Lesser, Ebbeling, et al. 2007).

Biased science can sometimes appear in highly regarded professional publications like the *New England Journal of Medicine*, but the easiest route to publication comes via what I think of as "junk journals." The equivalent of diploma mills, these journals take advantage of academics' career pressure to "publish or perish" by accepting and disseminating any article, no matter how bad. The hallmark of a good journal is a process known as "peer review," in which experts in the field evaluate the study for quality and refuse publication to those studies that don't meet rigorous research standards. Peer review by no means guarantees a good article, but it is one of the best filters we have.

The junk journal industry produces a huge volume of scientific research, much of it poorly executed, that allows authors to add the reference to their resume. There are many journals that now exist to accommodate the seemingly infinite number of studies that would not survive true peer review.

A journalist recently wanted to shed light on this issue, so he conducted a very shoddy experiment with just a few people that he fed chocolate to daily. He looked at multiple variables over a short period, knowing that if you have a few people followed for a short period you will find some variable that, simply by chance, will appear as a significant variable. In this situation he found that the group that ate chocolate daily, again just by chance, lost more weight over the short period of his purposely flawed study. He then created a false name complete with Ph.D. credentials and paid a junk journal to publish this ridiculous article. Low and behold, seventeen different media outlets ran stories saying chocolate can reduce weight.

The Government/Industry Connection

You might think that the government wouldn't lie to us, mislead us, or hide information that could be crucial to our health. After all, the government is by the people and for the people, and therefore not susceptible to false marketing claims. Nothing could be further from the truth.

It is fascinating to watch the different food lobby groups testify before Congress whenever they are voting on a bill that pertains to how we should eat. At the United States Department of Agriculture (USDA) hearings on the Food Pyramid and MyPlate (the public nutrition education campaign that gets taught in schools and has many policy implications), the dairy, meat, egg and soda lobbyists were all present to protect their special interest. That interest being, of course, their bottom line rather than your health.

Surely the USDA listens to these industry shills with a grain of salt. After all, there's so much objective science that undermines their claims.

Unfortunately, the USDA is required by law to be sympathetic to their positions. The USDA is charged to not only make sure food is safe and good for you, but to also make sure that the businesses that produce food are profitable. Can you see how the USDA can find itself in conflict? Worse yet, when conflict does arise between what is good for us and what is profitable, guess who wins? Profit, just about every time.

The Death of Expertise

To recap: a certain percentage of scientific research has been hijacked by a commercial agenda seeking to convince us that harmful foods are health-promoting. And a slew of low-quality journals have come into existence to provide an outlet for unsupervised junk science. When debates occur in front of government officials, the truth is usually sacrificed to the profit motive. Given this environment of more misleading information than we can possibly keep track of and sort out for ourselves, a couple of influential groups have stepped into the breach to complete the catastrophe: journalists and health bloggers.

These folks rely on a website called PubMed, a free public search engine that indexes all the articles tracked by MEDLINE (Medical Literature Analysis and Retrieval System Online), a database maintained by the U.S. National Institutes of Health. On the surface, this database seems like a great thing—and it can be, if you use it right. Unfortunately, the full articles are not available via PubMed—just the abstracts (brief summaries of just a few paragraphs). If you want to see the full article, you often have to pay for the privilege. Furthermore, few reporters or bloggers will take the time to read the full article, complete with confusing scientific jargon and complex tables and charts. Even if they did, most are not equipped to understand the intricacies that go into judging whether a study was properly executed. Instead, the last line of the summary is sensationalized and converted into the front page of the morning news, regardless of whether that study has any scientific value or not.

Science writer Julia Belluz notes that reporters and scientists approach research quite differently. Reporters want to know "what's new," while scientists are trained not to trust brand-new results that contradict established findings. The result? Small, badly designed studies with anomalous findings are reported as medical breakthroughs, instead of outlier data that needs to be replicated with rigor before informing public discussion and policy. Belluz points to a 2003 review of how so-called highly promising basic research fared as it was translated into clinical experiments and implementation. Of 101 articles published between 1979 and 1983 that claimed a "novel therapeutic or preventive" technology, only five had been licensed for clinical use by 2002, with just a single technology in widespread use. If health journalists in the early 1980s were as trigger-happy as many are today, the public would have had their hopes raised for 96 miraculous new treatments and cures that turned out to be total duds.

Increasingly, journalists are becoming the new health gurus in our society. Those who can write and speak with charm and conviction hold sway, even getting invited to keynote supposedly rigorous professional meetings where they are treated like celebrities. And unlike true scientists, who are bound by professional ethics to always question their current theories and actively seek evidence to refute or refine them, the health journalists tend to jump on their horses and ride unwaveringly into the sunset of whatever fad they've taken a fancy to.

Example: The Terrible "Meat Eaters Are Healthier Than Vegetarians" Study

In a world where health journalists lack perspective, expertise, and time, and where many have their own axes to grind, any bad study can become grist for the public confusion mill. In February 2014, researchers from the Medical University of Graz in Austria published a study in an online journal (Burkert, Muckenhuber, et al. 2014) that bore shocking news: vegetarians are significantly less healthy than meat eaters. This "man bites dog" story was bound to attract media attention: it looked authoritative, including lots of complicated terms and numbers and charts, it told a counterintuitive story, and it made millions of meat eaters feel better about their dietary choices.

Sure enough, the media did pick up on the story. On April 1, 2014 (a date chosen without any apparent irony), Benjamin Fearnow, a reporter for CBS News Atlanta, wrote an article headlined "Study: Vegetarians Less Healthy, Lower Quality of Life Than Meat-Eaters." The article repeated the published findings:

"Vegetarians were twice as likely to have allergies, a 50 percent increase in heart attacks and a 50 percent increase in incidences of cancer. . . . Vegetarians reported higher levels of impairment from disorders, chronic diseases, and suffer significantly more often from anxiety/depression."

Similar articles reporting on the Austrian study began appearing in print and online (a Google search in March 2015 returned over six thousand results for the phrase "Austrian study vegetarians less healthy lower quality of life").

Knowing what I know about thousands of articles that reach the opposite conclusion, my BS alarm starting ringing. Despite this, I didn't immediately dismiss the original study. Perhaps there was something new and valuable that I could learn from it. So instead of relying on the article abstract or other journalists' work, I found and downloaded the actual article from PLOS ONE journal. You can do the same; unlike most published research, the article is under an open-access license. Here's an easy web link that will get you there: j.mp/bad-veg-study.

The study looked at over 15,000 people. Since the point of the study was to compare the relative health of meat eaters and vegetarians, I would expect that it would have included a decent amount of vegetarians. Shockingly, only 0.2 percent of participants were vegetarians. Just 343 vegetarians. With such a low number there was no way to perform an adequately powered statistical analysis, so the authors didn't try. Instead, they compared the few vegetarians they had with age-matched meat eaters. Some of the vegetarians had no age-matched counterparts, so they were dropped from the study. Now we're down to 330 vegetarians.

Okay, we're clearly off to a bad start. But we can salvage the study to some extent. If we take these few vegetarians and compare them with meat eaters and follow both groups for years and see how they do, we'll certainly learn something of value. Is that what this study did? Of course not.

The researchers conducted one telephone interview with the study participants to assess their health and eating habits. So do we know how long they have been vegetarian? No. Could they have turned vegetarian because they were sick? Of course. Many people facing a diagnosis of heart disease or cancer adopt a vegetarian diet. Despite the fact that the diet may have been used as treatment, it was misidentified as a potential cause. That's like saying that insulin injections cause diabetes, since we see lots of diabetics taking insulin injections. That's the problem with a static snapshot study (called a cross-sectional study): not only can't it distinguish causation from correlation, it's liable to infer backward causation as we see here. This was a one-day study, not a multiple-year prospective study like other articles I will share later in this section.

Well, at least we should be able to discern exactly what "vegetarian" means, right? We should at least know that these vegetarians are in fact eating vegetables, right? Again, no such luck. The researchers labeled people but never assessed their exact meal plan. There is no mention of how many fruits and veggies they were eating. In fact, the study found that vegetarians were less likely to pursue preventive health measures, which in itself could explain their poor health. Many ethical vegans who avoid meat for moral reasons consume unhealthy diets devoid of fruits and veggies.

Overall, we're looking at bad science. Had a student turned this in, I would have had to give it an F, regardless of the findings, based just on the poor experimental design. Their conclusion is not worth the paper this would have been printed on, had it actually been printed. Instead, this utter waste of time wound up in an online journal. The methods and findings were not subject to debate at a large scientific conference, where it certainly would have been laughed off the plenary floor.

In the end, this study would have been never looked at again, except that media loves a good controversial study that supports our prejudices. Now, mentions of this article are showing up all over the Internet as if a Nobel Prize winner from Harvard Medical School had just completed a thirty-year prospective study and published the results in the *New England Journal of Medicine*. Do you still wonder why we're so confused?

Example: Misleading Paleo Weight-Loss Study

Another study that garnered lots of media attention purportedly "proved" that a Paleo diet can help people lose weight and prevent diabetes. On the surface, the study looks legit. It's full of medical jargon and features incredibly careful, precise, and well-considered outcome measures. The average layperson would not be able to understand it; therefore, the responsibility for analyzing and critiquing the study falls upon science journalists. Unfortunately, most journalists and bloggers simply reported the conclusions and paid no attention to the ridiculous study design.

The study, published in 2013 in the *Journal of Internal Medicine,* is titled "A Palaeolithic-Type Diet Causes Strong Tissue-Specific Effects on Ectopic Fat Deposition in Obese Postmenopausal Women." The researchers, all from prestigious European institutions, fed a Paleo diet (30% protein, 40% fat, and 30% carbohydrate) to 10 obese but otherwise apparently healthy postmenopausal women for five weeks. The women lost an average of 10 pounds and lost some fat from their livers. They also improved on some other measures, including blood pressure, cholesterol, and triglycerides. This suggests, according to the authors, that a Paleo diet can be protective against diabetes, as fatty liver appears to be a precursor to that disease.

Sounds reasonable, right? It's only when we go a bit deeper do we discover the craziness of the entire study and its design. First, there was no control group. Why is this important? Because the Paleo diet used in the study had an interesting characteristic: the women consumed 25 percent fewer calories on the Paleo diet than on their previous diet.

Here's a useful piece of scientific jargon for you: Big Deal.

That's the correct response to this study. A group of women ate 25 percent less and lost weight? Big Deal. Drop 25 percent of calories on *any* diet and you will lose weight. Lose weight and your cholesterol, blood pressure, and triglycerides will improve. Remember Professor Haub and his 1,800-calorie junk food diet?

A control group that also dropped caloric intake by 25 percent would have achieved the same results, at least. Even had they been eating Twinkies and drinking Coke, they would have seen improvements in those measures just through caloric restriction. The results had nothing to do with the Paleo part of the diet.

Remember the title of the article? It included the phrase "strong tissue-specific effects." This sounds important, right? It turns out that the calorically restricted diet led to fat loss in the liver, but not in the calf muscles (the other place the researchers measured). The article interprets this fact to mean that the Paleo diet has some sort of specific magical effect on fat in the liver; hence its effectiveness in preventing diabetes.

The truth is, any weight loss will bring about fat loss in the liver. What's more interesting is that there was no fat loss in the muscles. That's the fat you want to lose to become healthy. Another fact—probably the most important fact to come out of the study—was this: "Whole-body insulin sensitivity did not change." In other words, there was absolutely no effect on the mechanism that causes diabetes. This makes perfect sense, given that there was no decrease in intramyocellular (muscle) fat. We will discuss this in the diabetes chapter, but fat in the muscle determines how sensitive you are to insulin, and hence how susceptible you are to developing diabetes. Here, the subjects lost weight and yet they were not able to lose fat from their muscles.

To their slight credit, the researchers did acknowledge the possibility that their entire study was pointless near the end of the discussion section: "This suggests that macronutrient composition is important, although the *possibility cannot be excluded that the same result would be obtained with different food choices of identical macronutrient compositions*" (italics added).

This is the problem with PubMed. Journalists and bloggers reference articles but don't actually read the full articles. They rely on misleading abstracts that hide the design flaws and real findings of the study, and they generally lack the time, training, or incentive to uncover and report the truth.

Example: Death by Journalism

As I mentioned earlier, journalists are replacing scientists and clinicians as the public's go-to source of health advice. For example, a June 2014 *Time* magazine cover instructed us to eat butter!

There are hundreds, if not thousands, of scientific articles showing that saturated fat from animal sources is hazardous to your health. In fact, Finland has greatly reduced its huge rates of cardiovascular disease by specifically decreasing butter, as well as increasing fruits and veggies (Laatikainen, Critchley, et al. 2005). How can the honorable *Time* magazine and so many other media outlets get it so wrong?

The *Time* article was based on two meta-analysis studies. A meta-analysis combines the data from many smaller studies and looks for trends. Ideally, meta-analyses correct for small sample size and chance findings by zooming out and evaluating the preponderance of evidence. Unfortunately, the meta-analyses selected by the *Time* reporter did not show that butter and other sources of saturated fat are good for us. Instead, they concluded that the relationship between saturated fat and heart disease may not be as strongly correlated as previously thought.

Many scientists have shown that these articles ignore a large body of evidence to the contrary (Pedersen, James, et al. 2011). In fact, they made significant scientific errors (Kromhout, Geleijnse, et al. 2011; Stamler 2010), not to mention the fact that the authors received money from meat and dairy organizations.

Leaving aside these significant problems with those meta-analyses (which really were outrageously biased in the way they cherry-picked the studies to include) and with the studies they looked at (almost all of them performed a very sneaky trick called "overadjustment" to make the link between heart disease and saturated fat appear much smaller than it really is), *Time* magazine still took breathtaking liberties in concluding that we should eat butter. None of the studies, nor either meta-analysis, claim that fat is good for us, or that we should be eating more of it.

But if you were in the business of selling magazines, the cover proclaiming "Eat Butter" generates a lot more newsstand sales (and future food industry advertising) than "Eat Kale."

Understand this: while doctors are experts in their chosen fields, they are probably getting their nutrition advice from *Time* magazine and other mainstream sources. That's how I was prior to my recovery from proteinaholism. My profession needs to step up and stop believing the third-hand reports from "true believer" bloggers on secondhand articles from ignorant journalists about badly designed and questionably funded research studies.

The *Journal of American Medical Association* recently published an article about how to actually read and analyze a meta-analysis study. The article's authors advise, "Clinical decisions should be based on the totality of the best evidence and not the results of individual studies. When clinicians apply the results of a systematic review or meta-analysis to patient care, they should start by evaluating the credibility of the methods . . . the degree of confidence . . . the precision and consistency of the results . . . and the likelihood of reporting bias" (Murad, Montori, et al. 2014).

How to Tell Fact from Fiction

We're living in an age of information overload, and many people are taking advantage of this situation by promoting ambiguity and confusion around diet and health. As you've read this far, you may even entertain the thought that I'm just adding to your confusion. After all, in the next several chapters, I'll be sharing evidence that may contradict everything you've ever heard about the health benefits of protein.

To avoid that problem, I'm going to share my research process with you. I'll show you in detail how I make decisions about treatment protocols and patient recommendations based on the evidence, in spite of the noise created by irresponsible journalism and shoddy science. While you may not be able to access all the original articles, and you may not have the scientific background to evaluate and interpret every study, at the very least you can begin to ask the questions that can separate fact from fiction, and distinguish real science from profit-driven BS.

Here are my rules for being an educated consumer of health information.

1. Never believe anything you find in a newspaper, magazine, blog, or TV or radio story.

As we've seen, these second- and third-hand accounts are often based on sloppy perusals of abstracts rather than nuanced readings of the full studies. They typically suffer from conflicts of interest. And they cherry-pick what's new and controversial rather than what's old and established beyond doubt.

That's not to say you should bury your head in the sand and never read newspapers or blogs, or watch TV news. Rather, use those secondary sources as pointers to the original research. If you can't access the real study, you'll have to rely on scientists you trust to give you an accurate interpretation. (Hopefully, I've become one of those scientists you trust. If you follow me at Facebook.com/drgarth you can read my ongoing critiques of nutrition and health studies.)

2. Never trust a single source in isolation.

This goes back to the "orange pixel in the blue sky image" problem I discussed at the beginning of this chapter. You have to become aware of the breadth of research (in the rest of this section, I share that context with you). One paper cannot prove or disprove anything. No matter the study, I use it as a single data point within a complex algorithm for making medical recommendations to my patients. Don't fall for the pseudoexperts online who use single studies to prove points while ignoring the preponderance of evidence to the contrary. I'm not saying that every new finding is worthless; rather, be suspicious of outlier data and demand replication of the finding in larger, well-designed studies.

3. Consider the source.

Some researchers are more trustworthy than others. When you encounter a research article, look at the authors. What institution are they affiliated with? Where did they get their funding for this study? Many journals require authors to state any potential conflicts of interest; others are not so stringent. Sometimes researchers hide their funding by taking industry money for unrelated research so they don't have to declare it in any particular article. "Following the money" isn't foolproof, and unless you're a detective, you'll miss a lot, but it's a necessary step in determining credibility. Remember that funding almost invariably influences the outcome of a study, even if the researchers aren't consciously altering their design or conclusions.

You can also reference other articles they've written by finding their institutional biography online. Believe it or not, money may influence their results less than pride. There are academics who have devoted their entire careers to proving that low-carb diets are the healthiest choice. When you examine their history of published works, you find that pretty much everything is on the same topic. Once they establish "guru" status, it's mighty hard for them ever to see evidence that disproves their beliefs. I've found with many of them, God could descend from heaven and debunk their arguments, and they would still hold fast to their incorrect views.

Again, a history of holding a particular view doesn't automatically discredit it; rather, it alerts me to the potential of "pride bias." And please don't think I'm playing favorites here; the tendency to keep finding the results you expect applies to plant-based researchers as well.

4. Consider the study design.

In medical science, the randomized controlled clinical trial (RCCT) is widely assumed to be the "gold standard" of research. Before I argue with this view, let me explain what it means, working backward:

Trial: an experiment, rather than an observational study. In other words, a trial takes a bunch of people and does something to them, then reports on the result.

Clinical: in a clinical setting, with medical professionals monitoring the progress of the trial and the patient outcomes.

Controlled: including an additional group or groups that gets no treatment, or a variation of the main treatment, to make sure the reported outcome was a result of the specific treatment. For example, the Paleo weight-loss study discussed earlier in this chapter would have benefited from a control group of women who were given a diet identical in calories consumed, but different in macronutrient composition. This would have clarified whether the results were due to the Paleo diet, or simply due to caloric restriction and subsequent weight loss.

Randomized: where participants have an equal and random chance of being assigned to any of the experimental or control groups. Randomization ensures against creating groups that are so different at the start of the trial that any differences in outcome could be due to those initial differences.

If we are studying the effects of a new drug or surgical procedure or screening protocol, then the RCCT makes a great deal of sense. It works best when we want to introduce a single variable and keep everything else constant, to see if that variable makes a difference. But when we use the RCCT to decide the effects of various diets on chronic diseases, the model breaks down. There are too many variables that are important, and too many conditions to look at.

Also, it's impossible to randomize people to diets for more than a couple of months. People simply don't adhere to strict diets for the length of time it would take to see real changes in health. RCCTs typically try to overcome this problem by shortening the length of the trial. But there's a huge and often fatal trade-off: short trials can't look at clinical outcomes, like death, heart attacks, cancer, and onsets of diabetes. So researchers instead look at isolated lab values of biomarkers that are correlated with disease, may be predictive of disease, but do not necessarily equate to disease.

We previously discussed, in Chapter 6, one of the most famous diet RCCTs, which was the 2007 A to Z Trial, and it's a perfect example of the problem with using RCCT design to study diet. Set up as a one-year trial, the study randomized participants into one of four diets: Atkins, LEARN, Ornish, and Zone. The Atkins dieters were instructed to consume fewer than 20 grams of carbs per day for the first couple of months, and then fewer than 50 grams per day for the remainder of the trail. LEARN dieters included moderate exercise, 50 to 60 percent of calories from carbs, and less than 10 percent from saturated (mostly animal) fat. The Ornish diet-ers were told to keep their fat intake to 10 percent or less of total calories. The Zone was set up as a 40 percent carb/30 percent protein/30 percent fat diet.

After one year, the Atkins dieters had lost some weight, while the other three groups had not. The Atkins corporation jumped on the findings, and the media dutifully reported that a low-carb diet was crowned weight-loss champion. There were many problems with this study, and most of them derived from the RCCT design; specifically, the randomization. Participants who hadn't chosen the diets, hadn't bought into the lifestyles, and lacked any strong commitment to them simply didn't follow the study

Mean Dietary Intake and Energy Expenditure by Diet Group and Time Point*

	Atkins	Zone	LEARN	Ornish	P Value[†]
Energy, kcal/d					
Baseline	1888 (512)	1975 (567)	1925 (553)	1850 (541)	.52
2 mo	1381 (345)	1455 (464)	1476 (448)	1408 (453)	.52
6 mo	1538 (401)	1503 (348)	1598 (418)	1553 (530)	.64
12 mo	1599 (494)	1594 (523)	1654 (492)	1505 (437)	.43
Carbohydrate (% energy)					
Baseline	45.6 (10.5)	47.1 (9.0)	48.3 (9.2)	47.9 (8.6)	.31
2 mo	17.7 (11.8)[a]	42.0 (8.5)[b]	49.3 (8.6)[c]	63.1 (11.0)[d]	<.001
6 mo	29.5 (14.5)[a]	43.7 (9.2)[b]	48.2 (8.6)[b,c]	53.4 (13.4)[c]	<.001
12 mo	34.5 (14.4)[a]	45.4 (11.1)[b]	47.2 (8.9)[b,c]	52.4 (12.3)[c]	<.001
Protein (% energy)					
Baseline	16.6 (4.1)	15.6 (3.3)	16.7 (3.9)	16.3 (3.1)	.21
2 mo	27.7 (5.5)[a]	23.7 (5.8)[b]	20.1 (4.8)[c]	16.9 (4.3)[d]	<.001
6 mo	22.4 (6.3)[a]	20.1 (5.2)[a,b]	18.4 (4.6)[b]	18.1 (4.8)[b]	<.001
12 mo	20.6 (5.3)[a]	20.0 (5.2)[a,b]	18.5 (4.6)[a,b]	18.3 (4.0)[b]	.02
Fat (% energy)					
Baseline	36.2 (7.8)[a]	35.6 (6.5)[a,b]	33.2 (7.2)[b]	35.1 (7.0)[a,b]	.05
2 mo	54.7 (9.0)[a]	34.8 (6.6)[b]	30.2 (7.3)[c]	21.1 (8.0)[d]	<.001
6 mo	47.0 (11.9)[a]	35.7 (7.3)[b]	31.3 (7.8)[c]	28.3 (10.7)[c]	<.001
12 mo	44.3 (12.5)[a]	34.5 (7.8)[b]	32.9 (7.1)[b]	29.8 (10.5)[c]	<.001
Saturated fat, g/d					
Baseline	26.5 (11.1)	27.0 (10.9)	24.3 (11.0)	24.8 (10.3)	.34
2 mo	30.7 (9.8)[a]	19.3 (10.3)[b]	16.8 (9.8)[b]	10.3 (7.8)[c]	<.001
6 mo	28.1 (11.1)[a]	20.5 (8.0)[b]	19.0 (8.9)[b,c]	16.2 (10.1)[c]	<.001
12 mo	27.2 (13.3)[a]	21.6 (11.2)[b]	20.1 (9.8)[b]	16.9 (11.4)[b]	<.001
Fiber, g/d					
Baseline	17.4 (6.6)	17.8 (8.7)	17.6 (7.5)	16.6 (6.6)	.79
2 mo	11.0 (6.3)[a]	16.9 (6.7)[b]	17.8 (7.1)[b]	22.1 (9.4)[c]	<.001
6 mo	14.0 (6.3)[a]	15.3 (7.6)[a]	16.7 (6.3)[a,b]	19.3 (11.1)[b]	.001
12 mo	15.2 (6.6)[a]	16.7 (9.4)[a,b]	18.3 (7.8)[a,b]	19.3 (9.4)[b]	.03

* Data presented are unadjusted raw data with no imputations for missing data. Standard deviations are presented in parentheses. Sample sizes for baseline and 2, 6, and 12 months, respectively, are: Atkins, n = 77, 73, 71, and 68; Zone, n = 79, 73, 66, and 60; and Ornish, n = 76, 72, 67, and 56.

[†] By analysis of variance.

[a, b, c, d] When the analysis of variance (last column) was statistically significant (P<.05), all pairwise comparisons among diet groups were tested for statistical significance using the Tukey studentized range test. Pairwise comparisons that were significantly different from one another are indicated by superscripts as follows: when the values for two diet groups within a row do not share a common superscript, they are significantly different, whereas if the values do share a common superscript, they are not significantly different.

guidelines. A true plant-based diet that doesn't rely on processed junk food should provide at least 40 grams of fiber per day. The Ornish group got an average of just 20 grams. I'm not sure what these so-called vegetarians were eating, but it sure wasn't vegetables.

Oh, and remember that 10 percent fat guideline for the Ornish dieters? They sort of exceeded it . . . by about 300 percent. Before the trial began, the Ornish dieters were getting about 35 percent of their calories from fat. At two months, they had managed to drop that to 21 percent. And that was as compliant as they were ever going to get. At six months, they were up to 28 percent, and by the end of the study they were close to their original diet, obtaining a whopping 29.8 percent of calories from fat.

Yet the media trumpeted the Atkins victory over the "strict" Ornish diet. Of course, there was no Ornish diet under study. Instead, it was a group of people who steadfastly ignored the Ornish guidelines and ate pretty much whatever they wanted. That's what happens when you try to randomize people into lifestyles—they rebel. It's another important trade-off to remember: the more "airtight" the experimental design, the less it resembles real life and the less applicable the results.

Oh, and the following graph, taken from the A to Z Trial, shows that the Atkins dieters, like the others, were well on their way to putting the weight back on (a commonly observed outcome in a diet that's inherently unsustainable).

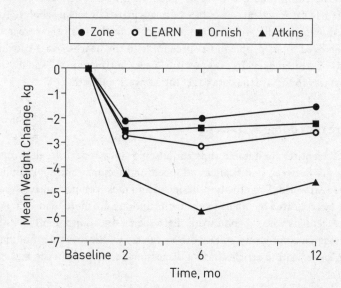

5. Question the choices of statistical analysis.

You might suspect that once the study is complete and the data have been gathered, that's the end of the scientific process. In fact, the way the data are analyzed and adjusted can introduce higher levels of clarity—and can also turn real findings on their heads. Mark Twain's phrase about the three main kinds of falsehoods ("lies, damn lies, and statistics") has never been truer than in nutrition studies.

Ideally, statistical analysis tells us the likelihood that a given result represents a true outcome, rather than random chance. For example, if you flip a coin three times and it comes up tails each time, is that enough evidence to declare the coin "fixed"? How about ten times, all tails? Fifty? Three thousand? Statistics help us put outcomes in perspective, so we don't over- or underattribute significance to them.

Statistical adjustment also allows researchers to find nuggets of truth that may otherwise be buried or obscured by other data. In the Austrian "vegetarians are less healthy" study, a useful adjustment would have been to examine how long the participants had been vegetarian, or whether their conversion had been motivated by a health scare.

The most misleading adjustments are those that mistakenly account for what are known as "confounding variables." Most of the studies included in the meta-analyses cited by the *Time* magazine article on saturated fat committed this error by adjusting for serum cholesterol. The problem is, saturated fat causes heart disease in part by raising cholesterol. By removing people with high cholesterol from the trial, the researchers removed those people most susceptible to the heart-disease-causing effects of saturated fat. This is known as "overadjustment bias," and it's the easiest way to torture the data to get the answers you want.

6. Are they doing real science?

Good scientists are humble and cautious. No study is perfect; all involve trade-offs between significance and speed, and accuracy and applicability to the real world. Even the best-designed and most comprehensive study must be replicated by others to ensure its findings are more than a chance blip. Scientists who do good work share their work transparently within the research community, so that others can try to disprove their findings.

Most scientific articles have a discussion section where the authors evaluate and discuss the relevance of the findings. These discussions usually include the authors' opinions of the shortcomings of the experimental design. It is critical to read and understand this to better understand the significance of the results.

7. Do the findings make sense in the real world?

Before I accept a result and use it to inform patient care, I have to analyze it based on my knowledge of the total body of research, the fundamentals of anatomy and physiology, and my own professional experience. I am in a unique position because I get to see how diet works in real life with real patients over months and years. Many studies are authored by nonphysicians, which is problematic when they come up with hypotheses without appropriate context and reach conclusions without real-life application.

When scientists lack clinical acumen about the subject of their research, they are in danger of completely missing the application of their findings. Recently I attended an Obesity Week scientific meeting where many of the experts in obesity research come to present their latest findings. One Ph.D. presented her work on insulin resistance. She hypothesized that insulin resistance is due to pancreatic beta cell dysfunction caused by high iron in diet. It turns out that when we eat iron it becomes oxidized, and oxidized iron is harmful to the beta cells of the pancreas, which can no longer secrete insulin optimally. Her experimental design was excellent and her animal studies and human studies were convincing. At the end of the presentation an audience member asked the presenter about her own diet. My mouth dropped to my shoes when she replied that she ate a low-carb/high-protein diet. What? A high-protein diet usually means high meat consumption, and high meat consumption means high iron consumption. Here's a brilliant scientist who is eating a diet that actually contradicts her science!

Even being a physician is no guarantee against this pitfall, as I know only too well. In my last book I recommended a high-protein diet, while in practice I saw people struggling with this diet, looking ill, and gaining weight.

One example where I paid attention to context was my experience with the laparoscopic (lap) band. The lap band, a device that essentially constricts the opening where the esophagus joins the stomach, came out in the mid-2000s. My knowledge of physiology made me suspicious about its efficacy, as prior attempts at placing foreign bodies on the stomach had failed. They would erode or cause motility issues in which the esophagus failed to empty fully or rapidly enough into the stomach. Also, I knew that the gastric bypass worked by altering gut hormones that controlled hunger, while the band did not alter hormone production. So I avoided using the band initially.

However, several surgeons published very promising data regarding the band's success. I now realize these surgeons built their practice around the band. They had financial incentive as well as academic pride vested in promoting the technology, both of which led to biased research and reporting. But after prolonged exposure to their copious and seemingly well-organized data supporting the lap band, I finally gave in and starting using them in my practice. I performed many lap band surgeries in the mid to late 2000s, always warning the patients about my reservations. As I expected, success was well below what was promised, and the rate and severity of complications was much higher. I stopped doing the bands. Meanwhile, the financially and ego-motivated lap band cheerleaders continued to publish articles with a positive spin. After several years, it was universally apparent that the real-life application failed to resemble what was promised by the science.

Honoring True Expertise

In addition to reviewing the studies, evaluating the research methods, and comparing the findings to my own clinical experience, I like to read and engage in discussion with physicians and scientists with years in the field. Social media fosters a pernicious distrust of true experts, often because those experts dismiss social media amateurs for what they are. An expert has reviewed all relevant studies and has analyzed them. Many times we do not see eye to eye, but I certainly can learn a lot from people with years of experience. In fact, one of the marks of a true scientist is an eagerness to go nose to nose with those who disagree. No Google search could ever provide you with the wisdom you can glean from a scientific meeting. Listening to the experts review the available data with the benefit of their deep and broad experience is a completely different experience than reading blogs and Facebook feeds. At these meetings we discover new research, share expert critiques of that research, and engage in lengthy debates, both in the auditoriums and later at the bars.

I can attest that there are in fact many experts who spend their waking hours exploring vital questions rather than padding their résumés or bank accounts, scientists whose only agenda is truth, wherever it may lead them. One such expert of the last century, Albert Einstein, once said; "Nothing will benefit human health and increase the chances for survival of life on earth as much as the evolution to a vegetarian diet." Of course, Einstein was merely speculating at the time. Since then, however, science has advanced considerable proof of the importance of, at the very least, increasing fruits and veggies and limiting meat and dairy. While it may appear that scientists are constantly disagreeing, there is in fact a broad consensus that including plants and limiting animals in our diets is the single best thing we can do for our health.

One reason you may not hear these things is that the true scientists simply don't have time to Tweet snarky, grandiose statements in 140 characters or fewer. A true scientist is always second-guessing and always learning. Let's look at how some real scientists, untainted by financial conflicts of interest or boastful pride, weigh in on the topic of human nutrition.

Kaiser Permanente is the country's largest health maintenance organization (HMO). HMOs make money by keeping people healthy, not through treatment. Unlike the traditional health-care models, Kaiser, a nonprofit, collects money from its subscribers and whatever costs for tests or treatments that need to be done comes out of the subscription fee. Therefore, Kaiser is motivated by a strong financial incentive to actually keep people well. After thoroughly reviewing the latest science, Kaiser researchers released recommendations to all their doctors emphasizing the importance of recommending a plant-based diet to their patients. The science was convincing enough for this very large health-care organization, whose 2014 operating budget totaled more than $56 billion.

In 2007, the World Cancer Research Fund teamed up with the American Institute of Cancer Research and the World Health Organization and got experts from around the world to review all research on diet and disease. They produced a huge report called "Food, Nutrition, Physical Activity and the Prevention of Cancer: A Global Perspective."

From the introduction: "This was a systematic approach to examine all the relevant evidence using predetermined criteria and assemble an international group of experts who, having brought their own knowledge and experience to bear, and having debated their disagreements, arrived at judgments at what all this evidence really means. We reviewed all the relevant research using the most meticulous methods, in order to generate a comprehensive series of recommendations on food and nutrition designed to reduce the risk of cancer."

So what did this huge, meticulous review of *all* the science by *the* world experts conclude? Among other things, reduce meat. There was a clear correlation between meat consumption and many forms of cancer. The report's experts recommended that diets be mostly of plant origin. While the report looked specifically at cancer, the researchers noted that the same diet promised protection from heart disease as well. And subsequent studies have already shown that following these guidelines does lead to less cancer (Vergnaud, Romaguera, et al. 2013).

The Academy of Nutrition and Dietetics (formerly known as the American Dietetic Association) recently released a statement that vegetarian diets "are healthful, nutritionally adequate, and may provide health benefits in the prevention and treatment of certain diseases. Well-planned vegetarian diets are appropriate for individuals during all stages of the life cycle, including pregnancy, lactation, infancy, childhood, and adolescence, and for athletes"(Craig, Mangels, et al. 2009).

The National Research Council, the American Heart Association, the American Institute for Cancer Research, and many more have emphasized the importance of cutting back on animal protein and eating more fruits and veggies. They may not say, "Go vegan," because they are trying to be middle of the road. The Harvard School of Public Health has published numerous excellent articles showing that animal protein and fat relates to disease. One of their top researchers was asked why they do not explicitly tell people to become vegetarian when the evidence so clearly supports this recommendation. His response in a Reuters interview was telling: "We can't tell people to stop eating all meat and dairy products. Well, we could tell all people to be vegetarians. . . . If we were truly basing this on science we would, but it is a bit extreme."*

Finally, "The Dietary Guidelines of America" released by the U.S. Department of Health and Human Services includes an article titled

---

* From the heights of research to daily doctor visits, this attitude that "You can't handle the truth" pervades the medical establishment. We the people would much rather grow cancers, develop heart disease, suffer with diabetes, and then take drugs and undergo surgeries than improve our diets. Such cynicism may be justified in some cases (not all that much in my personal and professional experience). Even so, doctors have an obligation to give their patients the facts so the patient may decide; "informed consent" is the basis of the patient's participation in the entire system. For doctors to fail to inform patients of the gentlest, safest, most beneficial action they can take to protect their own health is nothing short of criminal negligence.

"Finding Your Way to a Healthier You." Recommendations included focusing on fruits and veggies and supplementing them with grains and lean proteins, as well as fish, beans, and nuts and seeds. Despite the amount of industry pressure bearing down upon this committee, they still found the science compelling enough to stop recommending meat in favor of predominately plant-based alternatives.

Denialism

An enormous body of research shows that a diet high in animal protein can contribute to disease. Despite this evidence, there will always be naysayers: people who will never allow themselves to be convinced, regardless of the evidence. Highly vocal, they often dominate public conversation and confuse people with their cherry-picked, distorted, and outright false data. A 2009 scientific article explored this phenomenon of "denialism," and explained the classic methods used to promote head-in-the-sand refusal to see facts (Diethelm and McKee 2009). I'll summarize its conclusions on scientific denialism so you can better understand the noise you will hear from those who stalwartly oppose all forms of evidence.

1. Denialists believe peer-reviewed journal articles are some sort of conspiracy.

If there is an article that counters their belief, denialists will invent a conspiracy to slander the findings. For example, they contend that medical societies are conspiratorial organizations created with the express purpose of fooling the public. In fact, it is very difficult to get doctors and scientists to agree on anything, much less a global secret conspiracy. Yes, there are individual articles that, as I have mentioned, have been tainted by monetary influence. However, peer review will bring these to light. When you present an article at a scientific conference, you are required to list your financial interests.

2. Denialists like to denigrate experts.

Having been raised to respect experience and expertise, I find this stance extremely odd. When I argue with people online, if I refer to an expert in the field, the comment is often waved off as "appeal to authority." Why would you not want to hear from an authority who has studied a topic all of his or her life?

There was an interesting event online that will shine more light on this. A young schoolteacher published a blog aimed at discrediting the work of T. Colin Campbell, author of *The China Study*. The blog gained much publicity in Weston A. Price Foundation circles, and I have since heard many people claim that "the China study has been discredited" and reference this blog for proof. The blogger had basically looked at the raw data that Dr. Campbell collected and saw that one region of China ate lots of wheat and had a high amount of heart disease, which is counter to what was asserted in the book. She performed what is known as a univariate analysis, which simply doesn't work in research like that done by Dr. Campbell in China that looked at over eight thousand unique variables. She did not look at any other factors that could have caused the relationship. Turns out this region of China ate very few vegetables and lots of meat. An epidemiologist commented on her blog, "it was crude and irresponsible to draw conclusions based on raw, unadjusted, linear, and nondirectional data." The blogger responded with hostility to criticism from any "authorities," claiming her right to interpret highly complex scientific data without training or expertise as equal, if not superior, to theirs. Dr. Campbell responded to this hubris in measured fashion:

"I am the first to admit that background and academic credentials are not everything, and many interesting discoveries and contributions have been made by outsiders and newcomers in various fields. On the other hand, background time in the field, and especially peer review, all do give a one-of-a-kind perspective."

He explained that the biochemical effects he saw in his lab studies established fundamentals and concepts that lead to biologic plausibility that he went into the field to test. The China survey is just one point in a lifetime of study for a man who dedicated his career to investigating the effects of diet on health. It's simply irresponsible to brush off someone with so much knowledge and experience without trying to gain insight into their research methodology and proficiency with their statistical tools.

3. Denialists cherry-pick the articles that suit their prejudice.

They consider valid only those articles that support their existing point of view, and they ignore or denigrate the rest. As mentioned, true scientists doubt their own views and rigorously and mercilessly test their hypotheses. They also look at the full breadth of available information, actively seeking out opposing interpretations, before judging the validity of a single article (Murad and Montori 2013). Funny enough, should you present a bunch of studies to denialists, they will accuse you of cherry-picking.

4. Denialists create impossible expectations of research.

To a denialist, nothing is true unless the study is a randomized placebo controlled prospective study over many years. Earlier in this chapter, I defined the randomized controlled clinical trial. Denialists want to add one more feature to that trial: placebo control. In drug trials, it's vital to control for the placebo effect (patients often get better simply because they believe they're undergoing an effective treatment) so we don't mistakenly attribute effectiveness to a drug when the real benefit is due to the patients' beliefs. A common way of doing this is to give one group the active drug, and another group an identical-looking, inert sugar pill. Drug trials are usually "double blinded," whereby neither study participants nor researchers have any idea who is in the "experimental" group and who is getting an inactive placebo.

In nutritional research that is just not possible. As we saw in the A to Z Trial, when you put individuals on a diet and try to study them long term, there is a very good chance that some will quit the diet. The treatment and the control groups start looking very similar, causing the trial to fail (Willett 2010). And can you imagine trying to blind participants to what they're eating? You'd have to slap blindfolds on them and feed them through a tube. Obviously, the real-life value of such research would be nil.

Denialists' favorite type of research to criticize is epidemiologic research. Epidemiology is the study of populations over time to ascertain causes of disease. The denialist will tell you that epidemiologic studies show correlation but not causation and then dismiss the article. My question is, What in the world is wrong with finding correlation? If we couldn't use correlation, we'd never be able to claim that smoking causes lung cancer, emphysema, or heart disease. Because if an RCCT is the only standard of proof, we'd have to randomly assign a bunch of people to start smoking to see if they would develop those diseases.

Modern-day epidemiology uses all kinds of fancy statistical methods that can identify causal relationships as well as trends. If you are looking at, for example, the relationship between saturated fat and heart disease, you can eliminate other possible causes of heart disease using a statistical tool called "multivariate analysis." As long as you choose the right variables (like eliminating smoking as a possible contributor to heart disease), you can find correlations solid enough to inform private decisions, clinical practice, and public policy.

Modern-day statistical analysis is very powerful. The studies may show correlation, not causation, but if there is a significant correlation in a modern epidemiologic study, you better believe that where there is smoke there is fire. In fact, it is more common that the rigorous statistical methods actually erase correlations that actually exist than find false correlations (Jacobs, Anderson, et al. 1979). If a well-done, modern, peer-reviewed epidemiologic study shows a correlation, you should definitely take note.

As Dr. Walter Willett puts it, "Large nutritional epidemiology studies, with long-term follow-up to assess major clinical end points, coupled with advances in basic science and clinical trials, have led to important improvements in our understanding of nutrition and the primary prevention of disease" (Willett and Stampfer 2013).

5. Denialists misrepresent data.

They take statements out of context and deliberately misread conclusions. Critics of Gary Taubes, a popular low-carb author, note that he takes much of his "evidence" out of context. In fact, one of the articles he used to show that saturated fat does not cause heart disease actually proved that very same correlation.

Denialists gain influence not from wisdom or authority, but from repetition. Most people know that an unclouded, daytime sky is blue.

Now that we've established the rules of the research game, let's look directly at the scientific evidence. In the following chapters, you will discover the powerful correlation between animal protein and disease. You will encounter a large body of science that includes RCCTs as well as modern epidemiologic studies that have undergone the most rigorous of statistical analysis. You'll see that there's really no question that our love affair with animal protein is misguided, unsupported by evidence, and ultimately deadly.

CHAPTER 9

Diabetes: It's the Meat That Makes You Sweet

Let's start our review of the scientific literature on the effect of animal protein on human health with a real shocker: Meat consumption is a major cause of diabetes. Carbs are not.*

I know. That's a bold statement. Shocking, even. I wouldn't have believed it myself eight years ago. In fact, the president of the American Society of Bariatric Physicians doesn't know it today, as he actually stated at a recent meeting that we should be telling our patients not to eat fruits for fear of the carbs. Even the American Diabetes Association diet recommends including meat in the diet and instructs diabetics to count carbs. But they're wrong, and I'll prove it to you here.

I stumbled upon the meat/diabetes connection quite unexpectedly. I was studying the health of the Japanese because, while we are one of the most unhealthy cultures, the Japanese have traditionally experienced good health and longevity. I was most interested in the fact that they eat a very carb-heavy diet, including lots of white rice. Since I believed carbs caused diabetes, I figured that the Japanese were somehow genetically resistant to diabetes. This theory evaporated when I learned that the Japanese have recently experienced a rapid and dramatic increase in diabetes, from 9.9

---

* In this chapter, when I talk about diabetes, I am specifically referring to type 2 diabetes, formerly known as adult-onset diabetes.

percent in 1997 to 15.3 percent in 2007. Lower than the U.S. prevalence of 20 to 30 percent, but the Japanese government was still very concerned. Its Ministry of Health and Labor and Welfare officials studied the issue and noted that the Japanese diet has become increasingly Westernized. They specifically say that the increase in meat consumption and the decrease in fruits and vegetables may be the major factor behind the rise in diabetes (Morimoto 2010).

As I continued to research, it became apparent that the Japanese do not have a genetic resistance to diabetes; instead, they may actually be genetically susceptible. An excellent study was performed in Brazil, comparing Brazilian-born Japanese to previous generations that had immigrated to Brazil from Japan. They found that second-generation Brazilian-born Japanese had extremely high rates of diabetes, especially when compared to prior generations (Gimeno, Ferreira, et al. 2002). The picture became even clearer when I learned that Brazilians consume more animal protein than residents of just about any other country. In fact, the Brazilian government has been responding to the excessive meat consumption by releasing suggestions to the public to specifically limit meat intake (de Carvalho, César, et al. 2013).

Of course, this is a simple correlation, and by no means conclusive by itself. Many other factors could have contributed to the increase in diabetes. If meat truly has a causative role in the development of diabetes, then there would need to be a comprehensive epidemiologic study that shows this correlation while controlling for possible confounding factors. Additionally, just one study would not suffice. There would have to be multiple studies that draw the same correlation after extensive statistical analysis.

The first place I looked was the EPIC study. The EPIC (European Prospective Investigation into Cancer and Nutrition) study is one of the largest prospective cohort studies that has ever been done looking at the relationship between nutrition and disease. Hundreds of top scientists have followed 521,000 people recruited from ten European countries. They have used specialized, culturally relevant, food assessment tools to get a better understanding of how the food people eat affects their likelihood of developing disease.

After following thousands of people for twelve years, the EPIC researchers concluded that meat, and especially processed meat (bacon, lunch meats, etc.), is significantly associated with the development of type 2 diabetes, and fruit and vegetable consumption is associated with a decrease in diabetes development (Consortium 2013, 2014). The craziest finding in the EPIC data analysis was the fact that glucose and fructose consumption was actually correlated with *less* diabetes. Many authors, like Robert Lustig, talk at length about the harms of fructose. Lustig makes these claims largely based on rat studies and overfeeding studies, but in this very well-done epidemiological study, looking at real people, if you replace just 5 percent of the saturated fats in your diet with fructose (presumably from fruits) you reduce your risk of developing diabetes by a whopping 30 percent (Ahmadi-Abhari, Luben, et al. 2014).

This finding from a long-term study of over half a million people goes against just about everything you hear about diet in America. Maybe it's a good time to ask the question again: How is our meat-rich, carb-poor diet working for us? We are currently experiencing a diabetes epidemic, and the affected people are eating more meat and cutting out fruit. Are they doing any better? From what I see in my office, absolutely not.

When the low-carb denialists are forced to confront this evidence, they scream that correlation does not equal causation, and therefore there's nothing to it. But based on the theory that "where there's smoke, there's often fire," let's continue looking for correlation, this time in the United States.

If you're a health researcher, one of the most fascinating groups to study is the Seventh-day Adventists in Loma Linda, California. You may remember them from the Blue Zones discussion in Chapter 3. The Adventist religion adjoins its adherents to treat their body as a temple. As a group, they are much healthier than most other Americans. They do not drink or smoke, they exercise moderately, and they strive to eat healthy. Many Adventists believe that we should not eat animals. But—and here's where it gets interesting from a research perspective—there's a lot of dietary variation among Adventists even as their lifestyles are quite similar in all other respects. They comprise a mix of meat eaters, fish eaters, vegetarians who consume dairy, and a relatively large group of vegans. Because they are a fairly homogenous group, living near each other, practicing similar habits but different dietary choices makes them a perfect group to study.

In fact, the Adventist Health Studies have done just that. Researchers at Loma Linda University have prospectively followed thousands of Adventists for many years and released many papers detailing their findings. Like the EPIC study, they found that animal protein was significantly associated with diabetes. In fact, they found a graduated increase in the risk of developing diabetes depending on the amount of animal protein consumed. Vegans had an extremely low prevalence of diabetes (2.9%) followed by vegetarians who included dairy and eggs at 3.2 percent, pescatarians (adding fish) at 4.8 percent and meat eaters at 7.6 percent. The Adventist meat eaters had much less diabetes than the U.S. average, which is explained by the fact that Adventists tend to limit meat consumption, even if they don't identify as vegetarians. Crunching the numbers over time, researchers found that weekly consumption of meat over a seventeen-year period increased the risk of developing diabetes by a whopping 74 percent over that of vegetarians (Tonstad, Butler, et al. 2009; Rizzo, Sabaté, et al. 2011; Snowdon 1988; Vang, Singh, et al. 2008). This correlation held true even when controlling for weight (which was done by comparing vegans and vegetarians to the slimmest meat eaters). This was a surprise finding, given that vegans typically weigh less than meat eaters. Meat consumption still correlated with diabetes even in those who didn't gain weight from it.

Among the largest epidemiologic studies in America are the Nurses' Health Study and Health Professionals Follow-up Study, both conducted by researchers from Harvard University. There are two Nurses' Health studies. The original started in 1976 and prospectively followed up 122,000 nurses. The second has followed 116,000 nurses since 1989. The Health Professionals Follow-up Study has followed 51,000 male health-care professionals since 1986. So what did these studies show about the relationship between meat consumption and diabetes? Once again, there was a significant association between meat, processed meat, and development of type 2 diabetes. In fact, increasing meat consumption by just half a serving a day increased the risk of developing diabetes by 48 percent (Fung, Schulze, et al. 2004; Pan, Sun, et al. 2011, 2013; Ley, Sun, et al. 2014; van Dam, Willett, et al. 2002).

Another large prospective population study, the Women's Health Initiative, followed 37,000 women for eight years. Agreeing with the other studies just discussed, it again showed correlation between animal protein consumption and diabetes, especially the good old all-American hot dog and bacon (Song, Manson, et al. 2004). Like the EPIC study, it also found that sugar was completely unrelated to the development of diabetes (Janket, Manson, et al. 2003).

There are many epidemiologic studies from around the world that further confirm the animal protein–diabetes correlation, as well as many that show that plant-based diets protect against diabetes (Aune, Ursin, et al. 2009; Chiu, Huang, et al. 2014). In fact, one study in particular looked at fat versus protein and found that it was specifically meat protein that correlated with diabetes (Ericson, Hellstrand, et al. 2015). I do not know of a single study showing that people who eat meat are protected from diabetes. Correlation does not equal causation, but you have to admit that these data are certainly compelling, and this much smoke might indicate a dire need of a fire extinguisher.

Explaining Diabetes

Those who still believe in the carb theory of diabetes have a simple model of how those carbs spike our blood sugar and cause the pancreas to ultimately exhaust itself in an effort to maintain stable blood sugar. If we are to accept the universal epidemiologic evidence that animal protein, not carbs, cause diabetes, then we need a different explanation that makes biological sense. Does such a mechanism exist?

Let's start our search by looking at a documentary produced by the British Broadcasting Corporation (BBC). It profiled a pair of thirty-five-year-old twins who went on separate diets for a month. One ate very low carb and the other ate very low fat. By the end of the month, the low-carb brother complained of being constipated, having brain fog, and lacking energy. He did lose more weight, but much of it was water weight. Most interestingly for this discussion, he showed *increasing* fasting blood sugars. The producers found this shocking. The "carbs are the villain" theory of diabetes implies that eliminating carbs would increase insulin sensitivity, thus making the body more efficient in using insulin to regulate blood sugar. In fact it does not.

The reason is biologically complex, but I'll try to simplify it in a way that makes sense and still honors the complexity. Our bodies are literally designed to live on sugar. Every cell in our body takes in sugar and turns it into energy via a pathway called the Krebs cycle. Whether by divine design or evolution, we are literally created to process sugar and starch.

Here's where insulin comes in. Produced by the pancreas, insulin is essential to convey the sugar from the bloodstream into the cell. As a survival fail-safe, we do have an emergency pathway for energy if sugar is not available, but we most efficiently function using carbs. It is our brain's primary fuel. The cells of our body can use both fat and sugar, and do so to varying degrees, but when the going gets tough (running fast), sugar is the go-to energy source.

Low-carb promoters such as Robert Lustig and Gary Taubes actually demonize insulin, claiming that it is harmful and we should aim to produce as little as possible. Just from a commonsense perspective, this is ludicrous. Why in the world would we evolve such an efficient system that has worked forever if it were truly harmful? Why would we produce insulin in our body to begin with? But Lustig and Taubes go further in their insulin-fearing fantasy: they suggest patients eat protein to minimize insulin secretion. They seem to have missed the science that shows that animal protein actually causes disproportionately high insulin secretion compared to carbs. Beef raises insulin more than pasta (Holt, Miller, et al. 1997).

The problem is not insulin or sugar per se, it is the cells' decreased ability to respond to insulin. This is called insulin resistance. The muscle in our body is the greatest consumer of sugar and therefore the site where insulin must work effectively for us to remain healthy. When we eat meat, we are eating protein and fat. The protein raises insulin, which blocks fat mobilization from the cell and causes the consumed fat to enter the cell. When we eat an apple or a potato, there is insulin secretion but no fat to be placed into the muscle cell (Barnard, Roberts, et al. 1998; Lara-Castro and Garvey 2004, 2008; Watt and Hoy 2012). Insulin resistance is due to fat toxicity to the muscle cell (Anderson, Haynie, et al. 2015).

One of the main factors causing fat to be collected in the muscle is inflammation (Coletta and Mandarino 2011; Eckel, Grundy, et al. 2005), which causes damage to the muscle cells that result in fat accumulation. We have evolved from the bicarbonate-producing diet of our ancestors to our current high-protein, acidic diet. That increased protein consumption corresponds to greater intake of amino acids rich in sulfur (Sebastian, Frassetto, et al. 2002). Remember that amino acids are actually acids. When our body becomes too acidic, a state known as metabolic acidosis, our tissues become inflamed. Since our blood chemistry must remain within extremely tight margins for us to stay alive, our bodies go into emergency mode to keep the blood pH at safe levels. One mechanism by which the body fights to maintain pH is grabbing calcium from muscles and dumping it into the bloodstream. Calcium can neutralize the acid. This leaching of calcium from muscle cells to buffer the acid causes muscle wasting and leads to fat deposition in the muscle cells (Adeva and Souto 2011; de Nadai, de Nadai, et al. 2013; Souto, Donapetry, et al. 2011; Frassetto, Morris, et al. 2001; Fagherazzi, Vilier, et al. 2013). Gary Taubes, a hero of the high-protein/low-carb movement, recently published his labs to show that his lipids are within normal range. Not being a doctor, he failed to comprehend the fact that his bicarbonate level was a very low 19, which means he is in a state of acidosis, slowly but steadily harming his body and creating inflammation and disease. Gary, if you're reading this, it's not too late. Start by swapping out the beef for lentils and we'll have you back on a healthy track in short order.

Eating meat also causes inflammation because animals are rather dirty. You almost have to wear a hazmat suit to handle a raw piece of chicken because of fear of getting a bacterial infection like salmonella. According to a 2014 *Consumer Reports* study, 97 percent of chicken breasts purchased at American supermarkets contained such hazardous bacteria. Cooking at a high enough temperature kills the bacteria, but does not destroy the endotoxin produced by the bacteria, which is embedded in the muscle (protein) of the animal. When we consume meat, the saturated fat causes the endotoxin to be absorbed into the body and our immune system sets off a state of inflammation (Erridge, Attina, et al. 2007; Ghanim, Abuaysheh, et al. 2009). The inflammation leads, again, to fat deposition in the muscle cell.

Finally, stress hormones contribute to high sugars and inflammation. One study, often cited by people advocating a high-protein diet, took 21 overweight adolescents and had them do three different diets, each for one month. They ate the same amount of calories in each diet, but one was high protein/low carb, one was low glycemic index, and one was low fat. I suspect the authors wanted to show better weight loss with the low-carb diet, but they had no such luck. They did note, however, that the metabolic rate dropped the least with the high-protein diet and that became their conclusion in their article in the prestigious *Journal of the American Medical Association*. The supposed significance of a high metabolic rate is that it will lead to fat loss. (Of course, this study showed it didn't, but that didn't deter these avid high-protein proponents.) This finding was greeted with much fanfare by the high-protein advocates, but what they failed to see is that the high-protein group had very high levels of cortisol in their urine and higher levels of C-reactive protein, which is a measure of inflammation. Cortisol is a stress hormone that counters insulin's effect and raises blood sugar. It is also an independent risk factor for diabetes and heart disease (Adam, Hasson, et al. 2010; Holt, Wild, et al. 2007; Vogel-zangs, Beekman, et al. 2010). C-reactive protein, due to its significance as a sign of inflammation, has been independently associated with diabetes (Pickup 2004; Nanri, Moore, et al. 2007). So while they were celebrating the short-term, slightly better metabolic rate, they missed the fact that the overweight teenagers experienced inflammation that causes fat deposition in the muscle and likely eventual insulin resistance (Ebbeling, Swain, et al. 2012).

Once fat gets inside the muscle cells, it interferes with that cell's ability to develop new insulin receptors. With fewer insulin receptors it becomes more difficult to get sugar into the cell for processing, causing the sugar to build up in the blood. The pancreas then has to churn out even more insulin just to get the sugar into the cells. The very high insulin, which is not normal, will cause even more fat to enter the cells in a vicious cycle.

Combine this with the fact that the form of iron found in meat (known as "heme iron") causes oxidation, which affects the pancreas's ability to secrete insulin, and now you have full-blown diabetes with high sugars. Meat eaters tend to have higher iron stores, which are directly corre-lated with diabetes formation (Bao, Rong, et al. 2012; Jiang, Manson, et al. 2004; Reif 1992; Romeu, Aranda, et al. 2013). In fact, simply drawing large amounts of blood out of a diabetic does appear to improve insulin resistance just by reducing the iron (Hua, Stoohs, et al. 2001). Of course, given the choice between bloodletting and avoiding steak, I would think it's not a tough decision.

I should note that there is a chicken-and-egg disagreement among sci-entists as to which comes first, insulin resistance or insulin hypersecre-tion. In other words, do cells lose their ability to react to insulin, causing the pancreas to go into hyperproduction? Or does the pancreas initiate the process by overproducing insulin, which the cells deal with by decreasing their sensitivity to it. Those who favor the pancreatic-hypersecretion-first theory believe the phenomenon is caused by reactive oxygen species, cre-ated during consumption of meat and heme iron.

So we see that, popular belief to the contrary, the high blood sugars that *define* diabetes are not, in fact, the *cause* of diabetes. Rather, those high blood sugars are an aftereffect, a symptom. It also turns out that just lowering the blood sugars with medicines does not prevent the diseases of diabetes because it does not address the real issue. The problem is actually the fat and inflammation that is destroying the body's ability to utilize the sugar safely and efficiently.

The interesting thing is that people talk about carbs, and specifically wheat, as causing inflammation. If you actually take a group of people and feed them a high-fat meal versus a high-carb meal, you find the opposite: the high-fat eaters develop significantly increased inflammation after the meal, while the carb consumers do not (Esposito and Giugliano 2006; Esposito, Nappo, et al. 2003; Deopurkar, Ghanim, et al. 2010). The craziest study I have seen is one where researchers compared a group of people drinking 1.5 liters a day of sugary drinks to a group drinking 1.5 liters of artificially sweetened drinks. As would be expected, the sugary drink group consumed more calories and therefore gained more weight. But here's what's fascinating: even though they gained weight, they did not show any signs of increasing inflammation (Sørensen, Raben, et al. 2005). The sugar seems to have no inflammatory effect at all and, while being a source of extra calories, did not make these people sick.

Study after study has shown that people eating fruits, veggies, and especially grains exhibit remarkably low levels of inflammation. Not only do they have low levels of inflammation, but they also have considerably lower levels of diabetes than the general population. Numerous studies looking at carb and grain intake confirm that the more carbs you eat, the less inflammation, and consequently, the less diabetes risk you have (Valachovicová, Krajcovicová-Kudláčková, et al. 2006; Cozma, Sievenpiper, et al. 2012; Rankin and Turpyn 2007; Montonen, Boeing, et al. 2013; Barbaresko, Koch, et al. 2013; Ye, Chacko, et al. 2012; Muraki, Imamura, et al. 2013; Gao, Bermudez, et al. 2004; Galland 2010; Ford and Mokdad 2001; Cooper, Sharp, et al. 2012; Brunzell, Lerner, et al. 1971; Christensen, Viggers, et al. 2013).

Putting the Meat/Diabetes Link to the Test

I have shown you epidemiologic data and studies looking at individual lab values. I have used logic that says "meat causes inflammation, and inflammation causes fat deposition in muscles, fat in muscles cells leads to insulin resistance and eventually diabetes, so meat must cause diabetes." Certainly the preponderance of evidence points to this effect, but the gold standard in research is the randomized control trial that specifically compares a diet heavy with animal protein to one without animal protein. Studies on rats have shown that high-protein, high-fat diets (specifically diets that produce ketosis, a condition where the body is deprived of carbohydrates to the point where it turns on its emergency fuel source and metabolizes protein for energy) lead to inflammation and insulin resistance (Flanagan, Brown, et al. 2008; Jornayvaz, Jurczak, et al. 2010), but we really need to refine the search to humans.

Many studies have compared low-carb and low-fat diets for diabetes. There are several problems with these studies: the so-called low-fat group is not put on a truly low-fat diet, they still eat animal protein, and the end result the study authors look at is blood sugar rather than the much more important insulin resistance. If you do not eat any sugar, your blood sugar may be artificially low, but a high-protein diet devoid of carbs may still be causing inflammation and insulin resistance, conditions that may not be picked up by measuring blood sugar alone. Unfortunately, we currently don't have any randomized control trials comparing a plant-based diet to a high-protein Atkins or Paleo-type diet specifically with regard to diabetes.

However, researchers at the Imperial College School of Medicine in London did the kind of comprehensive testing that truly measures whether insulin resistance is present in plant eaters versus general omnivores (Goff, Bell, et al. 2005). They found 21 vegetarians and 21 omnivores and matched them for age, weight, waist circumference, and activity levels. They followed the 42 subjects for 7 days, making sure each group ate the same number of calories and their usual daily exercise activities were the same. Basically, the only difference between these groups was that one avoided animal protein. The researchers then performed comprehensive biological testing. Not only did they measure the amount of insulin produced, they actually did muscle biopsies to look at the amount of fat in the muscle. (How they talked their subjects into getting muscle biopsies, I do not know.) The results showed that despite eating a far higher carbohydrate load, the vegan group had lower insulin and had less fat in their muscle cells. Of course, based on what we've seen so far, their results should be edited to "*because* they ate a far higher carbohydrate load."

This study suffered from one big weakness, however: it was not a controlled intervention. Despite all the matching, it's quite possible that the two groups were still different in significant ways that weren't taken into account. It is one thing to compare vegans to omnivores but to actually make a group of people eat either a vegan diet or another type diet is much more difficult. People tend to be set in their ways, and having them stick to a diet plan is not always successful. But, if we are going to prove actual causation, we must show that taking people on a usual diet and making them remove the animal protein causes their insulin resistance to disappear.

Dr. Neal Barnard did just such a study. He and his colleagues took 100 diabetic, overweight people and randomized them from their usual diet to either a vegan diet or a reduced-calorie, low-fat American Diabetes Association (ADA) diet. The ADA diet was purposefully calorie reduced and was a very moderate diet. It was low in fat and moderate in protein and carbs, leaning to low glycemic carbs. The vegan diet was not limited in calorie intake at all. The subjects could eat as much as they wanted of fruits, veggies, and legumes. Oils and nuts were limited. Both group were intensively counseled over a 74-week period. Barnard measured A1C, which is a long-term measure of how well blood sugar is controlled, as well as weight and LDL cholesterol. My only regret about the study is that they did not look directly at insulin resistance. It's an invasive procedure, however, and it appears Americans are less interested in agreeing to muscle biopsies than the British. Nevertheless, the results showed that the vegans ended up eating many more carbs, yet had significantly better blood sugar control compared to the ADA dieters. The vegans also had much lower cholesterol. Despite the fact that the vegan group could eat as much as they wanted, they ended up losing slightly more weight as well (Barnard, Cohen, et al. 2006, 2009). It also appears that a vegan diet is superior to just a low-fat diet in controlling diabetes (Nicholson, Sklar, et al. 1999).

Of course, this study deserves the criticism I place on the low-carb studies, which is that researchers were simply measuring sugar levels. The difference in this case is that the vegan subjects were consuming sugars in the forms of carbs and yet still kept their blood sugar levels down. Their typical day's meals included oatmeal, pasta, cantaloupe, and various other fruits. Given that they were not avoiding sugar (as in Atkins) yet their blood sugars actually dropped, the only obvious explanation is that their insulin sensitivity must have been improving.

For the naysayers, I offer another interesting prospective study (Bloomer, Kabir, et al. 2010). In this study there was no separate control group; rather, the researchers used the participants as their own control by comparing how they would do on a vegan diet or their standard diet. They put 43 people on the Daniel Fast, which is essentially a vegan diet and not really a fast.*

The modern-day Daniel Fast is rich in fruits, vegetables, beans, seeds, and nuts. All junk food and all animal meats are avoided. The 43 study participants followed the diet with excellent compliance, showing that it really is easy to do. Despite being able to eat as much as they wanted, they actually ended up eating fewer calories. They also ate less protein and a higher percentage of calories from carbs. They ate more fat than in Barnard's study above, but the saturated fat consumption was obviously low since they were avoiding meat and dairy. It turns out that it is specifically saturated fat that creates the inflammation, not the polyunsaturated and monounsaturated fat found in many vegetables, legumes, nuts, and fruits (Rosqvist, Iggman, et al. 2014).

The participants on this Daniel Fast were studied extensively. During their vegan diet, they had a substantial drop in their blood lipid values and blood sugar and had trends to lower levels of inflammation and insulin. I find this especially interesting because these were not diabetics. These were basically well people (with few exceptions), yet they still showed improvements in their insulin resistance. Like the biblical Daniel, they became healthier during their "fast."

To summarize: type 2 diabetes is a serious disease that has reached epic numbers in the United States and worldwide and shows no sign of slowing. The biology of this disease is complex, but evidence is mounting that the typical high-protein diet may to blame, and our avoidance of carbs only makes things worse. If we avoided animal protein and instead increased consumption of fruits and veggies, we could substantially prevent and treat most of the type 2 diabetes we encounter. This may be in part be due to the high fiber in the plants, or the phytonutrients in the plants, but it is also due to the reduction in inflammation by avoiding animal protein and fat (Jenkins, Kendall, et al. 2003; Chandalia, Garg, et al. 2000; Watzl 2008).

---

* The diet gets its name from the biblical book of Daniel. According to chapter 10, verses two and three, Daniel was held in captivity in Babylon but was considered a valuable asset. He was offered the king's wine and meat, but refused. He ate only vegetables and pulses (legumes) and drank only water. The head of security was worried about the fact that Daniel would wither, but Daniel suggested that they conduct a little scientific experiment (to put it in modern terms). He asked that the guards also follow his diet, and after ten days, he and the guards had far better health and vigor than those who ate the rich food of the king.

CHAPTER 10

Hypertension: Protein Puts Us Under Pressure

I see thousands of patients a year in my bariatric clinic, and it's extremely rare to come across a patient who is not on medication. Most are taking multiple medications, the most common of which are antihypertensives (against high blood pressure, also known as hypertension). Many of my patients are actually taking more than one medication to control their blood pressure.

The NHANES (National Health Examination and Nutrition Survey) 2005 report estimated that in the United States, a whopping 42 million men and 28 million women have prehypertension, and 17 million men and 18 million women have actual treatable hypertension (National Center for Health Statistics 2005). It is estimated that over one billion people suffer from hypertension worldwide. These are astonishing, epidemic numbers for the condition the CDC calls "the silent killer."

Given the fact that hypertension is a direct cause of the number one killers, heart disease and stroke, as well as kidney disease, you would think we would do everything in our power to control our blood pressure. In terms of pharmaceutical treatments, that is in fact the case. Drug companies have developed eleven different classes of antihypertensives, each with multiple different medications. People are liberally placed on the meds by their doctors, and once on, they seldom come off.

I've got a question for you.

If you found out you had hypertension and your doctor told you that to avoid heart attack, stroke, and renal failure, it's crucial you should go on a couple of antihypertensives for life, you'd do it, right? Even if the side effects included blurred vision, cloudy urine, confusion, cough, dizziness, drowsiness, headache, depressed mood, nausea, vomiting, diarrhea, upset stomach, and mild skin itching or rash (those are all common side effects of the antihypertensive lisinopril, the third-most-prescribed drug in America), or headache, swelling of the lower extremities, dizziness, drowsiness, tired feeling, stomach pain, or flushing (side effects of amlodipine, the fourth-most-prescribed antihypertensive). And the less common side effects include risks of arm and back pain, fast or irregular heartbeat, loss of appetite, shivering, and trouble sleeping.

But what if your doctor offered you a choice: either take the meds, and probably a few other meds to deal with whichever side effects you experience, or switch to a plant-based diet, whose side effects include decreased risk of diabetes, cancer, heart disease, stroke, diabetes, and a host of other conditions?

That would kind of be a no-brainer, wouldn't it?

Yet while the facts show that a plant-based diet, low in animal protein, is very effective in controlling blood pressure (as we'll see in this chapter), I'm guessing that no reader of this book who received a diagnosis of hypertension was ever told to change his or her diet.

Evidence for a Diet/Hypertension Link

Medical science has known for quite some time that vegetarians, who avoid most animal proteins, tend to have lower blood pressure (Sacks, Rosner, et al. 1974). Several excellent population studies have looked at the relationship between animal protein and high blood pressure.

The Western Electric Study followed 1,714 male employees of the company for eight years and carefully examined correlations between their health and diet. Researchers found that the more animal protein and fat people ate, the more at risk they were for developing hypertension. Meanwhile, they found that consuming plant proteins had the opposite effect, actually lowering blood pressure (Stamler, Liu, et al. 2002).

It's testimony to the strength of the relationship that this study was able to find it at all, given that researchers were looking at a group of middle-aged men with fairly similar diets that were not very healthy and did not completely eliminate animal protein. The Adventist Health Study, which I discussed earlier, actually looked at healthy meat eaters versus vegetarians and vegans who cut out all animal protein. Again, the vegetarians and vegans showed less hypertension than the meat eaters (Pettersen, Anousheh, et al. 2012).

As we've seen, the EPIC study is one of the largest and most thorough of epidemiologic studies. The Oxford branch of the EPIC study looked at a population of meat eaters that was healthier than average (partly because their meat intake was much lower than that of the general population) and compared them to a rather unhealthy group of vegetarians. I say this because they had a fairly low fiber intake, consumed little calcium, and had a high incidence of not supplementing vitamin B_{12}. Despite this seemingly unfair comparison, the unhealthy vegetarians still had significantly lower rates of hypertension than the healthy meat eaters (Appleby, Davey, et al. 2002). Again, the effect was so pronounced as to show itself even in a less than optimal comparison.

One of the best-regarded hypertension studies is known as INTERMAP (INTERnational study of MAcronutrients and micronutrients and blood Pressure). This was a cross-sectional evaluation of thousands of people around the world looking specifically at the relationship between diet and blood pressure. An in-depth analysis of 4,680 people found that vegetable protein had a significant blood-pressure-lowering effect (Elliott, Stamler, et al. 2006). This was unexpected. The inflammation from animal protein could easily be causing the hypertension, but why would vegetable protein lower blood pressure?

Part of the explanation is certainly the fiber advantage of a high-vegetable diet. Fiber has been independently associated with lowering blood pressure (Whelton, Hyre, et al. 2005). An intriguing theory is that since animal protein and plant protein have different amino acid profiles, it may be the different amino acids that actually cause a different vascular effect.

Dr. Jeremiah Stamler looked at INTERMAP study and was struck by data about the participants' urine. He found that glutamic acid was inversely related to blood pressure: the higher the glutamic acid in urine, the lower the blood pressure. Stamler noted that glutamic acid, an amino acid found in much higher quantities in plant than animal proteins, is converted to glutathione, which is a very potent antioxidant. He theorized that this antioxidant effect may be the reason that plant proteins are so effective at lowering blood pressure (Stamler, Brown, et al. 2009).

Randomized Trials Complete the Picture

Of course, the epidemiologic data make a strong argument, but to truly show a causal relationship between animal protein and hypertension, or vegetable protein and the reduction of hypertension, we need to look at randomized control trials. In fact, there have been many. Studies have randomized people to just increasing fruits, to increasing soy, or to actually adopting a vegetarian diet, and all have shown the expected effect of lowering blood pressure. Other studies have shown that putting people who have high blood pressure on a vegetarian diet lowers their blood pressure, which goes back up when meat is reintroduced. Importantly, these studies control for weight and for salt intake, so that the only cause could be the meat (He, Gu, et al. 2005; Margetts, Beilin, et al. 1986; Rouse, Beilin, et al. 1983; Appel, Moore, et al. 1997; John, Ziebland, et al. 2002).

The NIH sponsored a series of studies looking at diet and hypertension, which led to the development of the DASH (Dietary Approaches to Stop Hypertension) diet. DASH is the current "best practice" diet for patients with high blood pressure and is recommended by the American College of Cardiology and the American Heart Association. In fact, the DASH was voted the most effective diet by the US World and News Report after evaluation by its panel of experts. Although the DASH studies never looked specifically at a vegetarian diet, one of the authors noted that the idea for the development of the DASH diet came from the observations that vegetarians had such low rates of hypertension. The Premiere Trial randomized 809 patients to the DASH diet or to a control diet with behavioral therapy. Again, the lower the animal protein, the lower the blood pressure (Wang, Yancy, et al. 2008; Lin, Miwa, et al. 2010). Consequently, the DASH diet is heavy in fruits and vegetables with limited meat consumption.

When it comes to hypertension, the data speak loud and clear. The typical high-animal-protein diet will likely lead to high blood pressure and will, unnecessarily, subject millions to lifelong medications with a nasty array of side effects. I hope that more doctors will become familiar with the evidence, so they stop withholding the best choice of treatment to their patients. In the meantime, I hope that you will spread the message, so that patients everywhere can make better choices once given all the facts.

CHAPTER 11

Heart Disease: Skip the Meat, Keep the Beat

Six hundred thousand Americans will die of heart disease this year, more than from any other single cause. An additional 720,000 will experience a heart attack. Yet on the news, we hear much more about the two people in America infected with Ebola than our runaway number one killer. More perspective: roughly 15,000 people in America died of AIDS in 2010, but the Centers for Disease Control and Prevention (CDC) spends more money on AIDS awareness than heart disease prevention, roughly $10,000 per infected person with AIDS versus $3.50 per person suffering with heart disease. Our curious apathy toward heart disease extends beyond marketing, into research priorities themselves. The National Institutes of Health (NIH) will spend far more studying an array of different diseases that affect far fewer people than they will on heart disease.

The crazy thing about these statistics is not just the discrepancy between impact and effect. It's also the fact that heart disease is almost entirely preventable. As Dr. Caldwell Esselstyn says, "Cardiovascular disease is a toothless paper tiger that need never exist. And if it does exist, it need never progress. It is a food-borne illness. Change your food, change your life."

There are several reasons heart disease doesn't receive its fair share of public attention and research funding. First, and probably most influential, is the fact that heart disease has become so prevalent, we just accept it as a part of aging. Grandpa dies of a heart attack at age seventy-eight and we think he died of "old age." Meanwhile, dying at seventy-eight of heart disease would be considered a tragic loss in Okinawa.

Even the so-called French paradox may have its origins in the fact that heart disease is considered just a part of aging. The French paradox states that the French have less heart disease while eating more fat. Truth be told, they actually eat far more fruits and veggies than most Westernized cultures, which offers them protection against their heavy diets (Dauchet, Ferrières, et al. 2004). But Pierre Ducimetiere, a French statistician, exposed the real explanation of the French paradox: it's simply not true. Pathologists in France were less likely to identify heart disease as a cause of death on the death certificate. Why this happened is hard to say. Possibly they were proud of the paradox and subconsciously tried to lend further credence to it. I suspect that in part, it's due to our modern conception that heart disease represents an inevitable part of aging. An "old" person passes and they sign the death certificate as natural causes. Recent changes in reporting protocols show that the French have fairly comparable heart disease to other Western countries, and the original French paradox may simply have been, after all the hype, nothing but a clerical error (Ducimetiere 2008).

Second, heart disease has a slow, insidious onset. In our younger years we don't think about the fact that we are adding plaques to our vessels on a daily basis. Autopsy studies have demonstrated that children as young as twelve already show the beginnings of heart disease. Unlike the more shocking infectious diseases like Ebola or HIV, onset isn't sudden and life-changing. This is not a disease that will suddenly overwhelm us. We'll take pills for now to delay that first heart attack, get a "rite of passage" stent in our fifties, and maybe change our eating and exercise habits when we're older. For now, bring on the steak. Heart disease is simply not exotic enough for us to pay attention to.

Third, as I've said many times already, there is so much conflicting data on what to eat to prevent heart disease that confusion has led us down a dangerous path. Just think of the 2014 *Time* magazine cover showing a curl of butter and claiming that science has gotten it wrong: we should eat more fat. The *New York Times* ran a similar article with the picture of a hamburger, suggesting that may be healthy (just hold the bun!). The Internet is rife with all kinds of propaganda claiming that fat, especially the saturated variety, is good. A popular new diet book goes so far as to recommend putting butter in your coffee!

I have watched this growing Internet and media sensationalism with shock and horror, like an extremely slo-mo traffic accident. I sometimes feel as if I am watching an episode of the *Twilight Zone*. It is just that crazy. The source for all this nonsense comes from two very flawed articles published in scientific journals (Siri-Tarino, Sun, et al. 2010; Chowdhury, Warnakula, et al. 2014). The fact is, there are thousands of articles showing that saturated fat is harmful to your heart, but they are apparently not sensational enough to qualify for the cover of *Time*. In fact, the Cochrane Collaboration reviewed available randomized control trials and found that saturated fat *is* related to heart disease (Hooper, Summerbell, et al. 2011). The Cochrane Collaboration, a nonprofit organization "free from commercial sponsorship and other conflicts of interest," is highly respected in the research field for its groups' very unbiased investigations and analysis. Yet, there was not a single media response to the findings of this respected and credible group. Instead, most emphasis has been placed on an article whose authors received money from the National Dairy Association, the National Beef Council, and Atkins Nutritionals (Siri-Tarino, Sun, et al. 2010). Hmmm.

And remember what we discovered in Chapter 9: terrible and misleading as the studies were, and funded as they were by corporate interests, they never claimed that fat is good for us. They don't come close to promoting buttered coffee. That conclusion was invented by newspaper and magazine editors eager to boost newsstand sales. These two articles simply question whether saturated fat is truly the culprit of heart disease. Let's now consider the studies' flaws in more detail.

First, there is an irresponsible amount of overadjustment in the statistical analysis. These studies were looking at whether saturated fat causes heart disease. To find a link, researchers sought to eliminate other factors that may have been responsible for heart disease. Two of the confounding factors they eliminated through statistical adjustment were obesity and smoking, as they are both known risk factors for heart disease. But they also used statistics to erase the effects of high cholesterol on heart disease. The researchers' rationale was that cholesterol is an independent cause of heart disease, and therefore a confounder. But there's a huge problem with this logic: saturated fat causes heart disease, in part, by raising cholesterol. So basically they ignored people who were suffering from the effects of saturated fat and focused instead on people who had the unique genetic fortitude to withstand saturated fat's heart-damaging effects.

Worse yet, some of the studies in the Chowdhury paper (Chowdhury, Warnakula, et al. 2014) actually included people who were on lipid-lowering medications. This is crazy. It allowed the researchers to conclude that saturated fat did not cause heart disease by looking at people who were actually taking medications that specifically block the effect of saturated fat!

There are many other statistical errors in these studies that have been brought out in the literature (Stamler 2010; Pedersen, James, et al. 2011; Kromhout, Geleijnse, et al. 2011). Unfortunately, responsible peer review in the scientific arena is not good fodder for Facebook, Twitter, and the blogosphere and is therefore hidden from the public.

In fact, there is considerable evidence that saturated fat causes heart disease, ranging from lab studies to epidemiologic studies to randomized control trials. Several of these studies show that if you simply switch saturated fat to polyunsaturated fat like olive oil, your heart disease risk will decrease significantly (Shrapnel, Calvert, et al. 1992; Hu, Stampfer, et al. 1997, 1999; Keogh, Grieger, et al. 2005; Mozaffarian, Micha, et al. 2010; Farvid, Ding, et al. 2014; Astrup, Dyerberg, et al. 2011; Clarke, Frost, et al. 1997; Tucker, Hallfrisch, et al. 2005).

Gary Taubes is one of the most influential promoters of the positive health effects of saturated fat. Interestingly, in his TV appearances, he rails against the use of observational studies to make conclusions, yet his book *Good Calories, Bad Calories* is loaded with observational studies. He tries to show that saturated fat is not associated with heart disease because some population studies, like the Western Electric study, did not show a correlation. The problem is that the Western Electric study, and others in his book, did not have a truly low-fat group to compare to (despite this, the author of the Western Electric study later concluded that saturated fat indeed increased heart disease). Caldwell Esselstyn likens this kind of research to automobile crash tests at 80, 90, and 100 miles per hour. Researchers would discover equal mortality rates at all three speeds and hence conclude that speed is not a factor in car crash mortality.

Taubes also points to a Swiss village where inhabitants consumed lots of dairy fat and had low heart disease. These people lived at a high altitude, which is known to decrease cholesterol levels. He refers to a study suggesting that that vegetarian Trappist monks actually have high heart disease but fails to note that these monks consumed lots of saturated fat in the form of butter. Finally, as do many who argue that fat is beneficial, he points to the Maasai. The Maasai, as I previously discussed in Chapter 7, are a tribe of Kenyans that eats lots of meat and dairy. Of course, they live at high altitude, walk all day long, and their cows graze on grass, all of which should help mitigate their heart disease. Unfortunately, these healthy factors didn't help all that much: the Maasai have low life expectancy, and autopsy studies show that they do, in fact, have heart disease (Mann, Spoerry, et al. 1972).

Many saturated fat advocates point to the fact that many people who die of heart disease have normal cholesterol at the time of their death. The implication is that cholesterol, known for years to be a definite risk factor for heart disease, may be falsely maligned. The problem is that many of these people die in the hospital after a prolonged illness. In late stages of life, especially when infirm, cholesterol levels will drop. Really sick people often can't eat and are often fed liquid nutrients intravenously. The fact that their cholesterol is low at the time of their death ignores the fact that it was likely high all their life and led to their current diseased state (Corti, Guralnik, et al. 1997).

Despite dangerously delusional books like Bowden and Sinatra's *The Great Cholesterol Myth* and Taubes's and other Paleo promoters' fantasies to the contrary, high cholesterol is most definitely a significant risk factor for heart disease. It's a bit of a complex discussion, as there are many types of cholesterol. The LDL (low-density lipoprotein) component of cholesterol is most concerning for creation of atherosclerosis (Shah, Casas, et al. 2013). Statin drugs have been a game changer as far as treating and lowering heart disease. It is now recommended that people with risk factors for heart disease stay on statins for life. Statin drugs work primarily by lowering LDL cholesterol levels, proving that cholesterol is a considerable risk factor for heart disease (Steinberg 2007; Steinberg, Glass, et al. 2008). If anything, the problem may be that levels of cholesterol that we consider normal may actually be high (Roberts 2010). The average cholesterol in the United States is 210. Vegetarians average about 161 and vegans (no animal products, including dairy) average about 133. Dr. William Castelli, the famed lead researcher of the Framingham Heart Study, noted that in the many years of studying tens of thousands of residents of Framingham, Massachusetts, they never witnessed a heart attack in someone with a total cholesterol level less than 150.

Taubes and other low carbers are fond of repeating that the low-fat diet has failed America. The truth is, we never went on a low-fat diet, but they did get one thing right: we did lower our saturated fat intake, and in so doing, decreased our cholesterol and heart disease. Certainly there have been medical advances in cardiovascular care, but it is estimated that half the improvement is due to our lifestyle changes (Goldman and Cook 1984).

Of course, this book isn't about fat, it's about protein. When we began our journey together, I stated that it is best to discuss whole foods rather than reducing them to their component parts, but to slay the protein myth, I would have to play the reductionist game. The problem when it comes to discussing heart disease is that it is almost impossible to separate saturated fat from animal protein. We don't eat fat. We don't eat protein. We eat meat. I will review studies that look specifically at protein, but remember that saturated fat is in all meat and all but completely absent from fruits and vegetables (except for the stearic acid and lauric acid in coconuts). The University of Copenhagen held a symposium and invited the top experts in the field of heart disease and nutrition to discuss the role of saturated fat. They concluded that the evidence does, in fact, implicate saturated fat as having a causative role in heart disease, but it cannot be just saturated fat alone. They hint to the fact that it is not just about the fat but the food in which it is contained (Astrup, Dyerberg, et al. 2011). Like Bonnie and Clyde, Frank and Jesse James, and Butch and Sundance, saturated fat and animal protein always work together to wreak their damage.

Ancel Keys, whose work we explored in Chapter 4, was the first to begin the reductionist debates by looking exclusively at fat. As you may recall, Keys noted that populations with lower fat intake had lower heart disease. At first he looked at total fat, but narrowed his focus to saturated fat in the Seven Countries Study. The correlation between saturated fat and heart disease was strong, and when you really look at the data with twenty-five years of hindsight, it's instantly apparent that butter, lard, and meat are associated with heart disease, while vegetables and, especially legumes, are associated with a decrease in heart disease (Menotti, Kromhout, et al. 1999). Since saturated fat and animal protein travel together, Keys's research implicates protein as well.

Keys's biggest detractors, you may remember, were Drs. Yerushalmy and Hilleboe. Accusing Keys of cherry-picking his populations, Yerushalmy and Hilleboe conducted their own 22-country study and reported that total fat was not associated with heart disease. Swept under the rug on the low-carb websites that celebrate this article is the fact that while Yerushalmy and Hilleboe may have exculpated fat, they did find a strong correlation between protein consumption and heart disease. Later, a 29-country study further supported the idea that animal protein, in fact, is highly correlated with the development of heart disease (Connor and Connor 1972).

While ethical and practical considerations keep us from performing food experiments on large populations, sometimes history does it for us. Several times during the twentieth century, large populations were forced to change their diets. During both World War I and World War II, Germany blockaded Holland and captured their ranches and their animals. Meat consumption in Holland dropped precipitously during both occupations. And heart disease dropped almost as fast. Of course, there were confounding factors, such as starvation, but cholesterol levels plummeted nonetheless (Schettler 1983). As the war ended, and people shifted back to heavy animal protein intake, heart disease promptly returned.

A similar situation was seen in Poland during the fall of communism. Heart disease had been rising dramatically in Poland during the 1970s and 80s. After the Berlin Wall came down and the USSR dissolved, there was an astounding drop in heart disease. Researchers attempted to determine the cause of this unexpected decrease. What they found was that the transition to a market economy had a dramatic effect on lifestyle. Poles reduced their smoking and increased their physical activity. Certainly there were also medical advances; however, researchers believe that lifestyle changes were the predominant reason heart disease decreased so rapidly. But it wasn't just cigarettes and jogging shoes. Once Soviet-era meat subsidies were eliminated, meat consumption dropped precipitously. There was also a rise in fruit consumption, which added to the 24 percent drop in cardiac mortality (Bandosz, O'Flaherty, et al. 2012).

One of the greatest examples of the power of diet to change a population comes from Finland. Traditionally, the diet in Finland was high in fat, specifically from consuming huge quantities of butter. Consequently cholesterol levels were high, and Finland had the dubious distinction of having the highest levels of heart disease in the world. Starting in 1972, the Finnish government took an active role in addressing this deadly problem. The North Karelia region had Finland's highest incidence of heart disease. Public health officials rolled out the North Karelia Project, an intensive, multidimensional, grassroots movement to decrease fat intake, increase fruits and vegetables, and cut out smoking. It took time, but the effects were dramatic. Heart disease dropped by 80 percent and Finnish men's life expectancy increased by a whopping seven years. The improvements were so impressive, the program was rolled out to the rest of the country, with similarly positive results. Investigators felt that the majority of these changes were due to the ability of the Finnish to cut back sausage and butter and switch to vegetable oils and low-fat milk (Laatikainen, Critchley, et al. 2005).

If decreasing meat in a population correlates with decreased heart disease, what happens if there is an increase in meat consumption? Recall from Chapter 7 the cautionary tale of economic development in Tunisia. Comparing the population in 2009 to the population in 1997, we find a rise of heart disease by 17 percent, due to increased cholesterol, increased blood pressure, increased diabetes, and increased weight. Physical activity dropped, but so did cigarette smoking. Most dramatic is the fact that animal protein consumption used to make up just 14 percent of total protein consumed and ballooned to over 27 percent. This is a substantial change and could certainly explain, in part, the rise of heart disease. In fact, the rural Tunisians are not suffering this rapid rise in heart disease because they are still eating a traditional Tunisian diet consisting mainly of wheat. The rural people ate half the meat and three times the wheat of their sick, Westernized city colleagues. We know from other studies that wheat appears to protect against heart disease (Liu, Stampfer, et al. 1999; Hu and Willett 2002; Mellen, Walsh, et al. 2008), despite the ludicrous, unsupported claims of *Wheat Belly*.

Again, these stories of countries and their changes in health are observational. To really understand relationships between animal protein and heart disease, we need better epidemiologic studies that use statistical methodology to remove other possible causes, and thereby give a more reliable correlation. Again, I turn to the EPIC study of European populations. The Oxford branch of this study did not look at protein in isolation, but it did compare unhealthy vegetarians to healthy meat eaters. To remind you: the vegetarians showed B_{12} deficiencies and ate paltry amounts of fiber for people who were supposed to be eating veggies. The meat eaters consumed a relatively low average of 64 grams of meat per day. The meat eating group included slightly more smokers, but they were controlled for in the study. The results showed a statistically significant 30 percent reduction in the risk of developing heart disease by eliminating animal protein from the diet (Crowe, Appleby, et al. 2013).

The Adventist Health Study, as previously described, is an excellent epidemiologic study that has studied thousands of people for many years. Again, the beauty of the Adventist Health Study is the ability to look specifically at people who consume animal protein, to be able to quantify the amount of animal protein consumed, and to compare to people who do not eat animal protein over many years. The results show clear correlation between animal protein consumption and the risk of heart disease after controlling for other factors (Snowdon 1988; Fraser 1999, 2005).

There are two excellent meta-analyses of vegetarians versus omnivores as they relate to heart disease (Key, Fraser, et al. 1999; Huang, Yang, et al. 2012). They reviewed studies that had been done in different countries around the world (Chang-Claude, Frentzel-Beyme, et al. 1992; Key, Fraser, et al. 1999). The conclusion was a significant decreased risk of heart disease and stroke in people consuming plant-based diets of about 29 percent over nonvegetarians.

A very complex statistical assessment was done on a database that followed 29,000 postmenopausal women in Iowa for fifteen years. Researchers concluded that if you substituted vegetable protein for animal protein, you could expect a 30 percent decreased risk of developing heart disease. Interestingly, if you replaced carbs with red meat there was a 33 percent increase in risk (Kelemen, Kushi, et al. 2005). The authors conclude, ominously, "Long term adherence to high protein diet without discrimination of protein source may have adverse consequences." In other words, meat kills.

These studies compared people who eliminated animal protein from their diet, but many population studies in many different countries show that simply eating less animal protein is associated with less heart disease. Studies in Japan, India, Sweden, and others have shown that if you eat more fruits and less meat your heart will thank you (McGee, Reed, et al. 1984; Micha, Wallace, et al. 2010; Nagura, Iso, et al. 2009; Marmot, Syme, et al. 1975; Osler, Heitmann, et al. 2001; Cai, Shu, et al. 2007; Patel, Vyas, et al. 2006; Shrapnel, Calvert, et al. 1992; Lagiou, Sandin, et al. 2007, 2012; Merino, Kones, et al. 2013).

I would be remiss if I did not mention that an analysis of the Nurses' Health Study in 1999 did not show a correlation between animal protein and heart disease (Hu, Stampfer, et al. 1999). The problem with the study was the fact that the high-animal-protein eaters were not eating much more animal protein than the low-protein consumers. When the difference in diets is small, of course we should not expect to see statistically significant outcomes. In fact, the low-animal-protein eaters' main source of "vegetable protein" was bread. Later analysis took a more whole foods approach and found there was, in fact, a strong correlation between meat and dairy and heart disease (Bernstein, Sun, et al. 2010). While the Nurses' Health Study itself failed to find a smoking gun, the scholars who ran the study have since published numerous papers recommending a prudent diet consisting of fruits, veggies, grains, and lean protein compared to a high-animal-protein diet, especially denouncing red and processed meat (Hu, Rimm, et al. 2000; Hu and Willett 2002; Hu 2003; Heidemann, Schulze, et al. 2008). In fact, Dr. Walter Willett, the chair of Harvard's Department of Nutrition, has stated that people should pick the best protein packages by emphasizing plant sources of protein rather than animal (Skerrett and Willett 2010). The most recent Harvard review shows that people who had a prior heart attack and then go on a high-protein/low-carb diet are at a significantly higher risk of dying from their heart disease than someone consuming a high-plant-protein diet (Li, Flint, et al. 2014).

Why do we see this amazing correlation between consumption of animal protein and heart disease? Well, diabetes, hypertension, and high cholesterol are leading risk factors, and we've already seen a large body of evidence showing that eating animal protein leads to these diseases. Importantly, inflammation is certainly a key causative factor in the formation of heart disease, and we know that a high-animal-protein diet raises cortisol and CRP (C-reactive protein), which is clearly correlated with heart disease. This is why your doctor will likely check these lab values when you get your annual exam (Ebbeling, Swain, et al. 2012; Vogelzangs, Beekman, et al. 2010). Part of the inflammation may be from the acidosis and part may be from the endotoxemia that occurs from eating animal meat laden with bacteria (Erridge, Attina, et al. 2007; Wiedermann, Kiechl, et al. 1999).

Of course, if you are eating less meat and substituting fruits and veggies, you are thereby ingesting flavonoids and antioxidants that can decrease the inflammation and thereby reduce the risk of heart disease. The added fiber can also help clear cholesterol (Nanri, Moore, et al. 2007; (Huxley and Neil 2003; Leenders, Sluijs, et al. 2013; Nagura, Iso, et al. 2009; Holt, Steffen, et al. 2009; Tucker, Hallfrisch, et al. 2005). Vegetable eaters certainly have lower cholesterol levels (Thorogood, Carter, et al. 1987; Gardner, Coulston, et al. 2005). There are even studies that show that plants have substances that interfere with clotting, a major risk factor for both heart attacks and stroke (Rajaram 2003).

More interesting is the fact that animal protein combined with saturated fat may have a direct effect on the wall of the vessel. In a study that has gained fame in nutritional research circles, individuals were fed either a high-fat or a low-fat meal and then subjected to an ultrasound exam. The study showed that a meal with lots of cream caused substantial constriction of the vessels, while the carb meal did not (Vogel, Corretti, et al. 1997). In fact, even a short-term low-fat diet can loosen the stiff vascular walls of a typical high-cholesterol meat eater (Pirro, Schillaci, et al. 2004). This occurs because the consumption of meat and fat interferes with the breakdown of the amino acid arginine. We depend on arginine to turn into nitrous oxide, an important chemical that causes our vessels to dilate. If this doesn't happen, then blood flow to vital organs can be restricted (Esposito, Nappo, et al. 2003; Böger 2003). We know that amino acids in meat can interfere with the production of nitrous oxide. I should note that the little blue pill, consumed by many men to promote romantic abilities (if you know what I mean), works on this nitrous oxide to increase blood flow. That macho man might not need to pop the pill if he's willing to skip the steak during that candlelight dinner.

Another problem with meat, as we discussed in the diabetes chapter, is that it is high in heme iron. Heme iron causes oxidation and is directly associated with development of heart disease (Kaluza, Wolk, et al. 2012, 2013; Yang, Li, et al. 2013).

Most recently there has been a lot of interest into the nutrients carnitine and choline, both found in high concentrations in meat and eggs. The interest comes from the fact that carnitine and choline can be broken down in the bowels to a compound called TMAO, which is directly related with the development of heart disease and heart failure. Here's what's curious: if you give steak to vegans, they do not create TMAO. Vegans apparently have bacteria in their bowels that will not convert the carnitine to TMAO. In fact, if you give meat eaters an antibiotic, their TMAO response to a meal is diminished. We know that eating meat greatly changes your bowel flora, and this may be just one more way that meat causes heart disease (Tang, Wang, et al. 2013; Wang, Klipfell, et al. 2011; Grant, 2014; David, Maurice, et al. 2013, 2014).

Randomized Clinical Trials

We have reviewed observational and epidemiological studies showing eating animal meat correlates with heart disease, and I have shown several pathophysiological reasons that might be the case. Now we must look at randomized control trials to see if we can show that this is not just correlation but actual causation. There are, in fact, many randomized control trials that have tested the hypothesis that plant-based protein can reduce heart disease by either decreasing risk factors or increasing blood flow.

An article in the *New England Journal of Medicine* (Anderson, Johnstone, et al. 1995) described a meta-analysis of randomized trials looking at replacing animal protein with soy protein. The results were dramatic. Soy protein significantly reduced LDL cholesterol and triglycerides, two known risk factors for heart disease. Similar studies have shown that substituting plant-based proteins is as effective as taking statins (but unlike statins, plants have only positive side effects). The much maligned soy protein turns out to be a key ingredient in lipid control (Jenkins, Kendall, et al. 2002, 2003; Harland and Haffner 2008). We know exercise helps reduce cholesterol, but studies show that decreasing protein in combination with exercise is far more effective (García-Unciti, Martinez, et al. 2012).

The Lyon Diet Heart Study was a huge study that randomized 423 people who had had a heart attack into either a standard diet or a Mediterranean diet (de Lorgeril, Salen, et al. 1999) and followed them for 46 months. The Mediterranean group did so well, the researchers actually ended the study prematurely to save lives in the standard diet group. This really put the Mediterranean diet on the map. In this study, the version of the Mediterranean diet they instructed people to use was very low in saturated fat and high in fiber. They told patients to eat more bread and grains, and less animal protein. Plant proteins were substituted for animal proteins for many meals. The results were spectacular. The people following these dietary recommendations decreased their risk of another heart attack by 50 to 70 percent. If there was a pill that could get these kind of results, it would sell by the millions.

A very clever study was done to test whether saturated fat truly has an effect on heart disease risk factors. Researchers gave participants a high-carb diet, including muffins. One group ate muffins made with saturated fat, a second group ate polyunsaturated fat muffins, and the third group ate muffins containing monounsaturated fat. They found much higher inflammation, and stiffer blood vessels, in the people eating the saturated fat (Keogh, Grieger, et al. 2005). And the high-carb diet had no negative effect on inflammation or vessel pliability.

An interesting "accidental" experiment took place in a study published in *Angiology Journal*. Researchers wanted to know whether intense medical treatment of risk factors could help treat heart disease. As part of the treatment, they recommended a low-fat diet. They found, however, that 10 of the 26 patients they were studying decided independently to pursue a high-protein, low-carb diet because they thought it would be better for them. Both groups received identical medical treatment but the high-protein group developed more inflammation, worse cholesterol, and worse blood flow on heart scans. The 16 patients who followed the prescribed diet did far better (Fleming 2000).

Doctors Dean Ornish (Ornish, Scherwitz, et al. 1998) and Caldwell Esselstyn (Esselstyn 1999; Esselstyn, Gendy, et al. 2014) have done some of the most dramatic studies on the effect of plant-based diets on heart disease. Ornish did a very elaborate study where he followed patients who had heart disease as measured by a cardiac catheterization (sticking a tube in a blood vessel, threading it to the heart, injecting dye, and inspecting the vessels). Half of the patients were randomized into a control group and received conventional recommendations, the usual lifestyle advice given to heart patients. The other half were put on a very low-fat (10% or less of total calories) vegetarian diet, instructed to perform moderate exercise, and practice stress management. After 5 years, 71 percent of patients had stayed in the intensive lifestyle management program, a number that confounded the predictions of many medical "experts" that patients would never agree to such "drastic" lifestyle changes when they could manage their conditions with drugs and surgeries.

Prior to publication of this study, the medical establishment assumed that heart disease could possibly be halted, but never actually reversed. Ornish, however, demonstrated that the elimination of animal protein, with the other lifestyle interventions, caused an 8 percent improvement in the stenosis of the vessels while the control group had the usual and expected 28 percent worsening of their vessels (Ornish, Scherwitz, et al. 1998). Esselstyn showed similar results with actual reversal of heart disease on a plant-based, no-animal-protein diet. His study didn't include the exercise or stress management components, showing that reversal of heart disease can be accomplished with a low-fat plant-based diet alone (Esselstyn 1999; Esselstyn, Ellis, et al. 1995; Esselstyn, Gendy, et al. 2014).

A later study showed the Ornish diet caused less inflammation and far better relaxation of blood vessels compared to Atkins and South Beach. The author advised that the Ornish diet was a far better choice for those who are obese and at risk for heart disease (Miller, Beach, et al. 2009).

The evidence to support cutting out meat consumption is very strong. From studies showing pathophysiologic changes (doctor-speak for "bad stuff happening in the body") associated with animal consumption that hypothetically could cause heart disease, to epidemiologic studies to randomized control trials, it's easy to see that the less animal protein, the happier your heart.

CHAPTER 12

Obesity: It's Not About the Carbs

Can you believe people actually avoid fruit in an attempt to lose weight? There has never been a single credible study showing that fruit consumption leads to weight gain, and yet this concept is as prevalent as any nutrition dogma. I have treated people for obesity for years and I can tell you, nobody is coming to see me because they ate too many apples or grapes. Why do people think fruit leads to weight gain? The quick answer from my patients is because of the carbs.

When I ask my patients what their downfall is, when it comes to weight loss, they unanimously blame carbs. Their diet log will read: eggs-and-bacon breakfast sandwich, Subway sandwich and chips for lunch, and a pork roast with potatoes for dinner. When asked the part of that menu that is causing them to gain weight, they blame the bread from the sandwiches, the chips, and the potatoes. It is always the bun, never the hamburger. Now don't get me wrong; there is nothing healthy about chips, loaded with fat. The sandwich bread is likely bleached flour with little, to no, nutrient value. However, the vast majority of the calories are coming from fat and protein. Pizza and donuts are considered carbs despite the fact that they contain as many (or more) calories from fat as carbs.

Let's discuss two examples. The first is for a Pizza Hut six-inch Personal Pan Meat Lover's Pizza (admittedly one of their more calorically dense and fat-heavy options). Of the 850 total calories, 430 come from fat.

That's 51 percent. Another hundred calories come from protein, leaving 320 calories from carbs.

Second, a Krispy Kreme Original Glazed Donut. According to the company's website (updated September 2014), a single donut delivers 190 calories, 100 of them from fat. That's 53 percent. Carbs account for 84 calories (44%), while protein comprises another 6 calories (3%).

Here's a recent conversation with a patient, a woman from Ghana, that really highlights the misconceptions about diet and weight loss. She has lived in the United States for many years, and during much of that time, struggled mightily with obesity. She has seen endocrinologists, dietitians, and trainers. She has done the Atkins diet several times and most recently went to a doctor who prescribed Belviq (the newest prescription medication targeting obesity). She sees a registered dietitian and a trainer regularly. Despite the meds, the medical oversight, and her sincere and steadfast efforts, she still has a body mass index (BMI) of 40, which classifies her as morbidly obese.

And as you'll see, she already knows everything she needs to make smarter decisions. It's only the proteinaholism that blinds her to the truth:

ME: *So what do you typically eat for breakfast?*

PATIENT: *Usually eggs of some sort and a protein.*

ME: *What do you mean by "protein"?*

PATIENT: *Well, it could be chicken or bacon or sausage.*

ME: *Hmm, those aren't really protein. I mean, some of those choices have more calories from fat than protein. So really, you could just as well say, "I have eggs and some fat for breakfast."*

PATIENT: *(Chuckles) Never thought about it like that.*

ME: *So what's for lunch?*

PATIENT: *Usually salad with a pro- um, I mean fish or chicken.*

ME: *OK, do you snack during the day?*

PATIENT: *No. My issues really are at night, when we eat more carbs from our traditional diet from Ghana. We eat lots of yams and stews. Lots of starches.*

ME: *Interesting that you view that as your bad meal when to me it's your best. Have you visited Ghana recently?*

PATIENT: *Yes. Funny enough, whenever I visit Ghana I lose weight. That is the only place I lose weight.*

ME: *What do you eat there?*

PATIENT: *Lots of yams, yam stews, lots of maize (corn), fruit.*

ME: *Are there lots of obese people in Ghana?*

PATIENT: *Not at all. In fact, when I am there I am one of the biggest.*

ME: *So do you see what I'm getting at? In Ghana you eat lots of starches and fruits, and people are thin and you lose weight. But come to America and eat American "health food," and you gain weight. As I look at your diet history, you have always tried diets that focus on high protein. You told me you try to eat lots of protein and it has never worked long for you. Yet you have completely avoided a diet that you enjoy and have lost weight on.*

PATIENT: *Well, I thought fruits and starches made you fat, and we need more protein. That is all I hear.*

In Ghana, the obesity rate is 5.5 percent, higher for women (7.9%) and lower for men (2.8%), compared to America's 34.9 percent rate of obesity. Higher rates of obesity were found among those who live in the more Westernized portions of Ghana and eat less fruit. Also, those who had not completed a secondary school education were much less likely to become obese than those who graduated from secondary school, high school, and college. This suggests that with higher earning power came the ability to buy meat and other rich Western fare. The Ghanaian traditional diet was the one most closely correlated with normal weight and is high in beans and starches, including maize, yams, fruits, and cassava roots (Biritwum, Gyapong, et al. 2005).

Traditional diets high in fruits, veggies and starches have worked for thousands of years, and continue to keep people slim and healthy. But our obsession with counting fat, carbs, and protein blinds us to this truth. My patient, an intelligent, motivated woman, could not see the obvious solution to her weight problem. I'm not sure yet if my "white coat" authority was able to undermine the grip of her proteinaholism and give her permission to return to her traditional, healthful diet—time will tell.

Let me make this abundantly clear: carbs do not make you fat, unless you are eating too many calories. In fact, the body is very resistant to turning carbs to fat. We are designed to burn carbs. Every cell in our body utilizes energy from glucose.

If you increase your carbohydrate consumption, your body will, in turn, increase its carbohydrate utilization. That's right; the more you eat, the more you burn. One fascinating lab study overfed test subjects, first with carbs and then, later, with fat. Through complex analysis the researchers found that the body increased its metabolism with the extra carbs, in attempt to burn the excess, but stored the excess of fat (Horton, Drougas, et al. 1995). Turning carbs to fat is a very inefficient process, costing energy that the body generally doesn't want to spend. The only time carbs will be turned to fat (called "de novo lipogenesis") is when carbohydrate stores are full, and the carbohydrate consumption causes calorie excess that exceeds your body's total energy expenditure. In other words, if you eat more calories than you burn, any additional food, whether carbs or protein or fat, will be turned to fat (Hellerstein 1999). Well, not quite: our bodies can actually store quite a lot of excess carbs as glycogen before turning it to fat. We can hold 15 grams of carbs per kilogram of total body weight in the form of glycogen and can add up to 500 additional grams before we even begin turning it into fat (Acheson, Schutz, et al. 1988). By contrast, our bodies do not have a place to store excess protein, which will be converted to fat. And any excess fat is immediately stored as fat, with no conversion necessary.

An elegant 2012 study placed overweight subjects on low-calorie diets but randomized them to different amounts of sugar or high-fructose corn syrup (HFCS). Just like Mark Haub, the professor who ate a high-sugar diet but kept his calories under control, these subjects all lost weight regardless of the amount of sugar or HFCS, simply because they kept their calories low. The researcher concluded that it is the amount of calories that matter, not the carbs or macronutrient breakdown (Lowndes, Kawiecki, et al. 2012).

The nutritional science literature is littered with thousands of studies comparing low-fat and low-carb/high-protein diets in regard to obesity. You can find, in some of the most prestigious journals, papers that provide evidence for low fat and others that support low carb. Many of these studies look impressive until you get past the abstracts and look at the actual numbers. Typically what you will find is that the so-called low-fat diet group was never on a low-fat diet. Many of the studies showing that low-fat diets don't lead to weight loss define low fat as 30 percent of calories, which is actually quite high. Typically, the participants' baseline diet contains 35 percent fat, so they are not making significant changes to their diet. Practically, they're probably just substituting a packet of fat-free cookies for a serving of fries. Meanwhile, the low-carb groups are making huge changes by severely limiting the amount of carbs they ingest. This limits their menu and food choices, which means they will eat less calories. In every low-carb versus low-fat study I have read, the low-carb group eats fewer calories. Again, keeping it simple: if you eat fewer calories, you will lose more weight. There's nothing earth-shattering about this finding; it's basic thermodynamics.

Of course, you could argue that it doesn't matter why the low-carb group is losing more weight, even if it's just calories in rather than some mystical theory about protein metabolism. And I might agree, if a low-carb diet were a sustainable way of eating. Unfortunately, as we've seen, the body thrives on carbs. It wants carbs. And when we deprive our body of carbs, it starts craving them like crazy. So when low-carb dieters finally exceed the limits of their resolve and binge on bread and pasta and pizza and donuts, it's not the carbs that are causing them to gain weight, but the excess calories. The saddest part, perhaps, is that the low-carb dieters end up blaming themselves, rather than realizing the diet itself is unsustainable. So many patients tell me, shame-faced, that they were successful on Atkins but didn't have the willpower to continue. By the time they come to see me, they've given up on themselves. I have to labor mightily to convince them that they are not failures; rather, the diet failed them by creating an unnatural state that their bodies will rebel against.

We've already looked at the A to Z Trial (Gardner, Kiazand, et al. 2007; Dansinger, Gleason, et al. 2005). To refresh your memory, this study compared the Atkins, Zone, Ornish, and LEARN diets. Initially, the Atkins group had the best weight loss, but on any low-carb diet you will burn up your glycogen reserve, which is stored with water. Basically, the rapid Atkins weight loss is just water weight. At the end of the year, all the groups had similar weight loss. Analysis of the study proved that it is not the macronutrient breakdown, but rather degree of adherence to the diet, whichever diet that may be, which determines weight loss (Alhassan, Kim, et al. 2008).

Many other studies have compared diets of different macronutrient levels, feeding people various levels of carbs, fats, and proteins. All the meta-analyses and review papers have concluded that, in the end, it is the total number of calories that matter (Freedman, King, et al. 2001; Powell, Tucker, et al. 1994; Alford, Blankenship, et al. 1990; Hu, Mills, et al. 2012; Bravata, Sanders, et al. 2003; Sacks, Bray, et al. 2009; Krebs, Elley, et al. 2012; Foster, Wyatt, et al. 2003; Shai, Schwarzfuchs, et al. 2008; Hill, Drougas, et al. 1993; Golay, Allaz, et al. 1996; Astrup, Meinert Larsen, et al. 2004). Science simply does not support the popular belief that protein causes weight loss and carbs cause weight gain, independent of calorie intake.

People who advocate high-protein diets claim that protein intake increases metabolism. They refer to the thermogenic effect of eating protein, which basically means that the body has to expend energy to process protein. This is actually true and makes sense when you think about it; as an inferior fuel source, protein makes our metabolism work harder to convert it into usable glucose. Studies have shown that basal metabolic rate increases when eating protein (Mikkelsen, Toubro, et al. 2000). The fact is, however, that this effect is tiny, maybe a 1 to 2 percent increase, which is about 20 calories. By contrast, carbs don't trigger this thermogenic effect unless you are overeating. And as we've seen, overeating on carbs causes an increase in metabolism. Carb are easily utilized, which is why there is no thermogenic effect (Horton, Drougas, et al. 1995).

Supporters of the high-protein diet will also tell you that protein is more satiating. That's a funny word for what really happens. If you eat a very low-carb diet, your body runs out of its primary form of energy: carbs. To stay alive, your body switches to an alternative energy source. The body will start burning fat for fuel, with chemicals called ketones created as a by-product. Ketones can make you feel ill. Complaints of nausea and abdominal discomfort are common on these diets and may be the reason people end up eating fewer calories. As far as protein itself having an independent effect on hunger, the data are cloudy. Studies comparing protein to carbs for satiety give protein the edge in blunting hunger, but these studies use isolated carbs, not fruits and veggies (Boelsma, Brink, et al. 2010). We know that eating pure sugar can make you hungry by affecting blood glucose levels. By not testing protein directly against fruit and vegetables, which have the sugars bound to fiber and therefore control hunger better, these satiety studies make protein look better than it really is.

Protein does affect hormones in the body that control hunger. It turns out, however, that it doesn't seem to matter if this from plant protein or animal protein (Bowen, Noakes, et al. 2006). In addition, the science does not show that protein has a dramatic independent effect on eating behavior (Martens, Lemmens, et al. 2013). We can go through all the studies you want analyzing how hormones like GLP1 vary with protein content of an experimental shake. In the real world, however, food choices do not seem to be governed independently by protein. In one study, researchers had test participants eat various different foods in equal energy amounts. They tested fullness after the meal and the amount of food eaten at the next meal. The high-carbohydrate potato actually had the highest satiety index (Holt, Miller, et al. 1995).

If protein is so satiating, and increases our metabolism, then why are we so overweight? After all, we eat more protein and less carbs than just about every civilized country and yet we lead the way in obesity, with roughly two-thirds of our population obese or overweight. The situation is so dire that we now spend $200 billion a year on obesity-related illnesses (Li and Heber 2012). The National Center for Health Statistics shared the NHANES data about American eating patterns on the CDC website. They concluded that between 1998 and 2008, total calorie intake has held stable, but our carbohydrate intake has decreased and our protein intake has increased. If protein calories keep us from gaining weight, that trend should have halted our growing obesity epidemic, or at least made a dent. But the data show no such effect; obesity increased significantly in men and adolescents over about that same time period (while women leveled off) (Ogden, Carroll, et al. 2006).

The Institute of Medicine has said that, if you are overweight, losing 5 percent of your weight is a success, and studies suggest losing 10 percent provides considerable cardiovascular benefit, but people want to lose far more weight. People come to see me and they want to lose extreme amounts of weight, and they want to do it quickly. Studies show that most people want to lose 32 percent of their weight and are disappointed with anything less (Foster, Wadden, et al. 1997). You can see why people would go on extreme low-carb/high-protein diets, ignoring the nausea and constipation, to try and lose as much weight as fast as possible.

The common belief is that diets don't work, and both science and many people's personal experience confirm this belief. It seems like everyone is always on a diet, yet we're always gaining weight. Looking at it with a clear eye, it becomes obvious that we are dieting ourselves to obesity.

Of course, some people do succeed in losing weight and keeping it off. In our society, they are extreme outliers, but they do exist. It makes sense to study these "positive defiants" rather than the millions who are failing to lose weight. In 1998, a National Weight Control Registry was formed to study people who lose a significant amount of weight and actually keep it off. I want to be clear that this is nowhere near a well-designed scientific experiment. Rather, it is an interesting study of people who have been able to escape the dieting pitfalls.

Analysis shows that most long-term successful "losers" have a few things in common. They get moderate exercise, they don't skip breakfast, they don't go on crash diets, and, importantly, they focus on low-fat diets (Shick, Wing, et al. 1998). Yes, many low-carb diets show better initial weight loss, but what we should be focusing on is the long term. After all, do you want to be lean for six months, or for the rest of your life? The initial weight loss, due to decreased water weight and calorie consumption from appetite suppression on low-carb/high-protein diets, is short-lived in most people. While this may be just an observation, one of the great researchers in nutritional science, George Bray, did a review of the literature and noted that decreasing fat intake really does correlate with weight loss (Bray and Popkin 1998), and many studies agree (Stamler and Dolecek 1997; Toubro and Astrup 1997; Howard, Manson, et al. 2006). In fact, while it is relatively easy to lose weight, the hardest thing to do is maintain weight. Dr. Rudolph Leibel, the codirector of Columbia University's Naomi Berrie Diabetes Center, has done excellent studies showing people lose weight easily but then hit a wall. The wall is partly due to lower metabolism and also due to some complex hormonal changes. Studies have shown, however, that similar to what we see in the National Weight Control Registry, low-fat diets do help people keep the weight off (Hill, Drougas, et al. 1993).

I've treated thousands of patients for weight loss in my years in practice, so I have a perspective born of personal experience, not just reviewing the research literature. I have become very skeptical of short-term weight loss. I used to prescribe a protein shake diet and patients saw incredible initial weight loss. The problem was that the weight would come back very quickly, and when they plateaued, they would be even heavier than before. Almost every patient I have ever seen has done Atkins, and every one of them gained the weight back (otherwise they wouldn't be in my office).

The Epidemiology of Protein and Weight Loss

Given that the National Weight Control Registry isn't a rigorously controlled study, and the population studies create "straw man" low-fat diets that are actually high in fat, and the lab studies are all over the place, what kind of research would settle the question of the best diet for long-term weight loss once and for all? Ideally, the best study would be to randomize people to two very different diets, one truly low fat and the other low carb/high protein, and follow them for twenty years to see how they do long term. Unfortunately, this study can never be performed. It is very difficult to get people to change their diet and stick with it for one year, never mind twenty. Our best bet is to look at how people who eat different diets do in general over many years. Again, people criticize epidemiology as correlation, not causation, but if multiple studies around the world all show the same results, it is worth taking note. If you want to lose weight, doesn't it make sense to model the lifestyles of large groups of people who already have what you want?

The EPIC study researchers, you'll recall, followed hundreds of thousands of people over several years and found that, contrary to popular belief, the more animal protein people ate, the more likely they were to become obese (Schulz, Kroke, et al. 2002; Halkjær, Olsen, et al. 2011). In fact, complex statistical analysis revealed that if individuals ate 22 percent of their calories from protein, they were 23 percent more likely to develop obesity than those eating only 14 percent of their calories from protein (Vergnaud, Norat, et al. 2013). Even more surprising is the fact that meat, especially chicken, was associated with weight gain over time (Vergnaud, Norat, et al. 2010). Before you fall for the low-carb excuse that there could be all kinds of reasons and biases and confounding variables that could produce these findings, the researchers controlled for every conceivable factor, even calorie intake. They made sure the different groups had equal calorie intake and yet chicken, our national health food, was still associated with the most weight gain!

The EPIC data have been used to look at a Mediterranean diet and have shown it to be a fantastic way of eating. The closer they looked, the more researchers found a Mediterranean diet to be an effective way to maintain weight loss. On close observation, they concluded that it was specifically the low-meat content that made the diet so successful at keeping obesity at bay (Romaguera, Norat, et al. 2010).

The Oxford component of the EPIC data allowed an interesting look at vegetarians and vegans and compared them to a healthy group of meat eaters. As we've seen, these meat eaters ate much less meat than the rest of the population in Great Britain. Controlling for many lifestyle factors, studies still showed that vegetarians and vegans tended to weigh less. When they looked at this group over time, researchers found that the more animal protein and the less fiber consumed, the more likely a person was to gain weight (Spencer, Appleby, et al. 2003; Appleby, Thorogood, et al. 1999).

The Adventist Health Studies provide a great opportunity to see how weight differs between people who consume animal protein and those who do not. Again, let me emphasize that the Adventist meat eaters are generally healthier than the population at large, and this database follows many people over many years. As expected, this long-term study of 71,000 people found the less animal protein eaten, the lower the body mass index (Rizzo, Jaceldo-Siegl, et al. 2013). They also note that the more animal protein eaten, the more nutrient deficient the diet was, which may be expected.

Many other studies have correlated how people ate over time with changes in their weight. Whether in Sweden (Newby, Muller, et al. 2003) or in America (Kahn, Tatham, et al. 1997), long-term prospective studies reliably show that the more animal protein and the less vegetable consumption, the more weight gain. The biggest study of how we eat comes from a database I mentioned earlier called the National Health Examination and Nutrition Survey, or NHANES. You may see people on the web (low carbers, I'm looking at you) jump to unfounded conclusions (and post them as pretty pie charts) from a cursory examination of the raw data. You cannot look at raw data and come to any scientific understanding. You have to use careful statistical analysis and control for factors that might result in a false correlation. Just because Switzerland has the most Nobel Prize laureates, and Switzerland produces and consumes the most chocolate, does not mean that the more chocolate you consume, the more likely you are to win a Nobel Prize. Researchers applied advanced statistical analysis to the NHANES data and stated that there is a clear statistical relationship between meat consumption and weight gain (Wang and Beydoun 2009). In panicked response, a high-powered lobbyist for the beef industry sent a letter to the editor of a medical journal. He argued that you see increased weight in meat eaters because they have increased muscle. Unfortunately for him, these studies looked at waist circumference, not just weight. Meat eaters were getting bigger bellies, not bigger pecs or biceps. Nice try, though.

Gary Taubes's book *Good Calories, Bad Calories* featured a lengthy discussion of the Chicago Western Electric study that monitored the diet and health of employees at that company. Taubes was trying to show that their saturated fat intake had nothing to do with developing heart disease, a notion we dealt with in the last chapter. What's relevant here is that the study followed 1,730 employees for eight years and looked at weight as it related to protein consumption. Animal protein was clearly and significantly associated with weight gain while plant protein actually was associated with weight loss (Bujnowski, Xun, et al. 2011).

Why Does Protein Cause Weight Gain?

You might be asking yourself how protein can be associated with weight gain when you have always been told to eat protein to lose weight. There are many possible answers to this very complex question. One comprehensive 2009 review considers mounting evidence that the chronic acid intake from high-protein diets may actually cause cellular dysfunction and eventual weight gain (Berkemeyer 2009). While this article is an interesting read (to me, at least), I think the answer is much more simple.

You may have heard of a term called "volumetrics." Barbara Rolls, Ph.D., a nutritionist at Penn State, invented this term to describe a very simple idea: if you eat food with low-calorie density, then you will not gain

Caloric Density

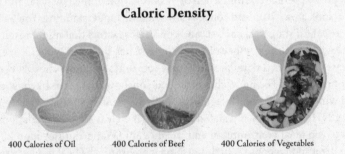

400 Calories of Oil   400 Calories of Beef   400 Calories of Vegetables

Stretch receptors are located throughout the stomach. When they are triggered by food, they send signals to your brain to tell you to stop eating. With high fiber, whole plant foods, you can eat the most quantity for the least amount of calories.

© 2012 Julieanna Hever, MS, RD, CPT • www.PlantBasedDietitian.com
Illustration by Sherri Nestorowich • www.sherrinest.wix.com/art

weight. The idea is that the stomach has stretch receptors that feed back to the brain when our stomachs are full.* If you eat food with lots of calories per weight, by the time your stretch receptors alert your brain that you're full, you have already eaten too many calories. However, if you eat food with a low amount of calories, you can stuff your face until your stomach tells you that you're full without overconsuming calories (Rolls 2000; Rolls and Bell 1999; Rolls, Ello-Martin, et al. 2004).

Fruits, vegetables, and beans are high in fiber, which is not absorbed into our bloodstream. So some of the weight of these plant foods does not translate into calories absorbed. Likewise, the fiber holds water and obviously water won't cause fat gain. So if you eat a giant 280 gram slice of watermelon, due to the fiber and water, you get only 85 calories. A 280 gram piece of chicken delivers almost six times the calories (480). If you could actually consume 280 grams of olive oil (20 tablespoons, in case you're crazy), you'd take in a whopping 2,380 calories.

This is why I tell my patients they do not need to count calories when they eat a plant-based diet. I don't care how many apples they eat, or how much kale they consume. I have never seen anybody get fat from broccoli or bananas. One patient didn't believe me and tried to prove me wrong by eating six apples a day. She still lost weight. Even the most dedicated overeater will become full before eating too many calories.

As an added bonus, the fiber in fruits and vegetables acts as a binder to the sugar they contain. I don't recommend drinking juices because they remove the fiber from the sugar. When you drink orange juice, the sugar goes into your system real fast. This doesn't make you fat, but it does make you hungry in an hour or so. Eat an orange, on the other hand, and the fiber turns the sugar into a slow release pill so you don't experience the same sugar rush. High fiber decreases the glycemic load of the food, and studies have shown that this really does decrease hunger (Lennerz, Alsop, et al. 2013). I believe this is why fiber is so well associated with weight loss. When you look at large studies, people eating the most fruits, veggies, and grains are eating the highest fiber and thereby eating lower calories and losing more weight than meat eaters (Mozaffarian, Hao, et al. 2011).

I have been using plant-based diets for weight loss for many years with considerable success. My goal is not to make everybody vegan, but rather

---

* In fact, scientists have invented an electronic device that can stimulate this nerve to create a full feeling. I don't know about you, but I would rather do it with food.

to greatly increase the amount of fruits, vegetables, grains, and legumes consumed, while decreasing our usual reliance on protein. I want my patients to turn their plate around. I tell them to dethrone the meat from its starring role in the center of the plate. I always hear that plant-based diets are hard to do, but it hasn't been for my patients. It's not just me; studies have found that vegetarian diets are very well tolerated in clinical settings (Berkow, Barnard, et al. 2010; Thedford and Raj 2011).

A plant-based diet liberates us from counting calories, but it goes further; I tell my patients not to count *anything*. Years of counting points and carbs, and weighing portions, has made them addicted to measuring. It is a huge relief for them to stop having to starve themselves and worrying about portions. I instruct them to eat the rainbow with a wide variety of fruits and veggies, without limits. If you are hungry, I tell them again and again, have an apple. Enjoy it fully and don't worry. I provide them with delicious recipes that allow large portions but with low-calorie content (which you can find in Chapter 17). Time and again they tell me how easy it is to eat this way. They gush over how delicious the food is, how they are never hungry, and how they feel fantastic. Remember, my business is helping people lose weight. If they didn't lose weight, I wouldn't be successful. Thankfully, this diet is extremely successful, which is why I recommend it.

One study that shows how easy and effective a low-fat, low-protein, high-carb plant-based diet can be is the Waianae Diet Study in Hawaii. Hawaii has seen a tremendous increase in obesity and metabolic diseases in the past several decades, but natives before Westernization did not suffer from these diseases. The researchers recruited 22 adults and placed them on a diet that would have been typically eaten by a pre-Western native for 21 days. They were told to eat as much as they wanted of native fruits and vegetables. The diet was about 78 percent carbs but only 11 percent protein and 11 percent fat. Despite the lack of limits, they ended up eating fewer calories while showing significant improvements in their cardiometabolic profile. They also lost an average of 10.8 pounds over the three weeks. Most important, the diet was very well received and tolerated (Shintani, Beckham, et al. 1994, 2001).

Of course, as many will surely point out, the Waianae Diet Study was not a randomized control trial, the so-called gold standard of research. Luckily, Dr. Gabrielle Turner-McGrievy has conducted two in-depth randomized control trials that confirm the striking results from the Waianae Diet Study. Her first study compared participants on a vegan diet to those on the National Cholesterol Education Program (NCEP) diet. This was interesting because the diets are somewhat similar. In fact, the NCEP diet is what many people would call a moderate diet. The individuals on NCEP did eat less fiber, more protein, and more fat, although by keeping fat below 30 percent of total calories it is still considered a low-fat diet by the dietary establishment. Despite the smallish differences between the diets, after two years the vegan group had achieved significantly more weight loss than the more moderate diet that is frequently recommended by doctors (Turner-McGrievy, Barnard, et al. 2007).

Dr. Turner-McGrievy conducted another interesting trial in which she randomized 63 overweight adults into five equal-sized groups: meat eaters, occasional meat eaters, pesco-vegetarian, vegetarian, and vegan. At six months the vegans showed significantly more weight loss than the other groups (Turner-McGrievy, Davidson, et al. 2015). Admittedly, this study was short term, but it did show that the vegan diet was well tolerated. If you wonder what would happen long term, the Adventist Health Studies have already shown that these results would likely continue, with the vegans losing and the meat eaters gaining the most weight.

If losing weight is one reason you're reading this book, then be assured that you've found the most effective, least complicated way to eat to help you achieve your goal. You can get started with the recipes and meal plan in Chapter 17. Once you experience the rapid healing and weight-loss benefits for yourself, you'll be hooked. Like so many of my patients. Like me.

CHAPTER 13

Cancer: Fleshing Out the Protein Connection

I don't think I have to tell you this, but cancer is a big deal. Nothing strikes fear into a person more than the "C word." In fact, while cancer is the second-leading cause of death, we spend double to triple on cancer research than on heart disease research.

Cancer can strike anybody at any age and any race. We have been in a war on cancer for four decades and yet cancer is poised to take over as the number one cause of death. We still seem baffled as to the best way to treat cancer, though our therapies are far more advanced than our ability to prevent. We talk a big game about prevention, but really when Western medicine says prevention, it means mammograms and colonoscopies. These are not preventive medicines, they are early diagnostic tools.

Why do we get cancer? You think I am going to say protein, don't you? I wish it were so simple. So many things have to happen in order to get a cancer. Genetics do play a strong part. We have found certain tumor suppressor genes and tumor promoter genes that are linked with certain cancers, but just having a gene doesn't mean you will get cancer. Something has to activate the gene. It could be an environmental toxin, it could be our food, it could be the sun, and obviously it could be a combination.

In fact, it is said that we always have cancers forming and dissipating in our bodies all the time. So maybe you go out in the sun and this causes a gene mutation in a cell. That doesn't mean you will necessarily get cancer. Our cells have an ability to repair DNA damage. We also have specialized cells that search the body for abnormal cells and extinguish them. The important thing is that we foster an environment where either we avoid the instigator or enable the repair.

So I cannot say that animal protein causes cancer. What I can say is that animal protein causes various reactions in the body that have been shown to be carcinogenic, and animal protein has been strongly correlated with cancer. In this chapter, we'll see epidemiologic evidence linking animal foods to cancer incidence and mortality. We'll also discover randomized controlled trials that prove a strong link between diet and cancer. But if we are going to say animal protein contributes to cancer development and progression, we first need to establish a mechanism of action, or probable cause.

Probable Cause

It's time to peer into the microscope and look at the mechanisms by which particular foods and diets may contribute to cancer progression or prevention. Identifying biological plausibility is important to weed out possible correlations found in the population studies that may be due to random chance. For example, if you study several hundred thousand people over twenty years and consider enough variables, you may find associations that are purely due to chance, such as wearing a yellow polo shirt on Tuesdays being linked with less prostate cancer. Here's a real-life example of a coincidence that looks real: you can predict stock market performance based on the winner of the Super Bowl. The market has had an up year following an NFC win and a down year after an AFC win over 80 percent of the time. Unless someone can find an explanatory mechanism linking the two data sets, we have to treat it as a whimsical coincidence. The following sections discuss the mechanisms connected to the development of many cancers.

Cooking-Derived Bad Guys: HCAs

Heterocyclic amines (HCAs) are chemicals formed in meat, or any animal protein, that is cooked at a high temperature or over an open flame (Sugimura 1997, 2000). You know those grill marks that commercials for meat products like to display? Well, if you scrape off that grilled substance and send it to a lab, technicians will find a formaldehyde-like substance called "heterocyclic amine."

2-Amino-1-methyl-6-phenylimidazo(4,5-b)pyridine (PhIP) is one such compound that has been well studied. The HCAs are implicated in many cancers, so it's reasonable to ask if it's the animal protein by itself, or the way meat is often seared or grilled, that is contributing to cancer development. One study of 1,600 people in North Carolina found that not only was meat consumption associated with colon cancer, but the strength of the association varied with cooking method. The worst way of cooking meat was pan fried and well done (Butler, Sinha, et al. 2003). This is likely due to that fact that the HCAs form when you burn animal protein.

Several animal studies link PhIP in cooked meat with prostate cancer. A 2005 prospective study of over 29,000 men confirmed that increased amounts of cooked meat lead to an increased risk of prostate cancer, and named PhIP specifically as a likely carcinogen (Cross, Peters, et al. 2005).

Another cancer closely linked to HCA, and PhIP in particular, is breast cancer. A large study of postmenopausal women in Long Island found that grilled, barbecued, and smoked meat was associated with an increased risk of breast cancer (Steck, Gaudet, et al. 2007). Again, the mediating mechanism here appears to be HCAs and PhIP. A 2011 in vitro (test tube) study published in *Toxicology* lent support to this hypothesis. Researchers exposed breast cancer cells to PhIP and watched what happened. The cells began dividing and actually became so invasive that they started to digest and then go through the basement membrane (the matrix of tissue that separates the epithelial layer from deeper tissue) (Lauber and Gooderham 2011). This is kind of a chilling finding, if you think about it; this one chemical found in cooked meats converted cancer cells from early stage to malignant. This was just a lab study, but research on actual humans does confirm this correlation.

An intriguing 2009 study reinforced the HCA/breast cancer connection. It sought to examine the breast tissue of women who had not been diagnosed with breast cancer to look for evidence of precancerous changes that might be linked to diet. There's one huge problem with this methodology, however: it's not ethical to perform breast biopsies on healthy women. The researchers solved this problem by enrolling participants who were undergoing breast reduction surgery; their breast tissue was already going to be removed. The women undergoing the surgery were interviewed about their diet, and their breast tissue was analyzed for the presence of DNA adducts (pieces of DNA that have bonded to a carcinogen and signal the beginning of cancer development). The study found that total HCA intake, and consumption of fried meat, beef, and processed meat were all correlated to precancerous damage to breast tissue (Rohrmann, Lukas Jung 2009). The scary thing is these women had no idea that this was happening in their breasts. They thought they had normal breasts, and all had negative mammograms, which are required prior to breast reduction.

While red meat, processed meat, and meat cooked at high temperatures appears to contribute to cancer formation via HCAs (and possibly other compounds, including polycyclic aromatic hydrocarbons (PAHs), fruits and veggies seem to mitigate those effects. In vitro studies show that eating fruits and veggies can block PhIP effects, a phenomenon that may have partially obscured the link between animal protein and cancer in the EPIC-Oxford study, which we will see in the next section. Since the meat eaters in that study were consuming unusually large quantities of fruits and veggies compared to the general population, they may have been somewhat protected from PhIP's carcinogenic effects (Edenharder, Sager et al., 2002). So the data in the EPIC-Oxford study may suggest animal protein does not cause breast cancer, or is weakly correlated, while in actuality the effect is being neutralized by the high plant content in the diet.

Heme Iron and N-Nitroso Compounds

We ingest two types of iron from food: heme iron and nonheme iron. Animal foods are the only sources of heme iron, which is often assumed to be nutritionally superior since we absorb it more efficiently into our bloodstream. Evidence is mounting, however, that links heme iron to various cancers, including colorectal cancer (Qiao and Feng 2013).

We're not exactly sure how heme iron contributes to cancer, but one promising theory links heme iron consumption to the creation of unstable N-nitroso compounds (NOC) in the body (Bingham, Hughes, et al. 2002). One of the EPIC studies showed that the more NOC produced, the higher the risk of gastrointestinal cancer; rectal cancer, specifically. A 2003 randomized controlled trial found that feeding people meat led to higher levels of NOC in their stool. When they were fed an equivalent amount of vegetable protein, their levels of NOC were much lower. And here's the fascinating part about this study: supplementation with 8 grams of heme iron spiked NOC levels, while adding ferrous (nonheme) iron had no such effect (Cross, Pollock, et al. 2003). So the "good-for-us" iron from meat may turn out to be the missing ingredient in turning nitrates into cancer-causing NOC.

An interesting 2010 study supports this theory. Researchers fed 14 participants a high-red-meat diet for 8 days, followed by 8 days of a combination of red meat and fish, then 8 days of a high-fish diet. Their stool samples were examined during each phase of the trial. The study found more NOC and heme iron on the red meat diet, and less on the fish diet (Joosen, Lecommandeur, et al. 2010). And another study by the same team found more NOCs and more DNA damage in the group eating red meat and processed meat than in those on a vegetarian diet (Joosen, Kuhnle, et al. 2009).

As with HCAs, eating more plants appears to reduce the effects of heme iron. Beets, for example, are high in nitrates, but there's no evidence that those chemicals are converting into NOC; beets have fewer amino acids than meat and are chock-full of antioxidants. It appears this may block the conversion of plant sources of nitrates into NOC. The Mediterranean diet consists of many foods with high antioxidant ability and also have the ability to chelate iron; that is, take it out of the bloodstream and remove it from the body (El and Karakaya 2004). Greens in particular are highly protective. This finding may also contribute to explaining the small differences found by EPIC-Oxford between meat eaters and vegetarians. The meat eaters were consuming a fair amount of plant-based food, which may have been partially canceling the toxic effects of heme iron.

IGF1: Another Smoking Gun

Insulin-like growth factor 1 (IGF1) is a human growth hormone produced in the liver and other tissues. We produce it all our lives, and in the proper amounts it helps us grow new tissue and synthesize new cellular DNA. We need IGF1 in the right quantities. Too little IGF1 is correlated with dwarfism, while if you are born with a disease where you make too much IGF1, then you develop acromegaly (giantism). You may remember the wrestler André the Giant. He had acromegaly. The large body and large forehead are a giveaway. The sad thing about people with acromegaly is they die an early death either from heart failure or from cancer. Studies show that people with acromegaly caused by high levels of IGF1 have high levels of breast, prostate, and colon cancer (Jenkins 2006; Epstein 2001).

The reason people with high IGF1 levels develop cancer can be explained. If you put cancer cells (or normal cells) in a culture dish and expose them to IGF1, the cells will activate and grow. Accelerated cell growth is part of cancer development. IGF1 can also promote cancer by inhibiting cell death. Cell death may not sound like a good thing, but it is. When normal cells become damaged, they activate a self-suicide process known as "apoptosis." Cancer cells lose this ability, which is one reason cancer can spread so aggressively at the expense of the rest of the body (Pollak 1998).

It's known that prostate cells are highly sensitive to IGF1 effects (Cohen and Peehl 1994). The 1998 Physicians Health Study associates increased IGF1 with higher rates of prostate cancer (Chan, Stampfer, et al. 1998). And it turns out there's a relationship between our diets and the IGF1 levels in our bodies. Restricting energy and animal protein intake causes IGF1 to fall. This is a crucial finding, as many studies show that calorie restriction slows aging and increases longevity. The trouble is, very few people are willingly to adopt a "mild starvation" diet to increase their life span. Fortunately, it appears that caloric restriction isn't necessary; it's the accompanying restriction in animal protein that decreases IGF1 and thereby increases longevity (Fontana, Weiss, et al. 2008).

The more animal protein we consume, the more circulating IGF1. Vegans, for example, have much less circulating IGF1 than meat eaters. And in addition to making our own IGF1, we can consume it in our diets. Milk cows are routinely treated with growth hormones to get them to milk-producing age as fast as possible. This IGF1 gets into their milk, and we absorb it into our bodies when we drink that milk (even when pasteurized) (Epstein 2001). Even hormone-free, organic milk contains IGF1 (after all, baby calves, for whom nature intended the milk, need to grow a lot over a short period of time). And its high protein content also increases IGF1 levels in humans.

One way that a vegan diet may protect against cancer is by limiting IGF1 synthesis and absorption in the body. A 2002 study, spurred by observations that Asian countries had lower incidences of cancer compared to Western societies, explored IGF1 as a possible cause. Researchers found that vegans had significantly lower levels of IGF1 and significantly higher levels of a protein that binds IGF1 and takes it out of active circulation. They concluded that a diet rich in essential amino acids (the ones found extensively in meat) was associated with higher IGF1 levels (Allen, Appleby, et al. 2002). And for "manly" men concerned about getting enough protein, another study found that despite having lower IGF1 levels, the vegan men actually had higher testosterone levels than vegetarians or meat eaters (Allen, Appleby, et al. 2000).

Several studies link IGF1 to breast cancer (Pollak 1998; Toniolo, Bruning, et al. 2000; Rollison, Newschaffer, et al. 2006). The Nurses' Health Study found a strong correlation in premenopausal women even though the dietary range of participants was quite narrow (Hankinson, Willett, et al. 1998). A 2010 meta analysis of 17 prospective studies found that increased IGF1 levels are associated with hormone sensitive breast cancer in both pre- and postmenopausal women (Key, Appleby, et al. 2010).

Breast and prostate cancer are just the beginning. IGF1 has also been associated with colon cancer and I am sure it has an effect on others as science is just starting to study this interesting hormone (Epstein 2001).

Carnitine, Choline, and TMAO

Another mechanism linking meat and prostate cancer (and possibly others) comes from ingestion of certain nutrients—nutrients some people actually supplement with. I mentioned carnitine and choline as possible causes of heart disease in the cardiac chapter. Well, there may also be a link when we look at cancer, especially prostate cancer. Eggs in particular are very high in choline. A prospective study of men already diagnosed with prostate cancer found that consuming high amounts of eggs and the skin of chickens doubled the risk of cancer progression or recurrence. Those men deemed "high risk" for recurrence were even more susceptible; their risk of recurrence or progression of prostate cancer quadrupled compared to men who ate the smallest amount of eggs and chicken skin (Richman, Stampfer, et al., 2010). And the Health Professionals Follow-up Study found that those men who ate the most eggs increased their risk of dying from prostate cancer by 70 percent compared with the men who ate the fewest (Richman, Kenfield, et al. 2012). Interestingly, the actual prostate cancer cells were found to have high choline levels. Why does this cause cancer? Researchers are not sure. There are several possible mechanisms that are being investigated (Richman, Kenfield, et al. 2011, 2012).

Reduction in Protective Bacteria

Butyrate, a substance formed when carbohydrates are fermented in the large intestines, helps with gene repair and apoptosis (cell death) (Bingham 1999). Both of these activities are protective against cancer and are specifically linked to reduced risk of adenomas of the colon, which are precancerous lesions. Nondigestible carbohydrates found in fruit, fructooliosaccharides, help promote bifidobacter, a beneficial bacteria that produces butyrate, which in turn protects the lining of the colon. A 2007 randomized controlled trial put people on first a high-carb, then a low-carb diet. The low-carb diet led to a significant reduction in butyrate production, which was accompanied by decreases in key protective bacteria (Duncan, Belenguer, et al. 2007). A 2013 study of people with adenomas found a relationship between fiber intake, butyrate formation, and subsequent risk of adenomas (Chen, Yu, et al. 2013).

A 2011 randomized controlled trial confirmed this relationship. Researchers placed 17 obese men on a "weight-maintenance diet" consisting of 12 percent protein, 37 percent fat, and 51 percent carbs (total calories: 2,824) for seven days. They spent the next four weeks on a high-protein/moderate-carb diet (28% protein, 37% fat, 36% carbs, 2,018 total calories), and the four weeks after that on a high-protein/low-carb diet (28% protein, 67% fat, 5% carbs, 1,923 total calories). Stool samples showed that the high-protein/low-carb diet "increased concentrations of hazardous metabolites" and significantly decreased concentrations of cancer-protective metabolites, including butyrate. The researchers concluded that despite the reduced calorie intake, which is known to be beneficial, long-term adherence to a high-protein/low-carb diet may increase the risk of colon cancer (Russell, Gratz, et al. 2011).

We know that diet has a rapid effect on our bowel bacteria. Worse yet, it has been shown that a diet heavy in meat alters the gut bacteria rapidly and allows colonization of certain bacteria that may cause inflammation in the bowels (David, Maurice, et al. 2014).

Methionine

Methionine is an essential amino acid, which means that humans cannot synthesize it and must get it in our diets. It appears in high concentrations in eggs, fish, and meat, and in some seeds and nuts, and in much lower levels in fruits, vegetables, and legumes. We need some methionine, but is too much methionine too much of a good thing?

Research has shown that restricting methionine increases longevity in rodents. It's been known for a while that caloric restriction increases life span; now we're starting to gain a better understanding of the underlying mechanisms. It's not all calories, but those from animal foods, that tend to shorten life. Methionine restriction appears to reduce cancer risk by preventing oxidation of mitochondria (López-Torres and Barja 2008), a phenomenon that's been documented in rodents and mammals, as well as in human cancers (Epner, 2001). Researchers are continuing to test the hypothesis that methionine restriction may increase life span in humans (McCarty, Barroso-Aranda, et al. 2009).

Some low-carb promoters, most notably Robert Lustig, see sugar as the root of all dietary evils and recommend attacking cancer by starving it of sugars. The problem with this approach is that all cells need sugar, so starving the cancer requires starving the whole body. Also, when people have to eliminate sugar and carbs they turn to meat, and therefore eliminate the antioxidants while increasing cancer-causing chemicals. Not good for curing cancer.

In an excellent 2003 article, researchers reviewed a number of in vitro (lab) and in vivo (in the body) studies showing that methionine restriction harms cancer cells but not normal ones. It appears that cancer cells must have methionine to reproduce. They suggest that methionine restriction may become a helpful additional therapeutic strategy in conjunction with chemotherapy (Cellarier, Durando, et al. 2003). Instead of starving cancer cells by starving yourself, adopt a plant-based diet that naturally lowers your methionine, an essential nutrient for cancer cells to divide, without harming your natural ability to heal.

Acidosis

As we saw in Chapter 9, an animal-protein-heavy diet creates a dangerous condition in the body known as acidosis. Evidence is beginning to emerge suggesting that chronic acidosis may act at a molecular/cellular level in ways that promote cancer formation (Robey 2012). So a low bicarbonate level on a blood test, such as the one Gary Taubes publicized to show the world how healthy he is, should be a wake-up call to take action to prevent cancer as well as diabetes.

Neu5Gc

Neu5Gc is a form of sialic acid that is found in animals, but not native to humans. Meat eaters can start expressing Neu5Gc after eating meat, however. After a person consumes an animal containing Neu5Gc, their body will incorporate it into the glycoproteins found on the surface of their cells. The problem is, even though the body is now expressing and assimilating Neu5Gc, it still doesn't quite recognize it as part of itself. When faced with a potential alien invader, the body creates antibodies, causing an inflammatory immune response (Tangvoranuntakul, Gagneux, et al. 2003). The ongoing antibody/antigen reaction may generate chronic inflammation that may contribute to carcinomas (Varki 2008). Cancer cells have been know to express Neu5Gc, which can only come from animals. Meanwhile, people who avoid animal proteins do not express Neu5Gc.

Hormone Plasma Levels

Some cancers are induced by specific hormones, including breast and prostate cancers. These hormonally induced cancers can be affected by diet, in that different foods affect the plasma levels of hormones in our bodies. Seventh-day Adventist males, for example, have one-third the mortality from prostate cancer as other Californians, and they consume 6 percent fewer fat calories. Vegetarians have different levels of various hormones than meat eaters, including lower estrogen levels (despite whatever nonsense you may have heard about soy). It's clear that we can reduce our cancer risk by changing our hormonal concentrations (Howie and Schultz 1985).

Also, we know that early onset of menses strongly increases the risk of breast cancer (Cheng Buyken, et al. 2012). It has been well established that children who eat more animal protein are at higher risk of developing premature puberty (Günther, Karaolis-Danckert, et al. 2010). Meanwhile, a diet low in animal protein but high in plants and soy exposes children to isoflavones, which are nutrients that have been shown to prevent early periods and to lower lifetime risk of developing breast cancer (Cheng, Remer, et al. 2010).

Slaughterhouse Chemicals

We don't know much about the effects of the many chemicals used during the raising, slaughter, processing, and packaging of the meats produced by our industrial farm system. That doesn't mean there isn't reason for concern: one study found that men working in a poultry slaughtering/processing plant got cancer of the penis almost nine times more frequently than the general population (Johnson, Ndetan, et al. 2010). The animals are given lots of hormones and antibiotics and ingest food that has all kinds of pesticides and chemicals. These can all have an effect on our health.

Thermoresistant Viruses

The final animal-protein-based cancer mechanism we'll look at is thermoresistant viruses (that is, they don't die even when cooked at high temperatures). Population studies show a clear and consistent relationship between red meat consumed and colon cancer. Red meat appears to increase colon cancer much more than fish and chicken, despite the formation of similar chemicals when cooked, including IGF1, HCAs, TMAO. It's become clear over the past decade that some cancers are triggered by viruses. Some researchers suspect that certain viruses found in cows initiate colon cancer (zur Hausen 2012).

The Protective Role of Phytonutrients

Part of the problem with our current reductionist philosophy when it comes to food is this false notion that carbs are bad, which inevitably leads to avoidance of fruits in an attempt to eat more animal protein. While I think we have shown there are harmful ingredients in animal protein, there is also the opportunity cost that comes from filling your belly with animal protein instead of plants.

Phytonutrients (nutrients synthesized only in plants) can foil cancer development through a large array of mechanisms. A 1991 review identified many potential cancer-fighting compounds in plants, " . . . including carotenoids, vitamins C and E, selenium, dietary fiber, dithiolthiones, glucosinolates and indoles, isothiocyanates, flavonoids, phenols, protease inhibitors, plant sterols, allium compounds, and limonene." It concludes that parts of fruits and veggies are essential for our growth and maintenance and hypothesizes that cancer is a maladaptive response to their deficiency (Steinmetz and Potter 1991). Cancer as a deficiency in fruits and veggies? An interesting possibility. If you look at the NHANES data on what we eat, we consume a surplus of protein but are well below the RDA for fiber consumption.

Flavonoids are a large family of phytonutrients shown to have powerful positive effects on our health. So far science has identified about six thousand of them, but there's no reason to suspect there aren't thousands more. They include the anthocyanidins found in berries and other fruit, the flavones from parsley, lettuce, apples, and oranges, and the flavonols in onions, almonds, sweet potatoes, and garbanzo beans.

There's reason to believe that fruits and veggies reduce cancer risk in and of themselves, even if animal protein consumption is not reduced. The EPIC study showed that increased flavonoid consumption led to a decrease in gastric cancer in women (Zamora-Ros, Agudo, et al. 2012). A 2003 meta-analysis found "weak evidence" for the protective effect of fruits and vegetables for all cancers, but it was able to pinpoint some specific links, despite various flaws the authors identified in the individual studies. These included the finding that fruit consumption lowers the risk of bladder and lung cancer (Riboli and Norat 2003).

So what's the bottom line? If we eat our fruits and veggies, can we avoid cancer even if we don't dial back our animal protein consumption? Several studies suggest the answer is no. While fruits and veggies are crucial, it's just as important to avoid the toxins found in meat, eggs, and dairy. Colon cancer is strikingly rare in black Africans: the prevalence is less than 1 case per 100,000 people. For comparison, the rate among white South Africans is about twenty times higher. Researchers wondered about the huge discrepancy, and a 1999 study of low-risk black South Africans and high-risk white South Africans looked at many dietary factors to see which ones might be significant contributors. According to the authors, "The diets of all the black subgroups were characterized by a low animal product and high boiled maize-meal content, whereas whites consumed more fresh animal products, cheese, and wheat products. Blacks consumed below RDA quantities of fiber (43% of RDA), vitamin A (78%), C (62%), folic acid (80%) and calcium (67%), whereas whites consumed more animal protein (177% of RDA) and fat (153%)." The researchers determined that the low rates of colon cancer among black South Africans could not be explained by known "protective factors," as their diet consisted largely of boiled maize. Instead, they found, the difference was the lack of "aggressive" factors, specifically "excess animal protein and fat" (O'Keefe, Kidd, et al. 1999).

This finding is supported by an analysis of the Health Professionals Follow-up Study of 48,000 men (Giovannucci, Rimm, et al. 1994). They found a significant risk of colon cancer specifically linked to animal protein consumption, one that was independent not only of fruit and veggie consumption, but also of saturated fat, total fat, and animal fat. In other words, animal protein all by itself increased colon cancer in middle-aged American men.

A 2005 meta-analysis of 13 large-scale prospective studies following 725,000 men for between 6 and 20 years likewise found that fiber intake is only weakly correlated with decreased rates of colorectal cancer. It may be that avoiding the meat protein is a bigger deal than eating lots of produce (Park, Hunter, et al. 2005). And if you're still wondering if the problem with animal foods is simply an effect of factory farming, a 2009 study out of Uruguay found a definite association between meat consumption and colon, gastric, and pharyngeal cancer. Interestingly, their animals were grass fed and hormone free, just like the Paleo people recommend, yet the cancer risk was still strong (Aune, De Stefani, et al. 2009). The HCA, PhIP, acid, IGF1, and so on, occur in grass-fed meat as much as they do in animals from industrial farms.

Epidemiology of Cancer and Diet

So we have established a probable cause. But if this cause is accurate we should see an effect. There should be a causal link between animal protein and actual cancer. The best way to prove this would be to start a study of people and randomize them to a high animal protein or low animal protein group. We would then have to make sure they stay on the diet by providing them the actual food and monitor every bite they take. Both groups would have to live the exact same lives. Same exposure to toxins, same exercise, and so on. And this study would ideally go many years. Study length really matters; most cancers take decades to get big enough to cause symptoms and thus get our attention. One article estimated the latency period between diet and cancer development at 15 to 20 years, except for prostate cancer, which required 28 years to manifest (Grant 2014). As we saw in Chapter 9, it's quite rare to study a population for decades. It's expensive, it's difficult, and perhaps most important, it's potential career suicide for less established scientists working under constant pressure of "publish or perish." But, if we are following two groups for only two years, it is unlikely that, if one of the diets is causing a cancer, that cancer would rear its ugly head in just two years. In fact, if a person in one group did develop a cancer, was that cancer from the experimental diet or the diet they ate before the experiment began?

All is not lost, however. There are many studies that look at the interplay of animal protein and cancer, following hundreds of thousands of people for many years, in many different countries. These studies tend not to randomize to a diet since it hard for people to stick to a diet. Instead they follow people who already eat a certain way and compare those that eat lots of protein versus those who do not. Lots of issues still arise. There is something called a healthy volunteer effect, where people who volunteer for a study tend to be healthier to begin with (Struijk, May, et al. 2015). Because they are healthier we are less likely to see differences between groups, especially if not a long-term study. The other issue with this is we tend to see little difference between the study groups. If two groups are actually eating a similar diet that only differs a little in amount of meat, we are less likely to see an actual significant difference in the study.

Finally there are plenty of confounding factors, meaning while animal protein may cause cancer, it may also be that one group has more smokers, or one group is heavier. Thankfully, we have very advanced statistical analysis that can eliminate these biases that may influence the data. The problem with the statistics is that scientists tend to overadjust. They are so concerned with eliminating bias that sometimes they actually eliminate a real correlation.

The point here is that there are many great long-term studies that draw attention to the link between animal protein and cancer. People may say that this is just a correlation, but I will tell you that if there is a correlation in multiple studies from multiple parts of the world, and these correlations have been put through vigorous analysis, then you better believe there is something to the connection.

You cannot just look at one individual study. You have to look at the entirety of the research, from the lab studies, to the randomized trials to the epidemiology.

For instance, let's look at prostate cancer. Many studies document the fact that there is a much lower incidence of prostate cancer in Asia compared to America (Jemal, Center, et al. 2010). There could be many reasons for this. It could be genetic, although migration studies of people moving to America show that, despite their genes, they actually get prostate cancer. Migrations studies are fascinating. We tend to think that cancer is all genetics but we find that cultures that have low rates of cancer seem to get the "big C" when they move to America. Take breast cancer, for example. Asian countries typically show low incidence of breast cancer, but Asian communities in the United States soon develop breast cancer at the same rate as other Americans (Deapen, Liu, et al. 2002). Breast cancer is also rapidly increasing in Asian and African countries as they adopt Western lifestyles and diets (Kelsey and Horn-Ross 1993).

So if the prostate cancer difference is not genes, could it be due to not testing for prostate cancer appropriately? This is true in parts of Asia, but Japan does have an active PSA testing. In addition, as Japanese men move to America, their rates of prostate cancer approximate ours.

So if it is not genetic, could it be environmental? Certain pollutants could be to blame but the best way to get polluted is in what you eat. Looking at diets in Japan versus America, Japanese eat far more soy but far less overall protein, more fruits and veggies, and far less meat. So they are not being exposed to all the carcinogenic chemicals we discussed earlier.

I would assume that the phytochemicals in fruits and veggies would be protective against prostate cancer, but a study looked at a large population in Europe and found that the amounts of fruits and veggies eaten didn't seem to make a difference in occurrence of prostate cancer (Key, Allen, et al. 2004). In fact, while the Adventist Health Study does show plant eaters have lower rates of prostate cancer, they still have large amounts. This could be due to dairy consumption. Milk and dairy are still consumed by vegetarians. So maybe it is not how many plants but rather how few animals that matters.

The Seventh-day Adventists offer us a great ability to further investigate this dilemma because, as we have seen, they have a fairly large group of vegans that we can compare to vegetarians and to meat eaters. It turns out that vegans have lower prostate cancer compared to vegetarians, and vegetarians have lower cancer rates than meat eaters (Fraser 1999). So maybe it is the lack of animal protein. This is a maybe. These epidemiologic studies show correlation but not necessarily causation.

However, there are other factors out there that can lead us to a better idea of causal relationships. As we have seen, we know that if you put cancer cells (or normal cells) in a culture dish and expose them to IGF1, the cells will activate and grow. Does this mean that IGF1 causes cancer? Not necessarily, but we do know that people who have acromegaly caused by high levels of IGF1 also have high levels of breast, prostate, and colon cancer. And we have shown that high IGF1 levels are associated with prostate cancer independent of having acromegaly.

To delve deeper we know that IGF1 release in the body is enhanced by consumption of animal protein. As we have seen, vegans have much lower circulating IGF1 than meat eaters. We also know that growth hormone given to cows gets into milk and is absorbed when we drink the milk even if it has been pasteurized. So could a vegan diet given to prostate cancer patients reduce the growth of cancer by reducing IGF1?

Well, Dr. Dean Ornish had the unique opportunity to test this hypothesis (Ornish, Weidner, et al. 2005). In 2005, he and his colleagues did a study in which they randomized 93 early-stage prostate cancer patients into a low-fat vegan diet (along with his lifestyle modification program) or a "standard of care" control group and followed them for a year (Ornish, Weidner, et al. 2005). During that whole period, those eating the low-fat vegan diet consumed more protective and fewer harmful dietary factors than the control group. Once put on the vegan diet, they ate more fiber (59 grams at year's end, compared to 31 at baseline), more lycopene, a cancer-fighting phytonutrient (34,464 mcg/day vs. 8693), and fewer saturated fats (from 20 grams/day down to 5) and cholesterol (from 200/mg per day down to 10) (Dewell, Weidner, et al. 2008). Again, note that the lycopene came from whole foods, not pills.

They then specifically looked at the progression of their cancer by monitoring their serum prostate-specific antigen (PSA), a measure of the presence of prostate cancer. They could see that the experimental group was avoiding carcinogens and eating protective substances—but was it slowing down or reversing the cancer?

The first thing the researchers noticed was that none of the lifestyle group, but six members of the control group, had to undergo treatment for worsening PSA. After one year, they found that the plant-based patients' PSA levels had dropped by 4 percent, while the control group's PSA levels had actually increased by 6 percent. Then Ornish and his team performed a fascinating experiment: they took serum from both groups and mixed it with prostate cancer cells. To their amazement, the serum from the lifestyle group was eight times more effective at stopping prostate cancer cells from replicating when compared to the control group. That's right: the vegan diet and other lifestyle changes literally made their blood poisonous to cancer. And both findings, the PSA changes and the serum's ability to inhibit cancer growth, were associated with the degree to which the men adhered to the lifestyle protocol. The closer they got to "perfect" compliance, the better their numbers.

Ornish got curious about the mechanism by which his protocol reversed prostate cancer progression. He came across the work of Nobel Prize–winning scientist Elizabeth Blackburn, who discovered the health significance of chromosomal telomeres. Telomeres are caps that sit on the ends of our chromosomes and protect them from unraveling. You might think of them as the plastic protectors at the ends of shoelaces. Blackburn postulated that it's possible to determine a person's health, and even their potential life span, by looking at their telomeres. Originally, scientists thought of telomere length as fate: determined at birth, and unchangeable. Born with short telomeres? That's a shame; you're probably going to die young, possibly of an opportunistic cancer just waiting for a telomere to wear out.

Ornish has always assumed that most of us can change our health outcomes through our own efforts, regardless of the genetic hand we've been dealt at birth. So he teamed with Blackburn to test this theory. They recruited 30 men with low-risk prostate cancer that had been identified by biopsy, measured their telomere length, and put them on the vegan diet and lifestyle program for three months. Sure enough, the lifestyle modification lengthen the telomeres by 29 percent in just 90 days (Ornish, Lin, et al. 2008). This is incredible. Ornish showed that changing diet actually has an effect on a chromosomal level!

My point in this long diatribe is that you cannot look at just one study but need to look at the totality of the medical science to understand the underlying story.

The Epidemiology of the Protein/Cancer Link

In this section, I'll take you on a tour of epidemiological studies, that is, large-scale studies of populations. Some just take static snapshots, while others follow participants for years and even decades. All have been published in leading peer-reviewed journals and have used strict protocols to elimate bias. We'll examine the strengths and weaknesses of the studies, and slowly and carefully connect the dots and arrange the pixels to come up with a relatively clear picture, especially given our knowledge of the probable cause.

EPIC Evidence

As we've seen, the EPIC study is one of the most comprehensive large-scale epidemiologic studies ever conducted. It found that gastric cancer risk rose with increased consumption of total meat, red meat, and processed meat (González, Jakszyn, et al. 2006). The risk was even greater in people infected with *H. pylori* bacteria, a common infection now known as the main cause of ulcers (rather than stress or Advil). *H. pylori* itself may have a food connection, being better able to survive and flourish in the presence of high-protein diets. Further examination of EPIC data linked meat and processed meat consumption to colon and rectal cancer. The more fiber people ate, the less cancer they got. Fish consumption also appeared protective, but it's not clear if fish itself helps fight tumors, or if fish was simply replacing land meats and was therefore "less worse."

Other findings of EPIC: fruit helps prevent lung cancer, and saturated fat found in animal products may be associated with increased breast cancer (González 2006a, 2006b).

But then some researchers looked at a subset of the EPIC data and threw a big wrench in the works. The subset was known as EPIC-Oxford and consisted of a large number of vegetarians living in and around Oxford, England, where that sort of diet was much more common than other parts of Europe, and their meat-eating neighbors. In the EPIC-Oxford data, the incidence of colon cancer *rose* in vegetarians compared to meat eaters. True, the effect had dissipated in the 2014 data, but still. What in the world was going on?

The EPIC-Oxford data have been trumpeted by low-carb advocates as proof of the inferiority of a vegan diet. Funny that they always complain about epidemiologic studies, until one goes their way. But as we look at other studies, EPIC-Oxford really becomes an outlier.

A meta-analysis of several studies shows red meat and processed meat were associated with increase risk of colorectal cancer (Norat, Lukanova, et al. 2002). Another meta-analysis of multiple epidemiologic studies showed a 2.5 times greater risk of developing colon cancer in those eating animals. It also showed the less fiber, the more cancer, independent of whether the person was eating meat or not.

In 2007, the World Cancer Research Fund and the American Institute for Cancer Research published their report, "Food, Nutrition, Physical Activity, and the Prevention of Cancer: A Global Perspective." In the following four years, researchers conducted ten prospective studies based on the recommendations in this report (many of which advised reducing animal consumption and eating more fruits and veggies). A 2011 meta-analysis of these studies showed that red meat and processed meat definitely correlate with colorectal cancer. This was very high level data (Chan Lau, et al. 2011).

A huge prospective Korean study followed over two million people for seven years. It looked at people who ate meat four days a week and those who ate meat just once a week. Researchers found a large and significant effect of meat eating on risk of colorectal cancer (Kim, Park, et al. 2011). And keep in mind that even the "heavy" meat eaters in this study were consuming considerably less animal protein than the average American.

So why did EPIC-Oxford show increased risk? Well, several reasons. As you can see above, one of the protective effects of being vegetarian/ vegan is presumably eating more plants and therefore more fiber. However, this group of vegetarians didn't eat nearly the amount of fiber you would expect for plant eaters. Only 20 grams, which is only slightly higher than the meat eaters. Other studies on this group show that they don't take B_{12} and many don't take calcium. Not the healthiest group of vegetarians. We can only conclude that while they were not eating meat, they must have been eating processed junk food.

In addition, the meat eaters were actually quite healthy meat eaters, compared to rest of the country. Their meat consumption was very moderate to low, and they controlled for vegetable consumption, meaning those meat eaters who didn't consume any fruits and veggies were discarded. Furthermore, they controlled for weight. Weight is an independent risk of cancer, so controlling for weight is appropriate, but one benefit of a plant-based diet, as we saw in the last chapter, is weight loss. So by controlling for weight they are eliminating one way the plant-based diet protects against cancer.

Finally, there was definitely a healthy volunteer effect. We can tell this because as the data goes out longer, the increased cancer rate has diminished. Taking all this into mind, the EPIC-Oxford becomes a true outlier.

Breast Cancer Studies

One of the most feared and common cancers in America is breast cancer. What does the evidence show?

A 2003 meta-analysis of case/control and cohort studies showed that fat and animal protein intake were associated with increased risk for breast cancer. Saturated fat and meat specifically were identified as culprits (Boyd, Stone, et al. 2003). Another study, the Women's Intervention Nutrition Study (WINS) looked at women who had already been diagnosed with breast cancer. It showed that when these women decreased their fat intake (generally correlated with decreased animal food consumption), they lived longer without relapse (Chlebowski, Blackburn, et al. 2006).

On the other hand, two large-scale studies failed to find a link between diet and breast cancer. The Women's Health Initiative (WHI) did not show that women who reduced their fat intake reduced their cancer risk (Willett 2010). Comparing WHI and WINS is instructive. The women eating "low fat" in the WHI study were still getting 25 to 28 percent of their daily calories from fat, and there's reason to believe that the participants underreported their fat consumption. By contrast, the low-fat WINS cohort were getting just 20 percent of their calories from fat. The WHI simply didn't look at sufficient variation in diet to spot meaningful differences. The group who were supposed to eat a normal diet actually reduced their fat, so the two groups ended up looking too similar to find a difference.

The concept of "sick populations" is helpful here. First proposed by Geoffrey Rose in 1985 (Rose 1985), it posits that we won't be able to find causation in a trait that is universally present in a population. Take smoking, for example. We know that smoking is highly correlated with lung cancer. Now imagine a population in which everyone smokes. Lung cancer will be common, but won't afflict everyone. The scariest thing about the epidemic will be its apparent randomness. Scientists will look for genetic susceptibility, for lifestyle factors, for environmental factors, and they may make a few weak correlations here and there. But the smoking (literally) gun will be invisible, since there's no way to conduct a study that compares smokers to nonsmokers.

Another breast cancer study suffering from the same design problem was the Women's Healthy Eating and Living (WHEL) study, a randomized trial that examined whether women previously diagnosed with early-stage invasive breast cancer who reduced fat and increased fruit and veggie consumption also reduced their risk of additional breast cancer events and early death. The study randomized women into a diet intervention or a control group. The dietary changes had no apparent effect. One obvious problem with the study design was its focus on fat rather than protein. This meant that participants could still eat lots of lean meat that wasn't accounted for in the analysis. Another problem, albeit a positive one, was that the control group appeared to increase their fruit and vegetable consumption nearly as much as the intervention group.

Additionally, some of the WHEL study participants had cancerous masses greater than one centimeter in diameter and yet were not given an aromatase inhibitor, the standard of care. Recurrence of cancer in these women may therefore have been due to failure to adhere to proper protocol rather than the low-fat diet. Finally, the researchers committed a classic "response bias" error in their reporting. Only 45 percent of study participants in the low-fat group completed their food surveys, yet it was assumed that nonresponders complied with the dietary recommendations to the same extent as responders. Logically, we would expect that people who didn't comply with the reporting requirements would also be less adherent to the low-fat diet (Pierce, Natarajan, et al. 2007).

In one very large study run by the National Institutes of Health (NIH) and the American Association of Retired Persons (AARP), researchers followed 189,000 postmenopausal women for an average of four years. Those women who ate the most fat had highest likelihood of getting breast cancer. There was a fairly wide range of fat intake, which allowed researchers to see clearly the effect of dietary fat on breast cancer (Thiébaut, Kipnis, et al. 2007). And the EPIC study, which looked at 334,000 women over 12 years, found that diets rich in fiber, especially from vegetable sources, decreased breast cancer risk regardless of menopausal status (Ferrari, Rinaldi, et al. 2013).

One reason to lend more credence to EPIC, the huge Korean study, WINS, and the NIH-AARP study, aside from their sheer size and length of study, is the wide variation in diets. Researchers often divide study populations into quintiles, or fifths, for ease of comparison. Each quintile would contain the same number of participants. Let's imagine a study of 1,000 people asking if animal protein consumption is related to colon cancer. The data might look like this:

Quintile	Number of people	Avg daily animal protein intake (g/day)	Number of cases of colon cancer
1	200	0	0
2	200	20	4
3	200	35	6
4	200	52	7
5	200	75	7

As you can see, the variance in animal protein intake is quite high. Quintile 1 is comprised of vegans, Quintile 2 might be vegetarians or flexitarians who consume meat just a couple times a week, while Quintile 5 consists of heavy meat eaters. If there's a link between animal protein and colon cancer, this study is likely to find it. Therefore, in our made-up data, we can see a big difference in cases of colon cancer between the first and fifth quintiles. And indeed, the real-life studies that showed a significant relationship between animal protein or saturated fat intake and cancer incidence studied populations similarly varied in their dietary patterns.

Now suppose another study, using exactly the same methodology, chose a population that was less diverse. Pretend, in fact, that this study looked at just the people in Quintiles 3, 4, and 5 of the first study. Now the chart looks like this:

Quintile	Number of people	Avg daily animal protein intake (g/day)	Number of cases of colon cancer
1	120	30	3
2	120	45	3
3	120	50	5
4	120	67	4
5	120	80	5

The 600 people who were in the bottom three quintiles have now been divided into five quintiles. Because the bottom of the range of animal protein intake has been cut off, it now looks like there's either a slight connection or no connection between protein and cancer. Due to a statistical anomaly, some might even point to the fact that Quintile 4 has less colon cancer than Quintile 3 as proof that steak and butter are protective against colon cancer! WHI and WHEL are good examples of this type of study. They found no significant differences in outcomes because they examined no significant differences in dietary habits.

The best epidemiologic data comes from the Adventist Health Studies. They were well designed and collected trustworthy data. They were also long-term, prospective studies that looked at large groups of people. They looked at a community that was similar in many ways except for diet, making it easier to see the effects of dietary differences in the absence of other potentially confounding factors. Finally, since many Adventists were completely vegan, while others were vegetarian (eating eggs and dairy), pescetarian (adding fish), and omnivorous, the dietary differences between the quintiles was huge.

One Adventist Health Study found that vegetarians developed significantly less colon, prostate, and bladder cancer than meat eaters. Legumes and fruits were specifically found to be protective against pancreatic cancer (Fraser 1999).

These findings agreed with a couple of extremely large-scale and long-term studies, the Health Professionals Follow-up Study that followed over 37,000 men from 1986 to 2008, and the Nurses' Health Study, which looked at over 83,000 women from 1980 to 2008. These studies clearly showed that the more red meat and processed meat in the diet, the more cancer. And the cancer death rate was significantly lower in those who ate less meat overall (Pan, Sun, et al. 2012). And these striking findings may have underestimated the harm of meat, as the study appears to have systematically overadjusted for participant weight.

An 11-year study of 1,904 German vegetarians also contradicted the EPIC-Oxford finding that vegetarians didn't seem protected against cancer. Researchers found that being vegetarian was associated with a significant decrease in cancer deaths, especially those caused by cancers of the GI tract. Overall, being vegetarian reduced risk of death 50 percent in men and 25 percent in women compared to the general population (Chang-Claude, Frentzel-Beyme, et al. 1992).

One of the largest studies ever, another joint effort of NIH-AARP, looked at almost half a million people from 1995 to 2005 (Daniel, Cross, et al. 2011). Researchers found that when red meat was replaced by chicken and fish, the risk of certain cancers decreased by modest but significant amounts. Careful statistical analysis of the data set suggests not that chicken and fish are protective, but rather less carcinogenic than red meat.

So by going to a better source (less saturated fat, less heme iron, more omega-3) it appears that chicken and fish are good. What they didn't do, because they didn't have enough of a comparison group, is look at what happens if you substitute meat with beans. Now that would have some interesting results, I would bet.

Please don't get misled by people who use this data to promote fish and chicken consumption. First of all, there's a big difference between wild-caught fish and farmed fish. Wild-caught fish have long-chain fatty acids, which may provide a protective effect because the greater concentration of omega-3 decreases the important omega-6/omega-3 ratio, decreasing inflammation. But most of the fish we get in the United States are farmed. They get omega-6 fatty acids from their grain feed, rather than the omega-3s they would get from their natural diet of algae. These omega-6s are not anti-inflammatory and therefore are not protective against cancer (Larsson, Kumlin, et al. 2004). And even wild-caught fish are not an unmitigated health food; even studies that find significant protective effects recommend limiting consumption to two servings per week because of heavy metal, PCB, and dioxin contamination (Mozaffarian and Rimm 2006).

Chicken is no better, and probably considerably worse, than fish. Studies show higher rates of lymphoma in chicken eaters (Rohrmann, Linseisen, et al. 2011). Even EPIC-Oxford showed that for lymphatic cancers, including leukemia, multiple myeloma, and lymphoma, a vegetarian or vegan diet is highly protective (Key, Appleby, et al. 2009b). And while correlation does not equal causation, it is interesting to note that our consumption of chicken has spiked over the past few years , as have our lymphoma rates.

Let's look at one more meta-analysis, a 2012 study that specifically looked at cardiovascular disease mortality and cancer incidence in vegetarians compared to the general population. When you look at the study design, you can see several factors that would tend to bias the study toward showing no benefit to vegetarianism. It included several studies suffering from the "healthy volunteer" effect, in which the control groups were healthier than the general population. Also, some of the vegetarians included in the analysis were actually "semi-vegetarian." And it also included the EPIC-Oxford data. Despite all these strikes against, the meta-analysis concluded that vegetarians get roughly 18% less cancer than meat eaters (Huang, Yang, et al. 2012).

Research on Other Specific Cancers

So far we've been looking at the big picture around diet and cancer, paying specific attention to breast cancer. Now I'd like to summarize some of the epidemiologic research on other cancers.

Pancreatic Cancer

One study followed 190,000 residents of Hawaii for seven years. Named the Multiethnic Cohort Study, it tried to eliminate genetic variability as a factor by including men and women of African American, Japanese, Latino, Native Hawaiian, and Caucasian origin. By study's end, 468 subjects had developed pancreatic cancer. Researchers found that those who consumed the most meat, and specifically processed meat, were 50 percent more likely to develop pancreatic cancer than those who ate the least. Researchers noted that they could not find correlations between pancreatic cancer and saturated fat levels in meat and dairy, which suggests that the animal protein specifically is the problem. They hypothesized that the way the meat was cooked may have increased its carcinogenic properties (Nöthlings, Wilkens, et al. 2005).

Other Cancers of the GI Tract

Epidemiologic evidence from the EPIC study of over half a million Europeans showed that eating more veggies and fiber reduced the risk of stomach and colon cancer, while red and processed meat increased the chances of developing those cancers (González 2006a; Bingham, Day, et al. 2003). EPIC also found that consuming dietary fiber reduced the risk of colon cancer, especially on the left side. If the people eating the least fiber would double their intake, they would reduce their colon cancer risk by 40 percent. This finding highlights one of the biggest problems with our society's protein addiction: it makes us avoid fiber. Combining a high-fiber diet with the added benefits of reducing or eliminating meat is powerful medicine indeed.

An Australian study that followed 37,000 people for nine years showed that as red meat and processed meat consumption went up, so did rates of rectal cancer (English, MacInnis, et al. 2004). And the NIH-AARP study that looked at half a million men and women between the ages of 50 and 71 showed that high red meat and processed meat consumption was significantly associated with cancers of the colon, esophagus, and liver (Cross, Leitzmann, et al. 2007).

Renal Cell Cancer

That same NIH-AARP study showed the quintile highest in fiber, fruit, and veggies had a 20 percent lower risk of developing renal cell cancer. The foods that made the biggest difference were cruciferous veggies, legumes, and whole grains (Daniel, Park, et al. 2013). Another large study (following half a million people for an average of nine years) showed that meat intake is related to renal cell cancer (Daniel, Cross, et al. 2012). An analysis of the Health Professionals Follow-up Study showed that men who ate more fruits and veggies had substantially lower incidence of developing renal cell cancer (Lee, Giovannucci, et al. 2006). And a 2007 meta-analysis of multiple studies confirmed the association between meat and renal cell cancer. This study implicated poultry as well (Faramawi, Johnson, et al. 2007).

Bladder Cancer

Cruciferous veggies significantly decrease uro-epithelial cancers like bladder cancer, due to sulforaphane, a chemical found in cauliflower and other veggies (Michaud, Spiegelman, et al. 1999). In the Health Professionals Follow-up there is a clear decreased risk in developing bladder cancer in the people eating the most broccoli and cauliflower. A full 40 percent reduction in risk from the highest consumer to the lowest.

Lung Cancer

The NIH-AARP study also found that eating large quantities of red meat and processed meat increased the risk of lung cancer by 16 percent (Cross, Leitzmann, et al. 2007). The EPIC study likewise found a reduction in lung cancer risk from increased fruit consumption (González 2006a).

Epidemiologic Advice

When I share my dietary views on Facebook, the most common argument made by meat eaters who don't want to hear the bad news is this: "Correlation doesn't equal causation." Which translates to, "I don't want to accept the fact that thousands of published studies following tens of millions of people for dozens of years have found clear and dramatic linkages between eating animal protein and developing cancer because you can't prove a direct causal link." To which I can only reply, using my best Facebook manners, "SMH."* By that criterion of proof, we can't prove that cigarettes are harmful. We can't even prove that shooting someone with a gun can kill them because sometimes people get shot and live.

If you're addicted to an animal-rich diet and don't want to change, that's no business of mine. If you don't care about your long-term health, again, that's your decision. But if you want to eat in a way that gives you a great quantity and quality of life, please don't dismiss the very best evidence we have with a lazy appeal to 50-cent words.

In 2004, a hugely important article, "Diet, Nutrition and the Prevention of Cancer," was published in the journal *Public Health Nutrition* (Key, Schatzkin, et al. 2004). Two of the authors, Timothy Key and Naomi Allen, were involved in many of the studies we've looked at. Lending further credence to the article was coauthor Walter Willett, professor of epidemiology and nutrition at the prestigious Harvard School of Public Health. The article summarized everything known about the links between diet and cancer at that time.

From the article: "Among the diet-related factors, overweight/obesity convincingly increases the risks of several common cancers. After tobacco, overweight/obesity appears to be the most important avoidable cause of cancer in populations with Western patterns of cancer incidence. Among non-smoking individuals in these populations, avoidance of overweight is the most important strategy for cancer prevention."

As we've already seen, a plant-based diet helps people lose weight. Even if it didn't accomplish anything else, that's reason enough to adopt one. Getting to a healthy weight is probably the most important thing you can do to prevent cancer.

The World Cancer Research Fund, with the American Institute for Cancer Research, has been publishing updated reports on what's known about diet and cancer for decades. Their most recent report, written by a panel chaired by Michael Marmot of University College, London, came out in 2007. I give extra credit to this report, titled "Food, Nutrition, Physi-

---

* Shaking my head.

cal Activity, and the Prevention of Cancer: A Global Perspective," because it is supported by public donation and has no governmental or industry ties. Its primary goal is to promote changes that will decrease rates of cancer around the world: in the words of the report, to "review all the relevant research using the most meticulous methods in order to generate a comprehensive series of recommendations on food, nutrition, and physical activity designed to reduce the risk of cancer and suitable for all societies." To achieve this goal, the report first summarized, assessed, and judged the existing evidence, then translated these "evidence-derived judgments" into goals and policy recommendations to prevent cancer worldwide.

In the preface, Marmot lays out how the panel went about formulating their recommendations: "The process was to use a systematic approach to examine all the relevant evidence using predetermined criteria, and assemble an international group of experts who, having brought their own knowledge to bear and having debated their disagreements, arrived at judgments as to what this evidence means. Both parts were crucial: the systematic review and, dare I say, the wisdom of the experts."

The report was based on three years of study and debate, in which the expert panel reviewed close to one thousand papers. The findings that were released were considered unanimous among those experts despite the fact that they had disagreed over many of the smaller details. Marmot summarizes, "None of our recommendations is based on 'could be' conclusions. All are based on judgments that evidence was definite or probable." This is about as complete a scientific review as possible. You don't need to believe me, but I don't know how anybody can doubt such an intensive review by the world's experts. I am sure many will, though.

The report clarified two controversial issues. First, the cancer rate has been increasing. It's not simply a factor of better reporting or earlier detection. Second, only a small percentage of cancer is genetic. Most cases can be prevented by lifestyle and other environmental improvements.

Ready for the diet and lifestyle recommendations of the most comprehensive review of the literature by an unbiased panel of the best-regarded experts in the world? Here goes:

1. Be as lean as possible, within the normal range of body weight. [Aim for the lower end of normal body mass index (BMI). In this book, we have seen that a plant-based diet is the best way to maintain low body weight.]

2. Be physically active as part of everyday life.

3. Limit consumption of energy-dense foods. Avoid sugary foods. [In other words, eat foods low in fat and high in fiber and water content. Foods low in fat and high in fiber are plant foods, *not* animal proteins.]

4. Eat mostly foods of plant origins. [The personal recommendation within this public health goal is to have at least five servings of fruits and veggies each day, and include pulses and unprocessed cereals with every meal.]

5. Limit intake of red meat and avoid processed meat. [The public health goal within the recommendation is to consume less than 300 grams (⅔ of a pound) per week. Being completely vegetarian does reduce cancer risk, but we can't rule out the possibility that the difference is due to other aspects of a healthy lifestyle.]

6. Limit alcoholic drinks.

7. Limit consumption of salt. Avoid moldy cereals (grains) or pulses (legumes).

8. Aim to meet nutritional needs through diet alone. [That is, without dietary supplements.]

The panel found convincing evidence that fruits and vegetables decrease risk of cancer of the mouth, pharynx, esophagus, lung, stomach, colon, and rectum. Eating more plants probably reduces cancer of the pancreas, breast, bladder, and possibly in liver, ovary, uterine and prostate.

Since the report was published in 2007, additional information has come to light that add even more weight and specificity to the panel's recommendations. A 2013 study applied the first six of the recommendations to one of the EPIC databases (and added breastfeeding for women) and compared those who adhered to them closely with those who didn't. The results were staggering: people who answered "mostly yes" to those recommendations had a 34 percent lower risk of dying in the twelve-year period of the study than those who answered "mostly no." They also had a significantly lower risk of developing cancer or coronary artery disease (CAD) (Vergnaud, Romaguera, et al. 2013).

That the plant-based diet is protective against both cancer and heart disease makes sense, as the panel's recommendations are very similar to American Heart Association's (AHA) advice for achieving ideal cardiac health in its Strategic Impact 2020 plan. To prevent CAD, the plan recommended the following:

1. Get active.

2. Eat better: more fish, veggies, and fiber and less saturated fat and added sugar.

3. Manage blood pressure.

4. Lose weight.

5. Control cholesterol.

6. Reduce blood sugar.

7. Stop smoking.

Another 2013 study looked at cancer incidence in people based on their adherence to the AHA guidelines. The researchers looked at data from the Atherosclerosis Risk in Communities (ARIC) study of over 13,000 people who had been observed for up to 17 years for signs of heart disease. It turned out that those who followed at least five of the recommendations had a 50 percent decreased risk of cancer compared to those who followed none of them (Rasmussen-Torvik, Shay, et al. 2013). And the relationship held in the middle groups as well, with the study authors reporting "a significant, graded, inverse association" between the number of heart healthy behaviors and combined cancer incidence, with the exception of nonmelanoma skin cancers. So, the better the weight, the less the high blood pressure, the better your sugars, the more likely you avoid cancer. Best way to do all those things? Cut back on animal protein and increase fruits and veggies.

One more thing. I don't want you leaving this section entertaining even the wisp of a thought that you can get the benefits of eating plants by taking supplements. In a very carefully designed and run case/control study of premenopausal women with breast cancer, researchers found that vegetable intake was strongly and inversely related with the cancer, but when they included supplements or consumption of component parts in the analysis, the relationship was much weaker. The whole vegetable, not the extracted or synthesized nutrient components, proved protective (Freudenheim, Marshall, et al. 1996). The researchers weren't sure why whole plant foods were superior to supplements of vitamins C and E, folic acid, individual carotenoids, and dietary fiber, but hypothesized that those ingredients of plants may have worked together synergistically to reduce breast cancer risk. Also, they surmised, "other unmeasured factors" in whole plant foods may also fight cancer. So don't be fooled by your neighbor in a pyramid marketing scheme, offering you a pill that has all the vegetable and fruit you need. That is just silly.

Summing Up

So what are the conclusions we can responsibly draw from all the research I've shared in this chapter? Have we "proved" that a vegan diet can prevent or cure all cancers? No, we haven't. But we've done serious damage to the lazy and irresponsible dismissal of evidence on the grounds that "correlation doesn't equal causation."

We've seen that populations that eat less meat tend to have less cancer. Adventist studies show that vegans are more protected than vegetarians and moderate meat eaters. We know that vegans have lower levels IGF1 and PhIP, and we know people with high IGF1 are predisposed to a variety of cancers. Ornish and Blackburn have shown us that a low-fat vegan diet can control prostate cancer, not just by altering our hormonal balance but also changing our very chromosomes. Have we proved that we can cure or prevent prostate or other cancers by going vegan? Not yet. But where there is this much smoke, there has got to be a fire, and this one is a barn burner.

CHAPTER 14

Preventing Premature Death

Do plant-based eaters live longer? In a sense, this is the big question, especially in light of the flood of reductionist short-term studies that focus on biomarkers rather than outcomes. While high-fat advocates can point to elevated CLA levels in adipose tissue as a result of eating butter, they can't find a single study showing that butter improves longevity. In this chapter, we'll look at the evidence linking diet to mortality and discover that proteinaholism is killing too many of us far too soon.

Recently the National Institutes of Health asked the National Research Council and the Institute of Medicine to assess the health of Americans versus the rest of the world. Their findings were shocking. Despite being the richest country with one of the most advanced healthcare infrastructures, and despite spending more money on health care per capita than any other country in the world, we have the worst health. We die at an earlier age, have more obesity, heart disease, diabetes, and lead the way in many cancers. Our advances in medicine have limited our cancer deaths but only slightly.

The idea that high-protein diets are dangerous is not new. A 2001 review of the literature by the Nutrition Committee of the American Heart Association's Council on Nutrition, Physical Activity, and Metabolism noted that while high-protein, low-carb diets "may not be harmful for most healthy people for a short period of time, there are no long-term scientific studies to support their overall efficacy and safety." In their zealous pursuit of weight loss, low-carb dieters risk "compromised vitamin and mineral intake, as well as potential cardiac, renal, bone, and liver abnormalities overall" (St Jeor, Howard, et al. 2001).

In 2003, at the height of the Atkins craze, a couple of Australian scientists wrote a paper as a call to health professionals not to get taken in by the media frenzy. They warned that there was no good data to support the low-carb fad. To the contrary, the diet was linked to dangerous side effects, including "heart arrhythmias, cardiac contractile function impairment, sudden death, osteoporosis, kidney damage, increased cancer risk, impairment of physical activity and lipid abnormalities" (Bilsborough and Crowe 2003).

The passage of time has done nothing to allay these fears. A 2013 meta-analysis of four low-carb studies followed 272,000 people for at least one year and counted almost 16,000 deaths. Those who scored highest on the low-carb scale had a 31 percent increased chance of dying. Interestingly, the increased deaths weren't attributable to cardiovascular disease, but some combination of other factors (Noto, Goto, et al. 2013).

In 2003, Walter Willett, the esteemed Harvard epidemiologist, reviewed the insights gained from the first Adventist Health Study, including the fact that the average member of this community eats less meat, lives longer, has less heart disease, and is leaner than the average American. Noting, nonetheless, that the Adventists still suffer from high rates of breast, prostate, and ovarian cancer, Willett called for further study into the link between those cancers and the consumption of dairy (Willett 2003).

Willett refined his views in a 2013 review of recent findings in nutritional science. Unlike the low-carb advocates, Willett understands the value of large and long-term nutritional epidemiology, noting that these studies, along with advances in science and better clinical trials, "have led to important improvements in our understanding of nutrition in primary prevention of chronic disease." He summarized the cutting edge of nutritional science as follows: "Good data now support the benefits of diets that are rich in plant sources of fats and protein, fish, nuts, whole grains, and fruits and vegetables; that avoid partially hydrogenated fats; and that limit red meat and refined carbohydrates" (Willett and Stampfer 2013).

As we've seen before, one of the shortcomings of many studies that show weak or no relationship between animal protein consumption and disease and death is the small variability in diets. The best studies, for our purposes, compare disease rates in people with significantly varied diets, but similar lifestyles in other respects.

Several studies have found that vegetarians live longer than their non-vegetarian counterparts. The following studies compared the death rates (per 100,000 people per year under the age of ninety) of their entire vegetarian population to those of the overall populations in the same regions. The results are reported below as standard mortality ratios (SMRs). An SMR of 100 percent means that the study population has exactly the same death rate as the population at large, while an SMR of 50 percent means half the death rate.

SMR (%)	
EPIC-Oxford	52
Oxford Vegetarian Study	46
Heidelberg Study	48
Adventist Mortality	49

Now that we've seen the big picture, let's take an epidemiologic trip around the world and look more closely at all the evidence that animal protein decreases life expectancy. We'll begin where I began my own exploration: the Blue Zone island of Okinawa.

Blue Zones

As you'll recall, the Blue Zones are regions of the world noted for their healthy longevity. The Japanese island of Okinawa, which boasts the most centenarians per capita of any place on earth, is one of the best studied of the Blue Zones, with more than sixty years' worth of data. Today's centenarians, born before 1915, grew up eating mainly wheat, rice, barley, and especially purple sweet potatoes. They see food as medicine. Dan Buettner, in *The Blue Zones Solution,* tells how a 104-year-old Okinawan woman showed him her "medicine cabinet" of longevity-promoting foods: sweet potatoes, soybeans, mugwort, turmeric, and bitter melon. Traditional Okinawan cuisine also includes frequent dishes with seaweed and soybeans, and pork only on special occasions (Sho 2001).

Not all Okinawans make it to one hundred, of course. Regression analysis shows that Okinawan longevity is associated with maintaining a stable low weight from an early age, which they do easily given their predominately plant-based diet (Willcox, Willcox, et al. 2007).

While Okinawa and other Blue Zones attribute their longevity to more than just diet, they all share a dietary pattern upon which the rest of a healthy culture can be built. Lawrence Appel, director of the Welch Center for Prevention, Epidemiology, and Clinical Research at Johns Hopkins University, states that Blue Zones, now sadly limited to just a few dots around the globe, could become commonplace if we would follow a diet "rich in fruits and vegetables and reduced in saturated fat, salt, meats, refined grains, sweets, and full-fat dairy products" (Appel 2008).

Japan

The rest of Japan isn't doing so bad, either. According to the World Health Organization and the United Nations' 2012 reports, Japan has the highest life expectancy of any country in the world. The traditional Japanese diet is, of course, a high-carb, lower-protein diet with little meat consumption (mostly pork on special occasions). A 1999 prospective study that followed 700 elderly Japanese men and women for seven years found that those who ate a plant-based diet were more likely to be alive at the end of the study. They ate more starch, more plants, and less protein than did the typical American (Kumagai, Shibata, et al. 1999). A large prospective study followed 60,000 Japanese men and women for 13 years and found that fruit consumption was most protective against death. Fruit and legumes were specifically associated with decreased mortality from coronary artery disease (Nagura, Iso, et al. 2009).

Seven Countries

Remember Ancel Keys's Seven Countries Study? Well, the study is still going strong, and continues to collect data on the links between diet and health. A 2000 update showed a direct correlation between saturated fat, smoking, and low vitamin C intake and all-cause mortality (Kromhout,

Bloemberg, et al. 2000). Of course, the saturated fat mainly comes tied with animal protein, and the vitamin C is only found in plants.

Sweden

Researchers in Sweden performed a seven-day diet assessment of 924 Swedish men, then followed them for 10 years. On average, those eating closest to a "Mediterranean pattern" high in vegetables, legumes, fruits, and cereals lived the longest, while those on carb-restricted diets had the shortest life spans (Sjögren, Becker, et al. 2010). A longer Swedish study followed 43,000 women over 12 years and found that low-carb diets and high-protein diets both lead to increased cardiac and overall death. The combination of low carb and high protein was the deadliest (Lagiou, Sandin, et al. 2007).

Spain

The PREDIMED trial was done in Spain to follow over 7,000 people and randomize them to Mediterranean diet. It was originally designed to test the response to nuts and olive oil. Researchers did go back, however, and reevaluate the data. Not surprisingly they found that increasing amounts of animal protein increased the results of fatal and nonfatal events. This was especially noticeable when carbs were substituted with protein (Hernández-Alonso, Salas-Salvadó, et al. 2015).

Oxford Health

A group of vegetarian/vegans living in Oxford, England, have been the subject of several studies: the Health Shoppers Study, the Oxford Health Study and the EPIC-Oxford Study. The EPIC-Oxford data, while probably underestimating the benefits of a vegetarian diet and downplaying the risks of a high-protein diet due to previously mentioned issues with subject selection, nevertheless was able to find mortality differences. The vegans in the study had the lowest cholesterol compared to vegetarians, fish eaters, and meat eaters and suffered less mortality from heart disease, cancer, and all causes (Appleby, Thorogood, et al. 1999). Interestingly, the control group of meat eaters in this study had low mortality compared to the rest of England. Analysis showed that they ate meat infrequently, around once a week and yet still had higher risk of premature mortality compared with vegetarians (Appleby, Key, et al. 2002).

EPIC

Seeking to cut through the confusion, the *American Journal of Clinical Nutrition* published a well-considered review of six prospective studies looking at the relationship between low meat intake and longevity. Four of the studies showed a significant increase in longevity in people who ate less meat, one was trending toward significance but didn't quite make it, and one showed no difference. The review concluded by reiterating that cutting back on meat clearly seems to increase life expectancy and posits that the nonpositive findings could be due to a variety of study shortcomings, including overadjustment, muddy definitions of "vegetarian," measurement error, and the healthy volunteer effect, among others (Singh, Sabaté, et al. 2003).

It's true that original EPIC studies showed modest benefits of a plant-based diet in regard to mortality. As it has continued to expand (to Germany and Italy) and gather data over the years, the benefits of less meat and more veggies are becoming clearer, like increasing the density of pixels in a photograph. Now it's becoming ever clearer that low meat consumption is associated with longevity.

One very clever 2005 study looked prospectively at 170,000 people age 60 or more, with no heart disease, in the EPIC data. Researchers created a scoring system to judge how closely participants followed a mostly plant-based Mediterranean diet. Close adherence meant substituting unsaturated and monosaturated fats (like those found in vegetables, nuts, seeds, and fish) for saturated fats (from land animals), eating more veggies, and reducing meat consumption. When they ran the numbers, they found the higher the adherence to the Mediterranean diet, the lower the mortality (Trichopoulou, Orfanos, et al. 2005). Two years later, the same researchers confirmed their original findings in a look at 23,000 healthy

Greek adults studied for up to ten years. Both high-protein and low-carb diets, and especially the combination, increased risk of early death from cancer, heart disease, and all causes (Trichopoulou, Psaltopoulou, et al. 2007).

A 2013 study of 450,000 people in the full EPIC database found a significant correlation between meat and processed meat and all-cause mortality. While some of this effect was diminished by statistical overadjustment (for some reason, the researchers controlled for vegetable consumption and weight), processed meat remained a significant cause of death from cancer and heart disease (Rohrmann, Overvad, et al. 2013).

A consortium reviewed the totality of the EPIC data and distilled it into three key recommendations for a long life:

Recommendation	Average years of extra life conferred
Eat five or more servings of fruits and veggies a day	4
Don't smoke	5
Engage in moderate exercise on a regular basis	3

Doing all three adds ten healthy years, and doing all three while abstaining from alcohol adds a whopping fourteen years of healthy, active life.

How many Americans do you think follow all three recommendations?

Well, 76 percent don't smoke. Somewhere between 15 and 20 percent eat at least five servings or fruits and veggies a day. And 20 percent get moderate exercise on a regular basis.

But just 3 percent of Americans follow all three. That's an awful lot of lost years. And while we've been focusing on statistics in this section of the book, maybe now is good time for each of us to reflect on what that particular statistic represents in human terms. Think of someone you know who's lost a loved one too soon to a preventable disease. Think of someone who is fighting for their life. Think of someone suffering through a physical and emotional decline. And multiply that by millions to get a sense of the magnitude of this largely avoidable tragedy.

Not all Americans have unhealthy lifestyles, of course. There's enough variability in behaviors and outcomes that it's possible to draw conclusions from large prospective epidemiology studies of U.S. populations.

Adventist Health I

The Seventh-day Adventists in Loma Linda, California, are considered the longest-living population ever studied. The Adventists live up to a decade longer than the average Californian. Specifically, an Adventist at age thirty can expect to live 7.8 years longer, and for some groups of women the number increases to 10. As we've seen, many factors contribute to their stellar health outcomes. They're leaner, they eat more plants, they get exercise, and they don't smoke. But the single factor that stands out in all the statistical analyses is diet (Fraser and Shavlik 2001; Fraser 1999).

Researchers noted in 1988 that the first Adventist Health Study was uniquely valuable in that it combined a long-term perspective with a wide range of eating behaviors. The study found that meat is correlated with all-cause mortality, heart disease, and diabetes (Snowdon 1988). Meat consumption is correlated with all-cause mortality, heart disease, and diabetes. Egg consumption is correlated with mortality and heart disease in women, and colon cancer in men and women. And as milk consumption increases, so does prostate cancer.

AHS2

In 2013, death rates for the first 5.8 years of Adventist Health Study-2 (AHS2) were released. When vegans, lacto-ovo-vegetarians, pesco-vegetarians, and semivegetarians were combined into one group, they had a 12 percent lower risk of mortality than the nonvegetarian Adventists. After adjusting for body mass index (BMI), the finding dropped to 10 percent; given that diet has a strong impact on BMI, adjusting for BMI is probably masking the true effect of diet. Vegans by themselves had a 15 percent lower risk of death, but it did not quite reach statistical significance.

The difference in mortality rates can mostly be explained by one factor: a lower incidence of cardiovascular disease among vegetarian and especially vegan men. Vegetarian women had about the same rates as nonvegetarian women, a similar finding to the first Adventist Health Study. There was also a benefit for all vegetarians for death from renal disease and endocrine disease (principally diabetes). No differences were found for all vegetarians for infectious or respiratory diseases (Orlich, Singh, et al. 2013).

There are a couple of caveats to this study. For one thing, participants' diets were assessed only once, at the start of the study, and never reassessed. We simply don't know if participants changed their diets during the study, which obviously would have major implications for the results. The study length, only 5.7 years, is quite short for a mortality study of this size. Researchers expected that the short follow-up would bias the results against finding significant mortality differences between the groups. As the study goes out further we should see increasing benefit to plant-based diets.

A large, and very well-performed meta-analysis looked at all the studies that had been done on vegetarians. After pooling all the data, researchers found that vegetarians had a 29 percent lower risk of dying from heart disease and 9 percent decreased risk of dying from all causes (Huang, Yang, et al. 2012).

NIH-AARP

Other studies don't include vegetarians or vegans specifically, but still look at varying dietary patterns. One of the largest population studies done in the United States was the NIH-AARP study, which followed, for up to 10 years, half a million people who had been between the ages of 50 and 71 when the study began. Researchers found that red and processed meat were both associated with an increased risk of all-cause mortality, as well as death due to cancer and coronary artery disease. Eating white meat slightly decreased mortality, but this is probably a substitution effect: not that chicken is good for you, but in this study it proved less bad than red meat and processed meat (Sinha, Cross, et al. 2009).

Nurses/Health Professionals

The very large and long-term Nurses' Health Study and Health Professionals Follow-up Study also provide evidence that more plants and fewer animals in the diet equals increased life expectancy. A 2008 analysis of a

20-year follow-up for 72,000 women in the Nurses' Health Study found that what the researchers termed "prudent eating" led to a 17 percent reduction in all-cause mortality, and a 28 percent reduction in deaths from heart disease. How did they define "prudent eating"? High-fruit-and-vegetable consumption and low red and processed meat consumption (Heidemann, Schulze, et al. 2008).

In 2010, Harvard researchers combined data from the Nurses' and Health Professionals studies with a question specifically about low-carb dieters. As a group, those who ate low carb tended to not survive for the entire duration of the study. A closer look at this group revealed that the low-carb dieters who ate more meat were at significantly greater risk than the low carbers who consumed more plants (Fung, van Dam, et al. 2010). Remember, these studies have been criticized for having too small differences between quintiles, and for focusing on individual dietary factors (fats, carbs, etc.) rather than entire dietary patterns. Even with these shortcomings, analysis of the data show clearly that a dietary pattern consisting of lots of fruits and veggies, and less meat of all kinds is protective against premature death. Walter Willett, chair of the department that conducted the study, was asked his bottom-line diet advice by a journalist from the *Los Angeles Times*. His simple reply: " . . . when you get down to maybe one serving of meat or less per week the risk gets pretty low. If you really want to go for the lowest possible, it does look like not consuming red meat at all, or a couple times a year, is where you'd want to be."

In one of the latest efforts to understand the diet/death relationship from these two American cohorts, a 2012 study looked at 120,000 men and women who had been free of cardiovascular disease and cancer when they first enrolled in the Nurses' Health Study or Health Professionals Follow-up Study. Researchers assessed participants' diets through food frequency questionnaires that were updated every four years. They documented almost 24,000 deaths over the length of the studies (22 years for the men and 28 years for the women), and adjusted for major lifestyle and dietary risk factors. Even with all that statistical adjustment (probably including some degree of overadjustment), the study still found that adding a single serving per day of red meat increased a person's chance of dying by 13 percent. When the meat was processed, the risk jumped to 20 percent. And the effects were consistent across cardiovascular and cancer deaths. The researchers estimated that 9.3 percent of the deaths in men, and 7.6 percent of the deaths in women, could have been prevented if everyone in the study had eaten fewer than one serving of meat every two days. Substituting just about anything for the red and processed meat significantly reduced all-cause mortality (Pan, Sun, et al. 2012).

Iowa Women

The final epidemiologic data we'll look at comes from the Iowa Women's Health Study, which began following 29,000 postmenopausal women who were free from cancer, coronary heart disease, and diabetes when the study began in 1986. Fifteen years later, researches found a considerable increased risk of death from heart disease when red meat was eaten instead of carbs. The risk was almost as great from dairy foods (Kelemen, Kushi, et al. 2005). Interestingly, they noted that substituting vegetable protein for animal protein could have prevented 30 percent of the observed mortality. They concluded this intensive study with prophetic words, "Long-term adherence to high-protein diets, without discrimination toward protein source, may have potentially adverse health consequences."

Summary of Epidemiology

In 2013, two Swedish researchers, Susanna Larsson and Nicola Orsini, wanted to know if eating red and processed meat increased the risk of death, and if so, how much or how little meat made a difference. They performed an exhaustive PubMed search, finding almost 5,000 seemingly relevant articles. By the time they finished reading all the abstracts, they were down to 35 studies they looked at in detail. Of these, 27 didn't meet their criteria for relevance or quality, leaving just eight prospective studies that examined nine different populations. When they were pooled and analyzed, the researchers found clear evidence that total meat and processed meat consumption was associated with higher all-cause mortality. When they compared high and low meat eaters, they found that processed meat consumption was linked to a 23 percent increased chance of death. Total meat, which was defined as processed meat and unprocessed red meat, raised the risk to 29 percent.

There are a couple of interesting things about this data. First, the dose-response was found to be nonlinear. For nonstatisticians, this means that there wasn't a straight line relationship between eating meat and dying. The risks increased the most at the lowest end of the scale, where people are eating less than one serving of meat per day. In other words, the difference between no meat and a little bit of meat is actually much more significant than the difference between some and a lot. The authors write: "This finding suggests that all-cause mortality is elevated even at low intakes of processed meat and total red meat." People always talk about eating meat in moderation, but what is moderation? Most people would consider smaller portions of daily meat moderation, but according to this data, just decreasing animal protein slightly may not be enough.

Second, fully seven of the nine prospective studies adjusted the data for body mass index (BMI), which almost certainly erases some of the mortality attributable to eating meat, as we saw in Chapter 13. This means that the real effect of eating meat in reducing life span is even bigger than it appears in this meta-analysis. Researchers have removed overweight people from the study, and being overweight is significantly associated with cancer and heart disease. That is definitely overadjustment.

Why? What's the Mechanism?

Now that we've looked at the considerable evidence linking animal foods to early death, we're left wondering: Why? What's the mechanism by which animal foods shorten life. Is it the lack of fruits and veggies, or something about meat itself? Is it just through the diseases we've already looked at, like heart disease, cancer, and diabetes, or is there something about a protein-heavy diet that ages us faster in general?

Fruits and Veggies, or Just Less Meat?

The question about the relative importance of fruits and veggies, or just avoiding animal foods, is up in the air. As we learned in the cancer section, studies of South African natives revealed that they had very low rates of colon cancer despite low fiber intake, suggesting it is the lack of animal protein that protects them (O'Keefe, Kidd, et al. 1999).

On the other hand, a 2000 study in the *Journal of the American Medical Association* looked at 42,000 women who had participated in a breast cancer screening. Researchers followed the women for an average of almost six years. They used a food frequency questionnaire and gave each participant a "diet score" based on their adherence to what the researchers considered an ideal diet: heavy in fruits and vegetables, with some white meat and fish. They divided the women into four groups (quartiles) based on their scores, with the lowest group eating the standard American diet. The data showed a significant difference in mortality between the highest and lowest quartiles, even though the "best" group was still eating substantial portions of animal products. I'm left wondering what the results would have shown if they had included a fifth group that dropped the meat entirely (Kant, Schatzkin, et al. 2000). Nevertheless, the study suggests that fruits and veggies by themselves can extend life.

A 2013 EPIC study that followed almost half a million Europeans for between 10 and 18 years found that fruit and vegetable consumption was independently associated with decreased mortality (Leenders, Sluijs, et al. 2013). After all, fruits and veggies are loaded with fiber, antioxidants, and phytochemicals. They also buffer acid. We should expect that they would improve health.

The United Nation's Food and Agriculture Organization (FAO) and the World Health Organization (WHO) implemented their Global Strategy on Diet, Physical Activity and Health in 2002 to combat growing rates of chronic disease. Their experts estimate that 1.7 million deaths per year are attributable to low fruit and vegetable consumption, making it one of the top 10 risk factors for global mortality. The latest World Health Report estimates that low fruit and veggie consumption is responsible for 14 percent of GI cancers, 11 percent CAD, and 9 percent of stroke. Those numbers turn out to be very conservative, as their recommended amount of fruits and vegetables falls far short of optimal: just 400 grams per day, or less than a pound.

While vitamins, antioxidants, and phytochemicals are getting all the press these days, the single biggest contributor to the health benefits of plants may be that unsung hero, fiber. In 2011, a very large prospective study of the NIH-AARP cohort showed that fiber was inversely related with the risks of dying from cancer as well as pulmonary, infectious, and cardiovascular diseases (Park, Subar, et al. 2011). And, in a finding that will surprise a lot of gluten fearers, the fiber found in grain was particularly protective. Researchers surmised that grain fiber may actually lower inflammation, which is exactly the opposite of what you'd expect if the Paleo crowd is to be believed. Additionally, a 2012 EPIC study showed that fiber intake is correlated with lower mortality especially from CAD, digestive, and inflammatory diseases (Chuang, Norat, et al. 2012).

We may never arrive at a definitive answer as to whether it's the fiber, or the antioxidants, or the other phytochemicals, or something else entirely that accounts for the longevity effects of plants. Practically, I'm not sure it makes all that much difference. Eat your fruits and veggies, legumes, and whole grains, and just enjoy the mystery of their protective power.

Meat and the Science of Life Extension

At present, science doesn't really know that much about the aging process. The field of antiaging research is in its infancy, but the popular press about aging lends as much credence to shysters as to qualified scientists. One finding that seems pretty clear at this stage is that aging is a process of cellular degeneration. The better our cells are doing, the longer we're likely to live. At the moment, there are three promising mechanisms that can explain how animal protein may compromise the health of our cells.

Leucine Restriction

Most of our lab studies on aging are carried out on animals. The one reliable factor that increased life span was a calorically restricted diet that still provided sufficient nutrients (Dar, Dar, et al. 2012). Predictably, this finding wasn't met with much enthusiasm by most humans. Sure, mild starvation might help us live longer, but that's not exactly a deal we can get thrilled about. Fortunately, new evidence is emerging to shift the picture significantly. It appears that it's not so much the low calories, as the low protein levels in those low-calorie diets that increased life expectancy (Nakagawa, Lagisz, et al. 2012). Specifically, it appears that leucine, an essential amino acid found predominately in animal foods, may be the real culprit in cellular degeneration (Simpson and Raubenheimer 2009).

Leucine may wreak havoc on our cells by interfering with what's known as the mTOR pathway (which stands for "mechanistic target of rapamycin," in case you're thinking of trying out for *Jeopardy!*) (Gallinetti, Harputlugil, et al. 2013). Known as a master growth regulator, mTOR orchestrates complex biochemical interactions to keep our cells and tissues functioning at optimal levels. It's been found to be a major pathway controlling the rate of aging (Johnson, Rabinovitch, et al. 2013). When mTOR signaling goes awry, many disease states have the opportunity to develop, including cancer, heart disease, and diabetes.

Overmineralization of Cells

It's also been found that too-high concentrations of minerals can cause cell death. We've seen that heme iron, the type of iron found in animal tissue, is easily absorbed into our bodies. It's also easily oxidized, which is essentially a form of rusting inside our bodies. It's known that iron is toxic to pancreatic cells, and that dying cells often contain higher than normal levels of iron. Based on this evidence, it's reasonable to speculate that one reason vegans live longer than others is the low concentration of heme iron in their cells.

BUN

Another link in the chain between animal foods and early death is the effect of animal protein consumption and blood urea nitrogen, or BUN. BUN is a break-down product of protein metabolism and increases with increased protein intake (Young, El-Khoury, et al. 2000). A study looking at lab results found a significant increased risk of death in people with a BUN value greater than 15 (Solinger and Rothman 2013). One study found that having a BUN above 40 was associated with a 500 percent increased risk of death compared to people in the referent ("normal") range of 10–20 (Beier, Eppanapally, et al. 2011). Again, I want to caution the Paleo eaters: get your BUN checked. Gary Taubes's publicly released blood test showed a BUN of 24, which puts him at increased risk of early death.

IGF1

We mention in the cancer section that IGF1 is associated with cancer growth. A review of the literature showed that mice and human studies demonstrate that low IGF1 is associated with longer life and fewer age-related diseases. The researchers did their own study by looking at how people ate using an automated food assessment tool and then following death statistics from a national database. The results showed that under age sixty-five, low protein was associated with less premature mortality from all causes. Over sixty-five, interestingly, people actually benefited from higher protein. The older people with high protein had more diabetes, as we should now expect, but they did live longer (Levine, Suarez, et al. 2014). This may be due to the added protein protecting against loss of muscle, which we will address in the next chapter.

To sum up, the link between diet and longevity is a complex one, and there's a lot we don't know. But don't let the complexity, or the uncertainty, hide the main point: it's overwhelmingly clear that an animal-rich diet is associated with a shortened life.

Science is discovering new things every day. To stay on top of the latest nutritional knowledge, sign up for free e-mail updates at Proteinaholic.com.

PART FOUR

The Proteinaholic Recovery Plan

CHAPTER 15

How Much Protein Do We Need?

We know there's a big gap between how much protein we're eating and how much we should be eating, as evidenced by the epidemics of chronic diseases linked to protein overconsumption. What's perhaps even more troubling is that there's another gap, this one of perception. As you may recall from Chapter 5, a 2013 survey revealed that 57 percent of Americans say they are actively trying to get *more* protein into their diets, and 63 percent are making food choices based on "high-protein" claims on the packaging. So we're eating more than we should, but less than we think we should. Unless we can change this perception, our health problems are only going to get worse.

Of course, we don't want to go to the other extreme and become protein deficient. I'm not saying at all that protein is bad for us. On the contrary, it's absolutely essential. So the question we now have to answer is, how much do we actually need?

In this chapter, we'll look at the recommended daily allowance (RDA) for protein, and whether it reflects good science. We'll examine the claims of those who find the RDA insufficient, and who advocate for higher amounts of protein. We'll review scientific advances in nitrogen balancing and other methods of measuring protein intake and output. We'll consider groups that may need more protein than others, specifically infants, athletes, the elderly, and bedridden persons. Finally, we'll examine a few extreme outliers: raw fruitarians, who technically consume almost no protein. We'll see whether they are wasting away or thriving and weigh the implications for the rest of us.

Protein Basics

Before we can determine our true protein requirements, it's helpful to remind ourselves of some basic biology. First, protein is essential for human health because it builds and maintains muscle. If we're not wasting away, that means we're getting enough protein. It follows that our protein requirements are greatest when we're growing the most muscle. Second, we don't need protein specifically. We need amino acids, which are the building blocks of protein. Given all the essential amino acids that we cannot metabolize ourselves, we can make every protein that our bodies need from those raw materials. Third, the ingredient of protein that distinguishes it from carbs and fat is nitrogen. Scientists have used this fact to measure the amount of protein we metabolize by measuring the nitrogen we excrete in our urine and feces and comparing that to the amount of nitrogen we consume, a method known as nitrogen balance.

Nitrogen balance studies have shown that we are very good recyclers of amino acids. When we break down muscle, we don't just flush all that valuable nitrogen down the toilet. Instead, we metabolize the proteins into amino acids that become available for reuse, to make whatever new proteins are required. Author and clinical pyschologist Doug Lisle, also director of research for TrueNorth Health Center, jokes that vegetarians confronted with the ubiquitous question "Where do you get your protein?" should respond, "From human flesh"—our own, of course.

There's no shortage of amino acids in our bodies. It turns out that calories, not amino acids, are the limiting factor that determines rate and efficiency of muscle building for the most part. For our systems to function, and muscle to be built, we need protein and its metabolites but also energy from carbs and fat. Without it, our bodies will take the carbon skeleton of protein to make fuel for energy. It's like on *Star Trek* when the *Enterprise* shuts down most of its functions and channels all resources into "life support."

Kwashiorkor, a third world disease often described as protein deficiency, is actually a combination protein/calorie deficiency. When children suffering from kwashiorkor are treated with additional calories, often from cereal grains, their condition resolves itself (Calloway 1975).

Given sufficient calories, there's another factor that determines how efficiently we are able to recycle urea and nitrogen into absorbable amino acids in the colon: the biome that lives in our guts. A 2009 study found that vegetarians ingest more probiotics and prebiotics, and their flora is better at recycling nitrogen to make new proteins. It's therefore possible for vegetarians, even with lower protein intake, to produce all the protein they need since they are using colonic reabsorption more efficiently (Bergen and Wu 2009). It's even been found that our gut bacteria can make the so-called essential amino acids—the ones we're supposedly able to get only from food—and recirculate them into our system.

The body of a lean 154-pound (70 kilogram) man has about 11 kilograms of protein, 4.7 in muscle and 6.3 in bone and tissues. Conventional wisdom holds that we don't store protein, but there does seem to be a "labile reserve," stored in the liver and other tissues, that can be utilized rapidly when we experience starvation. This is why we don't need to consume all the essential amino acids at every meal. When we aren't eating enough protein, it's been found that we can recycle amino acids at 90 percent efficiency. Our body's protein reserves are in constant motion; on average, we're degrading and synthesizing about 250 grams per day.

Futhermore, there's a limit to how much protein our bodies can use. One study sought to determine the point at which more doesn't equal better. Researchers steadily infused pure synthetic amino acids, including radio-labeled leucine, into 8 healthy individuals for 8.5 hours. Muscle protein synthesis increased with the increasing amino acids but hit a max level. Then, despite increasing amino acids, muscle synthesis decreased (Atherton, Etheridge, et al. 2010). In other words, there appears to be a max level at which point more protein does not mean more muscle, and as we have learned in prior chapters, may mean more disease.

The Evolution of Protein Recommendations

Let's start our recap of the protein recommendation roller coaster in the 1880s, with Dr. Carl von Voit's highly inflated 118 grams/day, based on his observations about how much protein nineteenth-century heavy laborers were consuming, as well as his pioneering work in developing the nitrogen balance method. As I discussed in Chapter 4, by the turn of the century, buoyed by increased understanding and more sensitive technology, Chittenden and others demonstrated that our true requirements were about half of von Voit's recommendations.

In the 1940s, William Rose, a University of Illinois professor of nutrition, identified the eight amino acids that humans cannot metabolize themselves and therefore must obtain from diet. He called these "essential amino acids" and set a minimum requirement for human consumption.

By the way, each of these amino acids is well represented in just about all vegetable foods, including white potatoes, wheat flour, and corn. There's absolutely no way you could eat sufficient calories of a varied plant-based diet and become protein deficient.

The U.S. government created RDAs (recommended daily allowances) during World War II, to protect U.S. citizens from possible wartime shortages. The RDAs were not minimums, or average requirements; instead, they represent an optimal amount. In other words, the average requirement needed is far lower, but they wanted to make sure that the amount they suggested was the amount needed for over 98 percent of the country.

In 1955, the Food and Agriculture Organization (FAO) of the United Nations began issuing nutritional recommendations based partly on Rose's data. Nutritionists took Rose's optimal requirement and set it as their minimum, on the assumption that too little is worse than too much. They revised these recommendations in 1963 and 1981, when they set a minimum protein requirement of 0.6 grams per kilogram of lean body mass (body weight minus the fat). Their voluminous 2002 document, "Protein and Amino Acid Requirements in Human Nutrition," filled with scientific review articles, revised this number to 0.66 g/kg.

In 1971, Frances Moore Lappé wrote *Diet for a Small Planet*, a book that convinced many readers to become vegetarian. Lappé, a sociologist working on world hunger issues, mistakenly promoted the idea of protein complementarity. She wrote that unlike animal proteins, plant proteins are incomplete and therefore need to be carefully combined at each meal to prevent protein deficiencies. Whatever the book did for public consciousness about food and hunger, it also started a worrying craze that infected vegetarians and their concerned parents. Rather than just eating of nature's bounty, vegetarians were tasked with complex rules of food combining that made it seem like vegetarianism was the hardest thing in the world.

From Numbers to Food

What do these protein ratios mean on a practical level? We turn this ratio into grams of protein by calculating our lean body mass. For example, let's take a five-foot-ten man weighing 160 pounds—a pretty thin guy, by modern standards. That's 72.5 kilograms total, with a lean body mass estimated around 58 kilograms. According to the FAO, this man requires 0.66 x 58, or 38.2 grams a day. Using the higher RDA of 0.8, he requires 0.8 x 58, or 46.4 grams of protein per day.

For reference, here are the grams of protein in some common foods:

1 cup milk: 8

3-ounce piece of meat: 21

1 cup dry beans: 16

1 serving broccoli: 4.2

1 small head cauliflower: 5

1 cup cooked brown rice: 5

1 medium cooked potato: 4.3

1 8-oz bag potato chips: 16

1 slice Domino's cheese pizza: 12

1 cup of peas: 8

You can see that even a poor-quality diet will fulfill all our protein requirements. If all you ate three time a day was 30 Lay's Classic potato chips and 2 slices of Domino's plain pizza, you'd be consuming 48 grams of protein. Obviously, I don't recommend that kind of diet. The point is it's virtually impossible to be protein deficient on a nonstarvation diet.

In later editions of the book, Lappé retracted this statement and regretted that she had created a myth. She said humans are virtually guaranteed enough protein from plants if consuming enough calories (Lappé 1985). But by then the notion of complementary proteins was so deeply ingrained in society, it has so far proved impossible to dislodge. Vegetarians, we suppose, must jump through nutritional hoops to equal the "perfect" protein found in beef and eggs.

One of the most prolific and influential protein researchers of the last half century was Vernon Young, an MIT professor who pioneered a novel method of estimating protein requirements that we'll look at shortly. In a 1994 study, Young found that plant proteins compose 65 percent of all protein consumed globally, but in the USA that number was more than halved, to just 32 percent (Young and Pellett 1994). The WHO/FAO took Young's amino acid score into account as part of its recommendations on specific protein sources. Meats, for example, have more indispensable and conditional essential amino acids than plants, and in fact far exceed recommendations. Plants were found to adequately meet, and often exceed, protein requirements. Soy in particular was cited as an example of a well-utilized, complete protein. Researchers pointed out that the rat studies that are cited to "prove" that animal proteins are superior to vegetable proteins paint an inadequate picture when applied to humans.

In 1982, before becoming enamored with amino acid oxidation, Young chaired an FAO/WHO/UNU (United Nations University) Expert Consultation on Energy and Protein Requirements. Reviewing long-term studies, the experts found that consuming half of the RDA for protein was associated with poor immune response to antigens (in other words, the immune system was found to be weakened). At the RDA level, people preserved their fat-free mass and resting energy expenditure, and they maintained or improved their strength. They concluded that the median protein requirement was 0.68 g/kg (Anderson, Haynie, et al. 2015).

And in 2005, the National Academy of Sciences' Institute of Medicine (IOM) released their panel's recommendations in a huge book, complete with a large body of research to support their findings. The authors wrote: "Protein is a major functional and structural component of all cells . . . Thus an adequate supply of dietary protein is essential to maintain cellular integrity and function." And even given that strong admonishment, they still recommended an upper limit of 35 percent of total calories coming from protein and left the recommendation of 0.66 g/kg (Institute of Medicine 2005).

Current Recommendations

The U.S. government RDA sets the bar at 0.8 g/kg. Indeed, the community of researchers using nitrogen balance as their method of choice agree with these figures. A 2003 meta-analysis set optimal protein intake at 0.8 g/kg of lean body mass (Rand, Pellett, et al. 2003). This review of many studies also noted that nitrogen balance had more to do with energy intake than protein intake. In other words, the protein recommendation itself wasn't important; rather, the key was getting sufficient calories, and this is crucial. If you don't want to waste away, then eat enough calories. If you want to build muscle, then eat enough calories.

Based on that RDA ratio, the public CDC website lists our average daily requirements at 46 grams for women and 56 grams for men. This comes not only from nitrogen balance lab studies, but also epidemiologic studies, randomized clinical trials utilizing biochemical assessments, and animal studies. The Food and Nutrition Board of the National Research Council (part of the National Academy of Sciences), which is tasked with formulated RDAs, incorporated the nitrogen balance studies as follows.

They began by determining how much protein is lost per day by calculating nitrogen losses in urine, fecal material, skin, and hair. On average, they found, a man loses about 24 grams of protein per day. They added an extra 30 percent to cover 98 percent of the population to bring the total lost to 31 grams. We don't absorb and utilize every single gram of protein that we eat; a common estimate is 75 percent. So men need to eat 56 grams daily to make up for the 31 grams we lose.

In one of the best-designed studies, researchers explored the protein requirements of healthy older adults compared to younger adults. They put 23 younger and 18 older men and women on three different 18-day diets (with protein intakes of 0.5, 0.75, and 1.0 grams of protein per kilogram of lean body mass, respectively), with one week of unrestricted eating between each of the trials. They made sure the women were not menstruating during any of the 18-day diet trials. The participants ate their morning meals under supervision and had all their meals provided for them. The researchers collected stool and urine samples and calculated protein needs using nitrogen balance methodology. The study concluded that the RDA of 0.8 g/kg was sufficient to meet the protein requirements of young and old alike, that there was no difference in protein needs between the younger and older participants (Campbell, Johnson, et al. 2008).

Currently, nutritional biochemists are embroiled in a heated debate about human protein requirements (one that has approximately zero practical significance, as I'll soon explain). The MIT lab led by Young came up with a new (and to them, quite exciting) method of analyzing protein requirements, called "amino acid oxidation." Basically, by labeling amino acids with a radioactive marker they can determine the amount of amino acid actually utilized by the body. The calculations produced numbers higher than those seen in other types of studies. It's technologically advanced, using carbon labeling, which naturally appeals to many scientists, and has the appearance of objectivity and accuracy, but in all probably overestimates our protein needs. And even its inventors admit that its validity is uncertain.

Nevertheless, the MIT researchers have been pushing for an increase in the RDA for protein, and suggesting that meat has more and better amino acids than vegetables. As we've already seen in human nutrition studies, meat delivers excess protein while plants contain perfectly adequate amounts. And as we've seen, methionine and leucine can lead to cancer and aging, respectively.

In the end, their studies suggest we need to increase our requirements up to 1.0 g/kg. Even though the absolute number, 1.0 g/kg of lean body mass, isn't hugely different from the 0.66 of the FAO and the 0.8 of the RDA, these researchers do go on to imply that wheat must be combined with milk in order to make a complete protein (Young and Borgonha 2000). Remember, they are likely thinking about starving children in Africa, not our overfed populace.

Recently, a group of researchers from Toronto's Hospital for Sick Children echoed the MIT call to increase our protein requirements. Noting that there are structural problems with the standard lab methods of nitrogen balance, they attempted to adjust for these problems and determined that a true nitrogen balance result would be somewhere between 0.91 and 0.99 g/kg. They triangulated these numbers with their own amino acid oxidation studies and came to a recommendation of between 0.93 and 1.2 g/kg. Compared with the RDA of 56 grams for the average man, these new recommendations work out to 84 grams of protein per day. They concluded their discussion by pointing out an "urgent need" to change the recommendations (Elango, Humayun, et al. 2010).

At the risk of sounding obvious, I'd like to point out several huge problems with raising our protein requirements based on amino acid oxidation. First, even the inventors of the method admit that they can't guarantee its validity.

Second, it's based on the principle that too much protein is better than not enough. You'll recognize this as the thinking behind inflating the RDA from 0.66 to 0.8 g/kg. In general, I agree with the concept of "better safe than sorry." The question is, which scenario is more likely to make us sorry: erring on the side of not enough protein, or too much? As a culture of proteinaholics, we've always assumed that a lot is good, and more is better. But as the last six chapters have shown us, too much protein is at least as harmful as too little. And as we'll soon see, it's almost impossible to get too little.

Third, what's this about an "urgent need" to advocate higher protein consumption? In a rational world, medical researchers spend their time looking for solutions to actual human problems. Whether it be an epidemic of concussions from high school football games, or an increase in the incidence of type 2 diabetes among preteens, scientists dedicate their time and ingenuity to identifying causes and coming up with treatments. In the case of protein requirements, these scientists are hyperventilating about a solution in search of a problem. True, they are probably more concerned with the many malnourished people around the world. Much of these data are used to decide how much they need to be fed. But why does the RDA for America need urgent attention? If our protein requirements are really not being met, we should be seeing some protein-deficient people out there. So it's not unreasonable to ask: Where are they? This type of scientific activism is impelled by their excitement over their own statistical analysis rather than an actual public health issue. We simply don't suffer from protein deficiency independent of caloric insufficiency.

Fourth, the whole debate is completely academic. This is often what happens when you take science out of a human context. We already consume far more protein than even this latest recommendation, and we're arguing about raising by 15 percent a threshold that we're already exceeding by 200 percent.

We're Getting Too Much Protein, No Matter How We Slice It

According to U.S. government data, we're eating a lot more protein than the RDAs of 56 grams for men and 46 grams for women. In fact, we're eating far more than the inflated recommendations coming out of MIT and Toronto, which work out to 70–80 grams for men and 58–68 grams for women. The National Health and Nutrition Examination Survey (NHANES) found that men eat an average of 102 grams and women an average of 70.

The NHANES data may actually be underestimating our true consumption of protein. The FAO notes that the United States is one of the world's largest consumers of protein per capita and estimates our consumption at an average of 130 grams a day. Red meat consumption has remained stable, or dropped slightly, over the years, but pork, fish, and especially poultry consumption has increased.

Most people don't take the time to calculate their protein requirements to the gram; athletes and dieters often do. Unfortunately, many weight-loss and fitness bloggers confuse lean body mass with total body weight. Since all the recommendations are in the form of a ratio between daily grams of protein and lean body mass, this misunderstanding inevitably leads to dangerous overestimates of protein requirements. Take, for example, one of my typical bariatric patients, a 300-pound person with 170 pounds of fat. The person's lean body mass is 130 pounds, which converts into 59 kg. The correct RDA calculation is therefore 0.8 x 59, or 47.2 grams per day. If we made the mistake of assuming they need 0.8 grams of protein per kg body weight we would recommend this patient eat 110 grams of protein daily.

So how much protein do we need? Probably getting the RDA of 0.8 g/kg is more than sufficient. But maybe the answer is, why are we asking that question in the first place? The Institute of Medicine recommends that men eat 38 grams of fiber a day and women eat 25 grams of fiber a day. Yet, NHANES data shows that we only eat about 15 grams of fiber a day. We are extremely deficient in fiber, so why does nobody ever ask where you get your fiber from?

What About Those Who Need Extra Protein?

So far we've been talking about average protein requirements. Some people require more protein than others. Let's see what science has discovered about the protein requirements of infants, athletes, bedridden persons, and the elderly.

Infants

We can think of amino acids as the bricks that make up our muscles and other tissues. We need more bricks at the beginning of a construction project than during the maintenance phases; likewise, we need the most protein when we're babies just embarking on our journeys of growth and development. A full liter of breast milk contains, on average, 7–11 grams of protein. Healthy growing babies consume about 1.5 g/kg per day, or 50 percent more than the highest MIT recommendation for adults. Interestingly, breast-fed babies tend to take in less protein than those given formula, only about 7 percent of total calories, and don't develop problems as a result. In fact, breast-fed babies have better immune function, which suggests that the smaller protein intake isn't compromising their antigen response. Also, predictably, formula-fed babies tend to be heavier.

Athletes

This topic is a real tough one. My hypothesis is that the research has never asked the right question: How do we prevent muscle from wasting? Instead, every study focuses solely on building muscle in the short term. Sadly, the studies can't seem to decide the absolute amount of protein to improve performance and build muscle. Research shows that athletes do have higher protein requirements than the average person. But not all athletes are equal in this respect; one study showed that compared to sedentary people, bodybuilders required 5 percent more protein, while endurance athletes needed 67 percent more, just to maintain their respective muscle mass (Tarnopolsky, MacDougall, et al. 1988). One study of endurance athletes estimated their ideal protein intake by giving them three different diets of varying protein levels (0.6, 0.9, and 1.2 g/kg) and measuring whole-body protein turnover. Researchers found that 0.6 was too low while 1.2 made no difference compared to 0.9. The "Cinderella" number, therefore, was, found to be 0.94 g/kg (Meredith, Zackin, et al. 1989).

Interestingly, there are studies all over the place on protein synthesis and degradation. Very complex studies have been done looking at responses to high protein intake showing increased protein synthesis (Forslund, Hambraeus, et al. 1998). These studies look at complicated formulas analyzing oxidation of radioactively labeled amino acids. However, seldom do they provide real-world response. Does the higher protein group actually end up growing more muscle? Does the higher protein group run a faster marathon, or set a record at the bench press? While some studies show more protein synthesis with higher protein intake, others show that 1.0 g/kg is adequate with moderate exercise (el-Khoury, Forslund, et al. 1997).

A very large scale 2005 study produced by a joint US/Canadian Dietary Reference Intake Committee stated that "the lack of compelling evidence to the contrary, no additional dietary protein is suggested for healthy adults undertaking resistance or endurance exercise." Also, it found no evidence supporting a different protein requirement for vegetarians (Otten, Hellwig, et al., 2006).

Athletes need protein the most right after working out. Their muscles have been stimulated and are now ready to use protein to rebuild and grow. A 2009 study asked healthy young men to perform strenuous resistance exercise, the kind known to stimulate muscle synthesis the most. Researchers wanted to know what level of protein intake was needed during this "acute" phase to maximize muscle synthesis. It turned out that the magic number was 20 grams (Moore, Robinson, et al. 2009). A 2013 study found that postexercise protein consumption in excess of 20 grams leads to oxidation and ureagenesis, a fancy word for excess ammonia in the body. This indicates that the body is struggling to get rid of the excess protein, and that it's going to waste, at best, and more likely causing harm (Witard, Jackman, et al. 2013). In elderly men, 10 grams provided the maximum benefit (Esmarck, Andersen, et al. 2001).

A 2001 study found that adding protein in the absence of carbohydrates is pointless (Tipton and Wolfe 2001), although that is what you see happening at gyms every day. For a 2011 study, scientists fed drinks with varying combinations of carbs and protein to 8 healthy men, both during three hours of cycling and three hours of recovery. The researchers found that the carb/protein combination led to the greatest utilization and recovery (Hulston, Wolsk, et al. 2011), and yet I always see guys drinking pure protein drinks after exercising, worried that the carbs may make them fat.

A much better approach is to consume a reasonable amount of protein with carbs. The exact ratios are debated but likely you should have three to four times the amount of carbs compared to the protein. Though it flies in the face of the "bro science" that passes for gospel in many gyms, postworkout carbs are at least as important as protein in improving performance. Workout enthusiasts tell me, "Carbs will make me fat, so I stick to protein." What they're missing is that protein intake doesn't increase protein synthesis unless you include carbs. Muscles fed protein in the absence of carbs is like an engine full of gas that can't run because there's no oxygen.

In 2012, researchers performed an extensive meta-analysis of many studies that looked at the supposed benefits of protein supplementation in both young and older adults performing exercise. Unlike the above studies that looked at radioactive amino acid markers, these actually looked at muscle gain and strength. For young athletic males, supplementation did improve strength and gained muscle, 1 kilogram over twelve weeks more. Interestingly, with elderly participants, not a single study showed increased muscle with protein supplementation. Once all the studies were combined and analyzed, there was a statistically significant improvement but practically meaningless benefit to protein supplementation. The meta-analysis was far from perfect. The amounts of supplemental protein varied wildly, from 18 to 82 grams. Confounding factors were ignored; it's possible that the protein supplementation's mild positive effect was due to increased calories rather than protein per se. Also, many studies were omitted from the meta-analysis. Also keep in mind, these authors are not concerned with possible negative effects of high protein. I doubt they even think that exists. Their only concern is bigger and stronger muscles. If you are a bodybuilder or a high-level endurance athlete, these results may suggest some benefit to a postworkout smoothie that contains a protein supplement. However, the results are not so impressive that the average person needs to use a supplement after a power walk (Cermak, Res, et al. 2012).

In general, for the average person, the RDA is more than sufficient protein for an active lifestyle. For the very active weekend warrior, trying to get big or fast, 1.0 g/kg with 20 grams after workout may be ideal. For bodybuilders, I am not sure it is all that different but some do suggest 1.8 g/kg. Probably for the Olympic endurance athletes 1.8 may possibly be the right amount. I am being vague because the data is vague.

I will say this, I did an informal poll of vegan athletes. I found that most would do a postworkout smoothie with a plant-based protein supplement, but very few counted protein grams during the day. There were some surprisingly muscular men and women who told me they don't worry about protein at all. They just eat a varied plant-based diet.

I fall into this latter category. I never count my protein. I did measure for two weeks out of curiosity and I averaged between 60 to 70 grams of protein a day. I don't usually drink protein smoothies, preferring a meal after workouts. Since starting this lifestyle I have gained considerable muscle and keep getting faster. At forty-five I set a personal record in the marathon of 3 hours and 35 minutes, which is 21 minutes faster than the last two marathons I ran when I was forty.

The Bedridden

A sick person on bed rest has among the highest protein requirements in order to combat muscle loss. One clever 1990 study put healthy subjects on bed rest for seven days and fed them either a high-protein or low-protein diet during that time. The researchers measured leucine oxidation and turnover. The low-protein group formed less protein, but didn't suffer more muscle loss. The researchers suggested that the daily protein requirements of a person on bed rest may need to be as high as 1 g/kg, or 70 grams per day, for the average person, to preserve muscle (Stuart, Shangraw, et al. 1990). That's not much higher than the RDA and is a lot less than most of us are getting. Also, the two groups weren't getting the same number of calories, so any differences may have been due to fewer overall calories rather than specifically the result of decreased protein.

A 2004 study of 14-day bed-rest intervals found impaired anabolism (muscle building) and also recommended slightly higher protein requirements for the bedridden (Biolo, Ciocchi, et al. 2004).

The Elderly

Conventional wisdom holds that our protein requirements increase when we get older, all other things being equal, to avoid sarcopenia (muscle loss due to aging). But the research is not at all clear. One study's scientists fed older adults a diet of 0.8 g/kg protein and had them perform various levels of physical exercise. The researchers found that those who were exercising gained muscle, while those who were sedentary lost muscle. Big deal: they basically proved the old dictum, use it or lose it. They suggested that the muscle loss in the nonexercising group might have been prevented by giving them even more protein, but that was pure conjecture. What the study really showed was that the RDA was completely adequate in an elderly population that was exercising (Campbell, Trappe, et al. 2002).

Another study used more complex measurements to assess the effects of protein levels on muscle synthesis in exercising older adults. Researchers put healthy men and women ages 62–75 on low-, medium-, or high-protein diets and had them exercise. They found no difference in muscle synthesis among the three groups (Welle and Thornton 1998). Another study sought to prove the hypothesis that adding more animal protein to the diet would add muscle in people in their sixties and above. Researchers had 36 older people exercise and consume either 0.9 g/kg or 1.2 g/kg, the difference achieved through an increase in meat, eggs, and dairy. They found no difference in fat-free mass between the two groups after 12 weeks (Iglay, Apolzan, et al. 2009). Nitrogen balance studies show that healthy older individuals have the same protein requirements as younger adults, and that 0.85 g/kg is perfectly adequate (Campbell, Johnson, et al. 2008).

Preventing Sarcopenia

The 2013 PROT-AGE study found that older people need slightly more protein, recommending from 1.0 to 1.2 g/kg lean body mass. It appears to contradict the other studies that show no increased protein requirement for the elderly, but with one fascinating exception. Those elderly with severe kidney disease did not benefit from increased protein, as their kidneys could not process that protein excess quickly or efficiently enough as measured by glomerular filtration rate (GFR) (Bauer, Biolo, et al. 2013). We know that most older people with sarcopenia also have a low GFR, as well as hypertension, which can affect the kidney function. Given what we know by now about the effects of a high-protein diet, it's reasonable to hypothesize that a lifetime of heroic effort filtering that diet has worn out their kidneys. What if the cause of the sarcopenia epidemic (estimating to afflict up to 30% of the aging population) (Cruz-Jentoft, Landi, et al. 2014) is not a low-protein diet in the elderly, but from too much protein over their lifetimes? Here's a known mechanism: the excess protein converts in the body to excess acid, which the body buffers by leaching calcium from muscles. The result? Possibly sarcopenia (Adeva and Souto 2011).

Perhaps our paradigm has been upside down. Instead of treating sarcopenia by forcing chronically overworked kidneys to ever greater amounts of protein, we can prevent it by reducing our protein intake while we're young.

A 2012 study (Tieland, Dirks, et al. 2012) published in the *Journal of the American Medical Directors Association* also appeared to contradict the finding that we don't need more protein as we age, finding benefit with supplementation. Researchers took what they described as frail elderly people and randomized them to receive either twice daily 15 gram protein supplements or placebos. They concluded that the supplementation increased physical performance, but not muscle mass. When I read the whole study, however, I found a totally different story.

First, the average BMI of this "frail" population was 28.1, which makes them more overweight than frail. Second, the difference between the two groups could just have easily been explained by increased calories in the protein group, rather than the effects of the protein itself. Third, and most egregious, the actual results were misrepresented in the abstract and discussion. The effect of protein supplementation on performance, as measured by single leg press and leg extension reps, was actually the same between the two groups. The researchers boasted about the increase in leg strength in the protein supplementation group: " . . . physical performance had improved significantly following dietary protein supplementations."

The data show something else. The protein group did experience a significant improvement from start to end, beginning at an average of 124 and ending up at 169 kilograms. What the discussion completely ignored was the fact that the placebo group achieved a bigger improvement, from 116 to 162 kilograms over the 24 weeks! It turns out that the only significant contributor to leg strength was time, not supplementation.

Potential damage from excess protein in the elderly

There's no proof that the elderly need more protein than the rest of us, but we're beginning to see evidence that high-protein diets can actually be harmful. In a comprehensive review of the scientific literature, a 2013 paper concluded that excess protein may be especially toxic in the elderly as their kidneys cannot clear it rapidly enough (Dideriksen, Reitelseder, et al. 2013).

One study put this theory to the test by feeding a high-protein diet to a group of young people and a small group of elderly people. Neither group increased muscle synthesis, but the authors note that kidney function had decreased in the elderly. They expressed concern that the high-acid, high-purine diet (foods containing purines include organ meats as well as red meats, poultry, and fish) was taxing their kidneys to the point of damage (Walrand, Short, et al. 2008).

Outliers: Fruitarian Athletes

So far in this chapter we've been looking at the upper end of the protein requirement question: How much do we need to maintain and grow muscle mass and avoid compromising our immune systems? Given that excess protein has been shown to be so pervasively harmful, let's turn the question on its head: How little protein can we get away with?

One small group offers some anecdotal insight into that question: athletes whose diets consist entirely or almost entirely of raw fruit. Fruit is extremely low in protein, as you can see:

Fruit	Calories	Protein (grams)	% Calories from Protein
Apple	95	0.5	2.1
Banana	105	1.3	5.0
Orange	45	0.9	8.0
Mango	201	2.8	5.5

If we were ever to find a protein deficiency that wasn't also a calorie deficiency, it would be in raw fruitarians who are also endurance athletes. Minimum intake, maximum output. So what do we find?

Michael Arnstein is one of the top ultrarunners in the world, finishing 29th in the 2011 New York Marathon. To Michael, a 26-mile marathon is just a warm-up run; he enjoys 100-mile races over some of the toughest terrain imaginable (just look up Leadville 100, Badlands, and Desert Solstice 100 if your imagination isn't doing it for you). In December 2012 he achieved the sixth-fastest time in a 100-mile track race for an American. If anybody should be obsessing over protein, it's Michael. Instead, though, he eats thirty pounds of fruit a day; he estimates that 80–90 percent of his calories come from fruit, with the remaining 10–20 percent from raw vegetables like celery, lettuce, peppers (technically fruits), and beets.

He's not the only one, either. If you've spent time in the raw food vegan community online, you may have come across Durian Rider and Freelie the Banana Girl. Both extremely good athletes, they brag about eating thirty bananas a day, and not much else.

These athletes repair and grow muscle by eating fruit during and immediately after exercise, taking advantage of the perfect combination of carbs and amino acids, and avoiding the acidosis and kidney load that accompanies high-protein diets.

You may have seen a YouTube video* I did with my good friend Kristina Carrillo-Bucaram, also known as FullyRaw Kristina, who runs a co-op in Houston that sells boxes of local organic produce in the community (and who also runs six to eight miles a day). I often write prescriptions for her boxes to my bariatric patients, preferring to send them to the "farmacy" than the pharmacy. Kristina eats a predominantly fruit diet and appears to be the picture of health, but I wanted to check her labs just to be sure. Her protein levels and muscle strength were completely normal, prompting even me to wonder, *Where do you get your protein?*

It turns out that while fruit is relatively low in protein, it's got plenty of amino acids. And since we're so good at recycling our own amino acids, and since our gut bacteria seem to have the ability to synthesize the amino acids we may be lacking at any given moment, the amino acids in fruit are all we need to function in blissful protein sufficiency. Even when we eat badly, choosing processed junk over real food, we still get enough protein. It's practically impossible to design a protein-deficient diet that isn't also a starvation diet. If we're eating enough, we are eating enough protein.

This isn't theoretical speculation: most of the world's inhabitants get their protein from cereals like maize (corn), rice, and wheat. A comprehensive 1999 study conducted in the Indian states of Tamil Nadhu and West Bengal found that plant-based diets provided plenty of protein. Even when the bulk of calories came from maize, rather than the milk-protein casein, growth and weight in children were found to be normal, with no deficiencies identified. Their protein needs were higher than the WHO recommendations, but lower than that suggested by the MIT researchers. Protein supplementation beyond a plant-based diet was totally unnecessary (Millward 1999).

Perhaps the best way to think about our protein requirements is through a metaphor I mentioned earlier: amino acids are like bricks. They are obviously necessary for the construction of a brick wall, and they're needed when we want to extend the height or length or width of the wall. They're likewise required for ongoing maintenance, when we need to replace missing or broken or worn-out bricks.

---

* If not, you can watch it at http://j.mp/fullyraw.

But are more bricks always better? What if your house were built, and in fine repair, but a dump truck kept dropping loads of bricks on your front lawn and a forklift kept leaving pallets of bricks on your kitchen floor. At that point, those bricks would go from valuable building materials to dangerous nuisances.

That's the difference between enough and excess protein. Our bodies are exquisitely tuned to deal with the amount and type of protein we get from plants. Our GI tracts limit our intake. Our livers can detox only at a certain rate. Our kidneys work optimally when they aren't taxed by too much protein. A 1999 study sums up the trade-off well: " . . . the absence of strong evidence that high protein diets confer any advantage in terms of strength or health must be weighed against potentially injurious consequences" (Garlick, McNurlan, et al. 1999).

In this chapter, we've discovered science that shows we need far less protein than we think. And furthermore, despite Paleo protestations to the contrary, protein can and should come from plants, not animals.

Here's the thing about protein: it's vitally important for our survival. So important, in fact, I believe it deserves its name, meaning "of prime importance." It's so important that it's literally everywhere in our food supply, in more than sufficient quantities. Nature has made sure there's no way humans could suffer an accidental protein deficiency.

Here's one more metaphor to put the whole proteinaholic craze in perspective. You know what else we can't be deficient in? Oxygen. As long as we're breathing on planet Earth, we are taking in enough oxygen for all our needs. Luckily for us, the atmosphere of our planet consists of roughly 20 percent oxygen and 80 percent nitrogen (with a whole lot of other gases in very small quantities).

Now imagine a whole "low nitrogen breathing movement" that started insisting we were suffering from too much nitrogen in our air. They would write Paleo fantasies about how the air was mostly oxygen before the last Ice Age, and how we've become puny and weak since we started breathing this unnatural nitrogen-rich air. They would perform lab studies that showed breathing 100 percent oxygen for up to ninety seconds could enhance performance on treadmills and multiple-choice tests. They would blog endlessly about how astronauts thrived on 100 percent oxygen in space, neglecting to mention that those astronauts were living at reduced pressure.

They would start selling branded 100 percent oxygen canisters so we could carry a supply of "natural" air with us wherever we go. And they would then sell us the necessary supplements to help us deal with the effects of oxygen poisoning, like chest pains, fluid accumulation in the lungs, and collapsed alveoli.

Sounds ridiculous, right? But that's the low-carb, high-protein argument in a nutshell.

Here are my bottom-line answers to the question, How much protein should I get?

If you like counting, eat the RDA and don't worry about it.

If you don't like counting, then just don't worry about it.

If you are an elite athlete or bodybuilder, then there is evidence that a little more may be beneficial, but a little more is not what you are getting in the huge protein smoothies and multiple chicken breasts recommended by the "bro science." A smoothie with some fruits and hemp seeds is sufficient. If you cannot get away from the whey protein, 20 grams in a postworkout smoothie with fruit should be enough. Or like me, and many athletes you might find on websites like Veganbodybuilding.com, just don't worry about it.

Curious about your protein requirements? Have friends and family members who are getting way too much whey? Check out the protein requirement calculator at Proteinaholic.com.

CHAPTER 16

Reducing Animal Protein:
The Why, How, and What

I'm on Facebook pretty much every day, and I'm known for posting rants about food and health. One thing I've learned from reading the comments to these posts is that when people have strong beliefs, facts are pretty much irrelevant. And of all the things we have opinions on, we often hold on most urgently to our beliefs in what we should eat. It's actually easier to talk about religion than food. People have "faith" in their diet and rationalize their choices, no matter how much science is thrown their way.

People defend their diets so dogmatically partly because they are so hard to change. We are creatures of habit, seeking the foods that have comforted us throughout our lives. When I discuss diet with my patients, they frequently tell me just how delicious hamburgers are. If I mention a food like broccoli, their immediate knee-jerk reaction is to tell me how they are not vegetable eaters and cannot fathom eating broccoli. It is a texture thing, they tell me.

After years of helping people change their diets, I am still surprised at how readily we pigeonhole ourselves into certain mind-sets. I think of them more as mind blocks. We are not our tastes. Our beliefs, preferences, and habits are all just a result of early conditioning, social programming, and the grooves cut deep by repeated thoughts and activities over a lifetime.

We are not even who we think we are. I have seen people completely change their lives and challenge all that they thought they knew of themselves. Fast-food-eating couch potatoes transform into athletes who crave their apples and kale. You may have to see it to believe it, but I am blessed to get to see it daily.

I, myself, am a prime example of such a transformation. For the first thirty-five years of my life I was a hamburger-consuming fiend. I cannot even recall eating a single vegetable during all that time. Had someone suggested I put broccoli on the menu, they would have seen one of my own mental blocks in action. I would simply have replied that I was a meat eater and didn't like broccoli. I understand both how hard it is to change, and how easy it can become, once we have the courage to face our own limiting beliefs and self-definitions.

Of course, I didn't change out of the blue. I had hit a frightening wall; my health was spiraling downward even as I was being celebrated as a paragon of health. As I faced my own mortality a lot earlier than I was expecting, I began doing the research that I've shared in this book. The science, as I have shown you, was crystal clear: I had to change my diet completely if I wanted to halt my own march to disease and early death. I clearly remember reading one well-written article on the effects of a vegan diet on the endocrine system. The study found a vegan diet was correlated with reduced cancer, obesity, and heart disease. In the discussion, the author noted that the data was so overwhelming that he decided to go vegan. The article concluded, "I suspect the single injunction 'do not eat animal products' has the potential to do more for world health than all of the abstruse wisdom in all of the world's medical libraries" (McCarty 1999). That really stuck with me, that a researcher could be so convinced by the data that he would change his own diet.

I wasn't thrilled about it, at that point. Despite finding the solution to my own health crisis, I felt more desperate than hopeful, more depressed than excited. I had to change my diet; I had to give up everything I usually ate and switch to everything I never thought I would eat. In Chapter 3, I wrote about my own winding and bumpy road to change. In this chapter, I want to focus on the why, the what, and the how of going plant based. I'll relate the principles and tactics that I used not only to change my diet, but to learn to love my new way of eating. And since I've personally helped many of my patients take the same journey, I've learned a lot about what works in helping people recover from their proteinaholism and embrace plant-based eating. If you're ready to say yes to your health, this chapter and the next are the parts of the book where I'll show you how to transform your thinking, your diet, and your health destiny.

When you want to change anything significant, you need to ask and answer three primary questions:

1. Why should I change?

2. What should I do differently?

3. How do I go about changing?

The rest of this chapter addresses these three questions in detail.

Why Should I Change?

It is vital to establish your "why." "My doctor says I should" doesn't have a lot of motivating power in it. When you lack a powerful, personal, and meaningful reason to go plant based, you'll be helpless the next time someone offers you a pizza or a hot dog. You don't need goals to keep doing what you have always done; habit alone will keep reinforcing your behaviors. But when you want to change—especially when your new behavior puts you at odds with your environment—you'll need to arm yourself with personal motivation. When you can recall at any moment the deep reasons you're avoiding processed food and animal foods, it becomes much easier to make good choices.

I have my patients write down their goals and keep them readily accessible. Many of them carry index cards they can pull out when tempted by some food that will taste good in the moment but move them away from their big goals. You can also write down why you are changing your diet and tape the list of reasons to your bathroom mirror. That way you can start every day enlisting your conscious and subconscious as allies in your quest.

My own "why" was obvious. Here's my own goal statement:

I'm only thirty-five and I've just been diagnosed with high blood pressure, high cholesterol, and fatty liver. I also have terrible irritable bowel syndrome. To make matters worse, I'm supposed to be an expert at helping people lose weight. I feel like a hypocrite.

I want to live a long, healthy life. I want to enjoy my wife and my two beautiful daughters. I want to have energy to be with them, have fun with them, and take care of them. I want to see my daughters grow up.

I want to feel better right now. I want to be able to go out without constantly worrying about sitting close to the bathroom. I want to have an active social life unencumbered by embarrassment or fear.

I want to walk my talk as a doctor and weight-loss expert. I want to give my patients the right advice, which I myself follow. I want to help them lose weight and feel great about themselves. I want to be a role model, inspiration, and guide for my patients.

As I became healthier and slimmer, I started adding goals that would have seemed ludicrous at first: getting fit, running twenty miles a week, entering a marathon, becoming a competitive triathlete. As I mentioned, I'm still growing and figuring out how to spend the tremendous energy that my diet and lifestyle generate.

Let's go over some of the most powerful whys of a plant-based diet.

Health Whys

I constantly remind myself of the health benefits of a plant-based diet. We've seen, in great detail, how plant-based diets help protect against diabetes, hypertension, heart disease, obesity, cancer, and premature death. That is just scratching the surface. Studies show (and my personal experience confirms) that a plant-based diet also helps with inflammatory bowel disease. If you have ulcerative colitis, a vegan diet can keep you in remission and greatly reduce the need for harmful medication by lowering the inflammation in your body. I know people who suffer horribly from inflammatory bowel disease, and this should be a huge why on their goal list (David, Maurice, et al. 2014; de Silva, Olsen, et al. 2010; Adam, Beringer, et al. 2003; Chiba, Abe, et al. 2010; Jantchou, Morois, et al. 2010).

I also see many patients suffering with severe rheumatoid arthritis (RA). Like inflammatory bowel disease, RA is exacerbated by the inflammatory high-animal-protein diet. A plant-based diet can greatly ameliorate and sometimes cure RA (McDougall, Bruce, et al. 2002; Müller, de Toledo, et al. 2001; Elkan, Sjöberg, et al. 2008).

One of the most common disorders in our Western world is diverticulosis, in which the wall of the colon develops outpouchings and can burst.

Denis Burkitt noted that populations with high-fiber, low-animal-protein diets had low to no diverticulosis, and subsequent studies have proved him correct (Gear, Ware, et al. 1979; Korzenik 2006). In fact, long-term studies show vegetarians have a 31 percent lower chance of developing diverticulosis (Crowe, Appleby, et al. 2011).

The most commonly performed general surgery in this country is gallbladder removal. The typical patient is described as "fat, female, and forty," as if having these demographics predestines you to having your gallbladder surgically removed. We could greatly reduce the rate of this disease by adopting a plant-based diet. In fact, studies show the reduction in gallstone disease with plant-based diet happens regardless of whether or not you lose weight (Pixley, Wilson, et al. 1985; Tsai, Leitzmann, et al. 2004).

Meat breaks down in the body to purines and uric acid. These substance cause gout, which can be an extremely painful arthritic condition. Often the pain is so severe that even slightly touching the toe can cause the patient to scream. Possibly even more painful are the kidney stones that can form from uric acid. While I personally haven't had the "pleasure," I've heard that kidney stones are one of the most painful things you can develop. And I've seen too many patients writhing in pain on a hospital gurney to ever go back to my old diet. If you switch to a plant-based diet, uric acid drops precipitously and kidney stones and gout can be avoided (Choi, Atkinson, et al. 2004; Siener and Hesse 2003; Reddy, Wang, et al. 2002; Adeva and Souto 2011).

Cataracts are a horrible disorder, causing our vision to cloud as we age. I had always thought of this as an inevitable part of aging. In Chapter 15, of course, we learned that our rate of aging is highly influenced by what we eat. It turns out that vegans have a 40 percent lower rate of cataract formation over a lifetime, and this is compared to infrequent meat eaters in Oxford, England (Appleby, Allen, et al. 2011). Switching to a plant-based diet with no dairy or eggs is likely to lower the risk of cataracts even more.

Even mental illness has been linked to how we eat. Studies have shown that diets high in amino acids and high in fat are linked with worse mood, worse concentration on mental tasks, and higher rates of dementia (Brinkworth, Buckley, et al. 2009; de Castro 1987; Beezhold and Johnston 2012; Giem, Beeson, et al. 1993; Wing, Vazquez, et al. 1995).

Obviously, the list of health benefits can easily answer the question, "Why should I switch to a plant-based diet?" But in order to change the brain and eliminate our harmful habits, the why has to be very powerful. There are many other reasons I will touch on that can help clarify and amplify your desire to switch to a plant-based diet.

Bigger Whys: Environment and Kinship

Eating a plant-based diet is one of the most powerful actions you can take on behalf of the environment. A 2010 report from the United Nations Environment Programme's (UNEP) international panel of sustainable resource management states that as the global population increases, and dependence on animal products increases, our diet becomes more unsustainable. "Impacts from agriculture are expected to increase substantially due to population growth and increasing consumption of animal products. Unlike fossil fuels, it is difficult to look for alternatives: people have to eat. A substantial reduction of impacts would only be possible with a substantial worldwide diet change, away from animal products."

Professor Edgar Hertwich, the lead author of the report, said, "Animal products cause more damage than [producing] construction minerals such as sand or cement, plastics or metals. Biomass and crops for animals are as damaging as [burning] fossil fuels."

The Intergovernmental Panel on Climate Change recently reported that climate change is in fact real, and that humans are having a substantial negative impact. As of this writing, the California drought has become so dire that severe water restrictions have been enacted, with more likely to come. For the first time, we're becoming aware that fresh water is a valuable and quite limited resource. Animal-based diets increase demand for water and fossil fuels. Raising so many animals to satisfy our voracious appetites produces huge waste streams, which poison our atmosphere and our water. Up to 75 percent of our farmland is used to raise grains to feed the animals, and the water consumption required for such agriculture far overshadows any other uses (Pimentel and Pimentel 2003).

I also think it is important to look at the cruelty aspect of eating animals. Watch the PETA videos, as hard as they are to witness. My whys were initially all about health, but as I learned more about the effects of my diet choices on the environment, and the more I saw how cruelly these animals were treated, the less appetizing the hamburger became. Eating a plant-based diet, beyond all its health benefits, has also made me feel like I am part of something larger. I am part of a movement that really is based on love and caring for our planet and for the creatures that share the planet with us.

Luigi Fontana, codirector of the Longevity Project at Washington University in St. Louis, wrote a powerful and moving opinion piece on plant-based diets. This quote summarizes my why completely:

"At the individual level, reducing the intake of calories by increasing the consumption of a variety of minimally processed plant foods and by significantly reducing the intake of animal foods will significantly increase health span and reduce health care costs, environmental pollution, soil erosion, water pollution and shortage, CO_2 production and global warming, violent weather and associated planetary consequences" (Fontana, Atella, et al. 2013).

Understanding your why and keeping it close to your mind and heart can help you make serious inroads to change behaviors you spent a lifetime building and reinforcing.

The Why Nots (Myths)

I would be remiss if I did not address the "why nots" of adopting a plant-based diet. There are many myths about vegan diets propagated by people who don't know the research. The most common one asserts that a vegan/vegetarian diet is deficient in essential vitamins, which proves that it's dangerous and unnatural. I find this myth ironic in the extreme, given that I run lab tests on thousands of meat eaters and most of them are extremely vitamin deficient. I diagnose B_{12}, thiamine, iron, and especially vitamin D deficiency in meat eaters on a regular basis. I also have found high rates of osteoporosis in people coming to see me for weight issues who are eating high-animal-protein diets.

The B_{12} Myth

You will hear the claim that a vegan diet must be bad for you because it is a vitamin-deficient diet due to the lack of B_{12}. And, in fact, strict vegans do become deficient in one vitamin: B_{12}. As I mentioned, though, I do see B_{12} deficiency in some meat eaters too, and others corroborate this persistent observation (Tucker, Rich, et al. 2000). Until recently it was quite easy to get enough B_{12} from plant food. The problem isn't choosing produce over beef; rather, it's the inorganic, pesticide-laden soil in which most of our produce is grown. B_{12} is made by bacteria, not animals. The reason most meat eaters can get enough B_{12} is that meat is heavily laden with B_{12}-producing bacteria.

If you could grow vegetables in truly organic soil, without tons of pesticides, and you ate these vegetables with minimal washing, you would likely get more than enough B_{12}. In the interest of science, I tried this experiment on myself once. We ordered our produce from a very organic local farm. The veggies came complete with grubs, soil, and many insects. I hate to say it, but I was kind of grossed out by the number of insects I found as I washed the plants. I tested my B_{12} while consuming this produce and found that it stayed normal in the absence of supplementation. However, I had a hard time staying that close to nature. I still eat organic produce from Whole Foods and other supermarkets and farmers' markets, but now it comes to me cleaner. I take a B_{12} supplement once a week, when I remember, and I have never had a B_{12} deficiency, despite not eating any animal protein for many years.

One more observation about B_{12} deficiency. If you are deficient in B_{12}, it should have several clinical presentations, from neurologic disorders to anemias, in addition to just being a red number on your lab test. Also, if B_{12} is low, then homocysteine should rise, a phenomenon that has been documented in vegans in different studies (Elmadfa and Singer 2009). Now, high homocysteine, theoretically, should increase the risk of heart disease. So I'd like to know: Where are all the vegans with heart attacks? As we saw in Chapter 11, people who minimize or eliminate animal protein have less heart disease. So, although B_{12} is a concern with our modern-day food production, vegans are not experiencing large-scale nutritional deficiencies with clinically poor outcomes. Quite the opposite. And to put your mind totally at ease, you only need a small amount of B_{12}, 100 mcg daily, to keep your B_{12} at completely healthy levels. You can take a weekly supplement, which is easy and costs almost nothing.

B_{12} is the only real deficiency seen in vegans, despite what you may hear. The National Health and Nutrition Examination Survey (NHANES) used a healthy eating index to evaluate the diets of Americans. Researchers were able, through their surveys, to distinguish vegetarians and to analyze their diet compared to the rest of the public. They found that vegetarians and vegans got higher fiber, calcium, magnesium, iron, vitamin A, vitamin C, vitamin E, thiamine, riboflavin, and folate, all while consuming fewer calories and less cholesterol (Farmer, Larson, et al. 2011). Certainly it is possible to eat an unhealthy vegan diet, especially given the processed vegan food items available at the grocery. The one and only vegan I've ever treated for obesity had a penchant for the fake vegan-chicken nuggets and vegan cookies. I especially see poor diets in the so-called ethical vegans who abstain from meat due to concerns about animal cruelty but are not particularly concerned about health. That said, even ethical vegans still appear to have a far healthier diet than the normal American (Haddad and Tanzman 2003). Even if you simply compare low-carb versus high-carb dieters, you will find the high-carb dieters tend to eat fewer calories but more fiber, vitamin A, vitamin C, folate, carotene, magnesium, and potassium (Bowman and Spence 2002).

The Brittle Bones Myth

Vegetarians and vegans get more than enough calcium, yet one of the biggest why nots I hear is that becoming vegan causes brittle bones. As a nation, we've been completely brainwashed by the milk industry's marketing campaigns for well over fifty years. We are captivated by the milk mustaches on our favorite shirtless actors and athletes. We recognize and mostly believe the slogan "Milk, it does a body good." We're taught in schools and by our doctors that dairy is essential for bone health. Eliminating animal protein means eliminating dairy, which must mean brittle bones.

Looking at the science, however, we find this not to be true. In fact, we see the opposite: vegans appear to have stronger bones. Studying the effects of diet on bone health is very difficult as there are many variables. Contrary to dairy propaganda, it is not all about calcium. Potassium, magnesium, fiber, beta-carotene, and vitamin C may be equally important in bone health, and all are largely deficient in the typical American, high-protein diet (New, Bolton-Smith, et al. 1997).

Vegetarians may have stronger bones than dairy drinkers, and this may be due to a larger fruit and vegetable consumption (New 2004). A review of 34 studies showed that people who consumed animal protein had a higher risk of hip fracture when compared to vegetarians (Abelow, Holford, et al. 1992).

How can this be? Shouldn't milk make your bones stronger? Here's how: a high-animal-protein diet is, as we have established, a high-acid diet. The body has to compensate for this excess acid production by any means necessary; if our blood pH strays even slightly from normal, we begin to die. The typical Western diet produces 50–100 meq* of acid daily, and a

---

* This is the abbreviation for milliequivalents, a fancy scientific term used to talk about concentrations of a substance in a solution.

high-protein, low-carb diet will produce even more. The more protein consumed, the higher the concentrations of acid in the urine, along with an increase in calcium in the urine (Wynn, Krieg, et al. 2010). The calcium increases in order to buffer the acid to maintain a healthy blood pH. But where does the body get the calcium? Studies show that with high-protein diets, more calcium is excreted in the urine than is consumed (Reddy, Wang, et al. 2002). That is, the calcium is actually being leached from both bone and muscle. High-protein dieters compound the problem by limiting their fruit intake, thereby limiting other essential bone nutrients, leading to even more bone disease.

The EPIC study found that vegans who ate a minimal 525 milligrams of calcium daily (the equivalent of one Tums tablet) had the same fracture rates as their meat-eating counterparts (Appleby, Roddam, et al. 2007). Meanwhile, a well-run prospective study that followed 1,000 women over age 65 for 7 years found that the more animal protein eaten, the higher the rate of bone fractures and the higher the loss of bone density (Sellmeyer, Stone, et al. 2001). The comprehensive Nurses' Health Study also found that women consuming higher animal protein actually had higher rates of forearm fractures compared to people eating more vegetable protein (Feskanich, Willett, et al. 1996).

Even studies of vegan Buddhist nuns, known to have lower than average calcium intake, found that while the nuns had lower than average bone mineral density, they had equal rates of fracture compared to dairy-drinking controls (Ho-Pham, Nguyen, and Nguyen 2009; Ho-Pham, Nguyen, et al. 2009).

The bottom line is that there is ample calcium in fruits and vegetables, as well as many other bone-building nutrients. The bioavailability of calcium in greens like kale (that is, the amount of the nutrient that is available for our bodies to metabolize) is upwards of 50 percent, compared to just 30 percent in milk. Eat your greens and you don't have to worry about your bones.

The Anemia Myth

The other myth I am constantly forced to dispel is the idea that a plant-based diet lacks iron and will therefore result in anemia. In fact, vegetarians do tend to have lower iron stores, but as I have mentioned in earlier chapters, excess iron, and in particular heme iron, may be an indicator and instigator for disease. Excess iron poses an oxidative stress to the system (Reif 1992). Scientists studying aging have found iron stored in dying cells, which may indicate that excess iron and minerals may contribute to aging. While vegetarians and vegans may have lower iron stores, they do not have iron deficiency and certainly do not show increased incidence of anemia (Hunt 2003; Ball and Bartlett 1999).

The Hypothyroid Myth

Recently, an article on the web claimed that cruciferous veggies make you hypothyroid. The author says she went to her doctor and he explained that her vegetarian diet was making her hypothyroid (insufficient production of thyroid hormone). The article went viral, and many people posted it to my Facebook page, either because they wanted to hear my response, or because they wanted to show me the error of my ways. Why people believe what they read on the web I will never understand, but this particular article gained a lot of traction and worried a lot of vegetarians unnecessarily. It's completely false, a fact that didn't take a lot of research time on my part to confirm. Vegans are actually far less likely to be hypothyroid than their meat-eating compatriots (Tonstad, Nathan, et al. 2013). It is true that some cruciferous veggies and soy can bind iodine and thereby limit a substrate necessary for making thyroid hormone, but we should have ample iodine in our American diet. Some iodized salt on your broccoli and all is well. Strange that the doctor told the patient that she was hypothyroid because she eats vegetables. I wonder what he tells his thousands of meat-eating patients when they become hypothyroid.

The Low HDL Myth

Some people claim that a plant-based diet is harmful because it decreases HDL levels, commonly known as "good cholesterol." HDL is indeed a good thing: it's a carrier protein, used to shuttle dietary cholesterol out of the bloodstream before it can do harm. However, if you do not eat cholesterol (which appears only in animal foods), then you do not need HDL. Vegans do have lower HDL but, as we saw in Chapter 11, they have far lower heart disease levels. HDL turns out not to be a very good indicator of heart disease. Low-carb/high-animal-protein diets typically raise HDL and are therefore celebrated, but studies clearly show that the rise in LDL, the "bad cholesterol," is far more predictive of heart disease than a fall in

HDL (Briel, Ferreira-Gonzalez, et al. 2009; Ray, Wainwright, et al. 2012; Nicholls, Lundman, et al. 2006; Voight, Peloso, et al. 2012; Brinton, Eisenberg, et al. 1990).

Vegans Are Weak Myth

Finally, there is this preconceived notion that if you eat a vegan diet you will become a frail weakling. The reality is that, as word spreads, many athletes are adopting a plant-based diet for competitive reasons. Football players like Arian Foster and Tony Gonzales, boxers like Timothy Bradley, and UFC fighter Mac Danzig have all switched to plant-based diets in part to improve their athletic performance. The record-breaking sprinter Carl Lewis credited a switch to a vegan diet for some of his best times on the track, and Dave Scott is one of the best Ironman triathletes ever, winning an astounding six Ironman World Championships on a plant-based diet.

Rich Roll credits his vegan diet for changing his life, aiding him in overcoming addictions to fast food and junk food and fueling him on his way to becoming a top endurance athlete. His book *Finding Ultra* is a must-read for anyone who still doubts that a plant-based diet can support incredible achievement. Scott Jurek is considered on of the top ultramarathoners in the world, and his book *Eat and Run* reviews how he fuels with plants to win grueling 100-mile races. Finally, I have to credit the book *Thrive* by renowned triathlete Brendan Brazier as critical in helping me design a plant-based diet that gave me the energy to get off the couch and complete an Ironman triathlon. I could not have completely the 2.4-mile swim, 112-mile bike ride, and 26.2-mile run consecutively in the same day were it not for my change in diet.

None of these athletes appear even the slightest bit weak or frail. In fact, all of them describe how a plant-based diet actually helped them train more intensely than their rivals by shortening their recovery time. If you are more interested in pure muscle than performance, I invite you to visit Veganbodybuilding.com, where you will meet many vegan bodybuilders. I find it strange that people believe it's not possible to build muscle with plants.

"People eat meat thinking they will become strong as an ox,
forgetting that the ox eats grass."
—PINO CARUSO

What Should I Do Differently?

Now that we have covered the whys and why nots, let's look at the "what," specifically what should you eat. If you are religious, please turn in your Bible to Genesis 1:29: "Then God said, 'Behold, I have given you every plant yielding seed that is on the surface of all the earth, and every tree which has fruit yielding seed; it shall be food for you; and to every beast of the earth and to every bird of the sky and to every thing that moves on the earth which has life, I have given every green plant for food'; and it was so. . . ."

Or you could turn to the Book of Daniel in the Old Testament. Daniel, you'll recall from Chapter 9, was held captive by King Nebuchadnezzar. He was offered the king's wine and food, including meat, but instead thrived on vegetables, pulses (beans), and water.

If, instead, you are more inclined to be convinced by nature, I'll remind you of all the research presented in the Paleo chapter (Chapter 7) that outlines how we are perfectly designed as plant eaters, and how people who consume a plant-based diet tend to live longer and healthier lives. We are poorly designed to eat animal protein; we do not handle acid nearly as well as carnivores, and our jaws, saliva, and intestines are better designed to consume plants and fruits.

To put it as simply as possible, I tell my patients to eat the earth's bounty. Any food that can be grown from the ground or in a tree or a vine becomes fair game. Anything with a mother, or with eyes, should be eaten in a limited fashion, or avoided completely. You should also avoid or significantly decrease dairy, as it comes directly from an animal and is designed specifically for the young of that animal. Of course, you certainly can eat some animal protein and still be healthy, but the less you eat, the better off you are. If you do eat meat, make it a condiment. Turn the American plate around: let the veggies have the starring role and make the meat a side dish or a flavoring the way it's eaten in Blue Zone cultures.

I eat a far more varied diet than I ever did as a meat eater. People think I need massive amounts of willpower, imagining me suffering on a boring, bland diet and envying the plates of everyone around me. Nothing could be further from the truth. On the contrary, I eat a wide variety of meals that happen to be nutritious as well as delicious. Best of all, I feel healthy after eating them.

If you want to avoid the veggie burger diet (that really did take willpower and made me feel like my way of eating was a pale imitation of "real" food), concentrate on fruits, veggies, nuts, beans, whole grains, and seeds. I try to make sure I eat a whole fruit at least once a day, like a banana, apple, pear, peach, kiwi, and so on. I also always try to eat a serving of berries daily, sometimes on top of my morning cereal, sometimes as a snack or dessert. It doesn't matter what kind—all edible berries are awesome.

For veggies, I try to eat some raw veggies every day in a salad. I go for dark greens like spinach and kale. Romaine lettuce is great too. Mustard and collard greens are fantastic.

I also want to make sure I eat some cruciferous veggies; I usually put them in salads. Not to brag, but I have become quite the salad bar artist. Cauliflower, with its sulforaphane (a cancer-killing substance), makes a nice color contrast to the broccoli and bell peppers with which it shares the bowl. Top all that off with pumpkin seeds, loaded with magnesium, and some plain or infused balsamic vinegar, and you have a fantastic lunch.

We also cook veggies. I love steamed veggies; they're quick and easy to prepare, and steaming brings out their flavor nicely. I often add some wilted spinach to my whole-grain pasta. Throwing veggies on the grill gives them a nice smoky flavor. And don't forget your mushrooms, which I know are technically not vegetables, but fungi. Mushrooms are a great source of B vitamins and minerals, and there is even vitamin D in button mushrooms. The large portbello mushrooms have a meaty texture and make a great burger, topped with grilled or roasted or raw veggies and served on a whole-grain bun.

Don't be afraid of using frozen fruits and veggies. Often, they are more nutritious than the fresh ones. From the moment it is harvested, produce begins to lose its vitamins. Most of our produce travels thousands of miles to get to our stores, and a lot of nutrition is lost during that journey. Frozen produce is harvested, washed, and immediately frozen, locking in much of the vitamins. It also tends to be cheaper, even when organic.

I am not the least bit impressed by "superfoods," which for the most part are just regular plants with a hefty marketing budget. Sure, acai berries may have a lot of antioxidants—when you pick them fresh in the Amazon jungle. But by the time they are juiced, mixed with preservatives, and bottled for the long, hot journey to your local pyramid scheme distributor, they have lost much of their value. Meanwhile, the cheap and abundant blueberry is available at your local farmers' market, fresh and sweet and loaded with antioxidants.

I also avoid juices for the most part. It turns out fruits and vegetables are perfectly packaged. The sugars in fruit are designed to work almost like a time release pill, due to their relationship and binding with the fiber. When you juice, you uncouple this perfect package by removing the fiber. Studies show that fiber intake alone may be responsible for longer and healthier lives (Chuang, Norat, et al. 2012). Most Americans suffer from fiber deficiency. Most of us are constipated, and many suffer from GI problems such as diverticulosis or even cancer. Yet we sit in front of juicers and watch that all important fiber spit out the side of the machine as waste. The most ridiculous thing to me is a prolonged juice fast for detox purposes. Fiber is the most detoxifying substance we can consume. It literally scrubs your insides. You can't detox without fiber.

Healthy fats are also an important part of a well-balanced diet, so I make sure to add a serving of nuts and seeds daily. Studies have shown that a handful of nuts a day does not increase weight, and they can be a great source of minerals and electrolytes. If you have a tendency to gain weight, make sure you don't overdo the nuts, however. There are many well-regarded nutrition experts who promote a very low-fat vegan diet. Practitioners and researchers such as Caldwell Esselstyn, Dean Ornish, John McDougall, and T. Colin Campbell have demonstrated stellar heart health on a very low-fat diet. On these diets, nuts are minimized or even totally avoided because they are calorie dense. McDougall also points out, in his book *The Starch Solution* and in most of his talks, that "the fat you eat is the fat you wear." He's absolutely correct: unlike carbs, which are burned or stored as glycogen after eating, fat is readily stored as fat. In fact, if I were to take a piece of fat from your butt, I could send it to a lab that can determine exactly what you have been eating.

It is, in fact, another misconception that vegans do not get enough omega-3 fatty acids. We certainly need omega-3 in our diets, and fish do provide a ready source of omega-3 in the form of chemicals called DHA and EPA. Plants have a chemical called ALA, and studies suggest that vegetarians can convert ALA readily to DHA and EPA (Welch, Shakya-Shrestha, et al. 2010).

Omega-3 levels by themselves don't tell us much about health. This gets confusing but I'll try to simplify. Inflammation in the body partly depends on the ratio of omega-6 fat to omega-3 fat, which ideally is somewhere between 1:1 and 4:1. Unfortunately, in this country the omega-6 to omega-3 ratio is more like 15:1 (Simopoulos 2006). We can decrease our inflammation, therefore, by decreasing omega-6, or increasing omega-3, or a combination.

The main source of omega-6 in our diets is food cooked with vegetable oils. Cutting out fried food would certainly drop levels and bring the ratio back into healthy balance. I do very little cooking with oils. Any oil is a heavily processed food, and the processing is usually heat related and can greatly damage the oil. Oil is also the most calorie-dense food there is. Registered dietitian Jeff Novick pointed out to me that the nutrition label for PAM cooking spray lists zero calories and zero fat. How is that possible, given that PAM is pure fat, at 9 calories per gram? The answer can be found in the fine print, under serving size. Until recently, the serving size was given as a spray lasting one-third of a second. Under FDA rules, food manufacturers are allowed to round down to zero at certain threshold levels. The next time someone sprays PAM on a frying pan, get out your stopwatch and time them. I'll bet it will be many multiples of a third of a second. The new PAM goes one better; the latest label has decreased spray time to one-fourth of a second, which comes out to 0.2 grams of PAM.

Many of the excess calories we consume can be attributed to all the oils we cook with. When a restaurant lists the calorie content of its food, for example, it doesn't include the puddles of calorie-dense oil coating its slick grills.

Cutting back omega-6 helps balance the ratio, but how can you increase omega-3? You could eat fish, many species of which are high in omega-3. Unfortunately, we have overfished our waters and severely polluted them with runoff from our land animal agriculture. The result is fish with dangerously high concentrations of heavy metals in their fat. When I first started changing my diet, I still ate fish. I checked my labs and was shocked to find I had high levels of mercury in my blood.

When you buy fish in the supermarket or order it at a restaurant, you are usually getting farmed fish. Fish get their omega-3 from eating algae. The fish in farms are fed grains, not algae. So they have a lot less omega-3 than you probably think. Farmed fish also get diseases due to overcrowded conditions in their tanks, just like the animals in factory farms. The fish suffer from sea lice and are contaminated with PCBs and dioxin, chemicals that may have several toxic effects when we consume them. There is also mounting evidence that fish oil capsules can oxidize and that fish oil supplementation can increase prostate cancer (Brasky, Darke, et al. 2013) and may not prevent heart disease (Roncaglioni, Tombesi, et al. 2013).

Given that vegans have very low heart disease and inflammation levels, maybe just avoiding omega-6 is sufficient. Personally, I feel better adding a little omega-3 from seeds or nuts just to be extra sure. Despite the fact that nuts are dense in calories, studies show nut eaters tend to have lower weight (Casas-Agustench, Bulló, et al. 2011; Flores-Mateo, Rojas-Rueda, et al. 2013). Why can you eat extra nuts and still maintain weight is not quite known. Again, we're talking about a small handful. Don't binge eat them. Also, don't think honey-roasted peanuts. I am talking about raw or soaked almonds, walnuts, cashews, Brazil nuts, macadamia nuts, and others. It turns out that nuts are a large part of the healthiest diets in the world and have been associated with a decrease in chronic disease (Bao, Han, et al. 2013).

Nuts are high in plant-based protein, fiber, vitamins, and especially minerals like magnesium. Walnuts tend to have the best nutritional profile with less calorie density but the highest omega-3 concentrations. Seeds are also a great source of omega-3, as well as other nutrients. Ground flaxseed has plenty of omega-3, as do hemp and chia seeds. I use all three as toppings on my salad and oatmeal. Finally, if you have a nut allergy, you can just take algae supplements to increase your omega-3 intake (Geppert, Kraft, et al. 2005).

My diet typically consists of roughly 60–70 percent carbs. As we've seen, the healthiest societies have all eaten high-carb diets. Rice and potatoes are my go-to carbs. Remember, potatoes are among the most satiating foods you can eat (Holt, Miller, et al. 1995). Like the very healthy Sardinians, I eat whole-grain breads and pastas, and I strongly encourage my patients to overcome their fear of grains and do so as well. Whole grains are associated with lower heart disease and protect against cancer, diabetes, and even weight gain (Mellen, Walsh, et al. 2008; Slavin 2003; Ye, Chacko, et al. 2012). Most people believe the Mediterranean diet is one of the healthiest, yet they seem to miss the fact that bread is a major part of the diet, and partly responsible for its lifesaving properties (Gil, Ortega, et al. 2011).

While populations have thrived on grains for over ten thousand years, all of a sudden people fear them. Did we all suddenly become gluten intolerant, out of nowhere? It turns out this gluten intolerance may be way overblown. Researchers took a group of people complaining of gluten sensitivities and randomized them to a high-gluten, medium-gluten, or low-gluten diet, without letting them know which diet they were consuming. In the end, they all complained of GI symptoms equally (Biesiekier-ski, Muir, et al. 2013; Biesiekierski, Peters, et al. 2013). I suspect that most cases of so-called gluten intolerance are actually symptoms of having the wrong bowel bacteria to help process the food we should be eating. After all, our gut biome changes extremely rapidly when we eat meat (David, Maurice, et al. 2014), and vegetarians seem to have different, more benefi-cial bacteria in their bowels. Avoiding grains means you are avoiding fiber and fructo-oligosaccharides that feed the good bacteria in our bowels.

This may be the reason my irritable bowel syndrome completely van-ished after changing my diet. From a diet heavy in chicken and meat, I now eat pasta primavera and whole-grain breads with almond butters, and my GI system feels great.

If that is not convincing enough, grains are loaded with B vitamins, minerals, plant sterols, and omega fats. I am often shocked by the low B vitamins I see in my carb-avoiding, meat-eating patients. Atkins also noticed this, but he advised all his patients to take vitamins (which he hap-pily and profitably sold them). Why not just eat some whole-wheat pasta or Ezekiel bread (made with wheat, millet, barley, spelt, soybeans, and lentils) and save your money?

To make sure you're getting real whole grains, you have to get good at reading labels. The Whole Grain Council states: "Whole grains or foods made from them contain all the essential parts and naturally-occurring nutrients of the entire grain seed in their original proportions. If the grain has been processed (e.g., cracked, crushed, rolled, extruded, and/or cooked), the food product should deliver the same rich balance of nutri-ents that are found in the original grain seed."

When choosing grains, look for foods that have been minimally processed. I prefer long grain, uncut, basmati rice. I avoid most flours, especially bleached flours and polished rice, in which part of the grain (generally the healthiest part) has been removed. I also look for whole-wheat pasta. The term "whole wheat" in the ingredient list means that the product has a whole grain, since wheat is a grain. Be careful of terms like "multigrain," which generally means the product includes different grains, none of them whole.

As we approach the end of this long book, in which you've encountered mountains of evidence that high-protein diets are not only unnecessary but actually dangerous, are you still wondering, *Where do I get my protein?*

I hope not, but the protein myth is so powerful and omnipresent that I wouldn't be surprised if the question is still lurking somewhere in the back of your mind. Let's start with all the green veggies. My go-to salad green is kale, which contains about 2.5 grams of protein per cup. Since a cup of kale contains just 33 calories, my servings are quite large, typically two to three cups of salad at a go. So before I've added another ingredient to my salad, my protein tally is already up to 7.5 grams. There are 4 grams of protein in a cup of broccoli, which I throw on top, taking me to 11.5 grams. Next I toss in half a cup of mushrooms, adding another 1.5 grams, and some artichoke hearts at 3–5 grams, and my salad is up to 16 grams of protein. Finally, I top it off with half a cup of garbanzo beans (chickpeas) at 7.5 grams, a quarter cup of almonds at 7 grams, and a tablespoon of flaxseed at 2 grams, and now I get to tuck into a salad containing a whopping 32 or more grams of protein. Give me a side of a baked potato at 5 more grams, and I'm already two-thirds of the way to fulfilling my RDA (which as you'll recall, is already more than I really need). All this protein is plant protein, which I have pointed out, is distinctly different from meat protein. Plant protein does not increase inflammation, does not contribute carcinogenic materials, is not bound to saturated fat, and does not increase hormones that can affect cancer.

I knew I had fully recovered from my proteinaholism when I stopped asking myself, *Where is my protein?* I just eat a varied, plant-based diet, and I'm confident that all plants, even fruit, contain the amino acid building blocks I need. As we saw in Chapter 15, the people with the highest protein requirements are endurance athletes. Now I'm one of them; I am constantly training for triathlons and marathons and have only improved over time on my 100 percent plant-based diet.

I rely heavily on the legume, or bean family. Beans do have lots of protein, but I eat them because they are very high in fiber, loaded with great starch, filled with vitamins, and especially rich in minerals like magnesium and even iron. Oh, and they taste great. I am sure you have heard a Paleo follower tell you not to eat beans because they contain chemicals called lectins that can poison you.

Like most Paleo beliefs, this is a giant mistake built around a kernel of truth. Lectins are part of a bean's defense system, deterring animals from eating them before they get a chance to grow into plants. Luckily for us, lectins are easily inactivated by soaking the beans in water or cooking them (Cuadrado 2002). Furthermore, if beans are so dangerous, why have numerous studies shown that beans are an integral part of a healthy diet?

Beans were the single food most common to the Blue Zones, and the EPIC study found that legume consumption was the most important predictor of longevity (Darmadi-Blackberry, Wahlqvist, et al. 2004; Menotti, Kromhout, et al. 1999). In fact, studies have also shown that a bean-deficient diet can actually increase metabolic diseases and shorten life (Chang, Wahlqvist, et al. 2012).

I also love soy, which is a bean and part of the legume family. True, much of the soy in America is genetically modified, but organic soy is not, and it has great nutritional value. No, you will not grow breasts if you are a man. If that were true, I would be wearing a double D bra! Soy contains substances called isoflavones and phytoestrogens. Pseudoscientists from the Weston A. Price Foundation have spread the falsehood that these plant-based estrogens can stimulate breast growth, and even breast cancer. At face value this is a strange claim, since literally hundreds of millions of Asians eat huge quantities of soy and do not develop breasts or breast cancer. In fact, contrary to popular belief, soy not only does not cause breast cancer, but also may decrease the incidence of breast cancer, the rates of breast, and the risk of dying from breast cancer. It appears that soy is an important substance to eat if you get breast cancer to prevent recurrence (Nechuta, Caan, et al. 2012).

The stories told about soy are so wild that it's tempting to believe them; how could someone have made them up with absolutely no scientific basis? People have told me, straight faced, that feeding soy to my daughters will cause them to undergo early puberty. In fact, the exact opposite is true. The more animal protein consumed, the earlier the age of menses (Günther, Karaolis-Danckert, et al. 2010), and we know that earlier menses are a risk factor for breast cancer (Cheng, Buyken, et al. 2012). It turns out that the isoflavones found in soy are associated with delaying onset of puberty and possibly therefore reducing lifetime risk of breast cancer (Cheng, Remer, et al. 2010).

Finally, we have to talk about eggs. Eggs have recently enjoyed a strange and sudden rise to fame. The media's embrace of saturated fat has given eggs a "health halo." After being demonized for a couple of decades, they now dominate our diets. Eggs are among the most common foods listed on my patients' diet intakes. The scientific literature on the subject is all over the place, with some studies championing and others demonizing eggs. One problem is that much of the research is funded by the egg industry, and it's not always easy to follow the money trail.

Here's one fact that isn't up for debate: eggs are loaded with cholesterol. Some of the studies that have given eggs the okay have looked only at egg intake in healthy people. Many studies have shown that if you have high cholesterol, or especially diabetes, eggs are a very bad idea. The studies that do not find ill effects from egg consumption were looking at quantities of seven or fewer eggs per week. Most of my patients eat far more than that. The egg industry tells us eggs are good because they are high in protein, but I have already shown you we don't need the protein, and in fact the FDA does not allow the egg industry to advertise that eggs are a healthy food. Both because even one egg exceeds the recommended daily allowance for cholesterol, and because so many eggs harbor harmful salmonella bacteria, eggs are barely this side of legal.

If you've been around long enough, you may remember the commercial jingle from the 1970s, "the incredible, edible egg." Recently the Egg Board resurrected that jingle (you can even download it as a ringtone) because "edible" is the most complimentary thing they were allowed to say about their product. Think about that for a moment. Imagine getting a plate of food at a restaurant and asking, "Is this good for me?" And the waiter replies, "Well, it's edible." Not exactly the substance of a 5-star Yelp review.

Eggs have carnitine, which, as I have shown, can turn to TMAO, a known contributor to heart disease. Eggs are also high in the amino acid methionine, which cancer cells thrive on. The egg industry points to the fact that eggs are high in lutein, but so are carrots. Bottom line: a few eggs a week are probably okay if you're very healthy, but I prefer to avoid them (Spence, Jenkins, et al. 2010; Li, Zhou, et al. 2013; Nakamura, Okamura, et al. 2004; French, Jeffery, et al. 1994; Rong, Chen, et al. 2013; Djoussé and Gaziano, 2008).

How Do I Go About Changing?

Most people in this country have been on multiple diets, and most of them fail. Sure, you can lose weight in the beginning, but it is estimated that 95 percent of people will eventually get back to their starting weight. There are a million reasons why. Some have to do with actual genetic and physiologic reactions to diet, and some have to do with stubborn old habits. Change is always tough.

One of the biggest problems with dieting is our mind-set when we tell ourselves we're "on a diet." You can yell and scream at yourself not to eat that hamburger, but if you think about avoiding the burger because of the diet, then eventually you will fail. You may have tried a diet strategy that has become popular lately, that of the "cheat meal." If you eat good, healthy food all week, but get to eat a hamburger on Saturday, the hamburger lives on a pedestal in your mind. You don't allow yourself to appreciate the good food because you cannot wait to get to that juicy hamburger.

I don't want you to not eat a hamburger because I told you not to, or because you've read this book and now tell yourself not to. I want you to not eat a hamburger because you are absolutely disgusted by hamburgers to the point that you could never fathom the thought of eating one. And because you love yourself too much to put that burger into your beautiful, amazing body.

To elicit this kind of change in thinking in my patients, I rely on a psychological method known as cognitive behavioral therapy, or CBT. The central tenet of CBT is that once you understand how your thoughts are controlling your behavior, you can begin to question and replace them with habit-changing routines. The big revelation experienced by people who practice CBT is that they are not their thoughts. CBT has been used successfully for alcoholics and people addicted to drugs. Over the past couple of decades, it has been applied to weight loss, with stellar results. One of the world's top CBT experts, Judith Beck (daughter of the psychologist who pioneered the technique, Aaron Beck), wrote a book for weight loss, *The Beck Diet Solution*. The book is not a diet at all, but a framework and action plan for changing your thoughts around food and eating.

Even things like tastes and preferences are nothing more than thoughts. You may have thoughts like *I like ice cream, but I do not like exercising*. They seem like unchanging truths about you, but in reality they are just thoughts you have established over time. You can change your thoughts, and so doing, you can change your life. Some of the suggestions below might sound kind of corny, but trust me, they really work.

Write Down Your Goals

To start off, I want you to write down the whys we discussed above. Why do you want to change? Set your goals, and please write them down. There's a lot of evidence that writing them down is far more powerful and effective than just thinking them. Go get a pen and notepad and do it now. I'll wait.

Make those goals both broad and specific. Write down some long-term goals, like living a long healthy life with your family, living to see your children's weddings, and even your grandchildren's. You may also have some short-term goals, like fitting into a certain dress or pant size. You may be concerned about how your eating affects the environment. Write it all down. Carry these goals with you. Keep them at the forefront of your mind. I find most people live far below their potentials, mainly because they have no goals to guide them. Let this list be your GPS navigation system. Imagine the old voice in your head, the one that tells you to eat whatever you want and sit on the couch and watch TV, as a devil on your shoulder, dressed up in a comic red suit with pointy tail. Every time the devil whispers in your ear to eat a steak, imagine a little angel with a halo on your other shoulder, holding your goal list, reminding you of your aspirations.

Set your bar higher than you think you can accomplish. I am always amazed at how full of self-doubt and self-loathing people are. Hell, I used to be the same. We fear failure and settle in to a "comfortable" life as free from risk as possible. We don't try new things. We get in a rut. Are we happy in that rut? I certainly wasn't. When I was honest with myself, I knew something important was missing. I felt like I was just going through life, slowly dying for lack of a higher purpose. When I meet my patients for the first time, I get this exact sense from them. For years they have been doing the same things and getting the same results. They eat as they have always eaten and any suggestion that they could change is met with disbelieving stares. They can't imagine themselves living a heroic, powerful, amazing life. I hear, not the big dreams, but the little objections: "I can't exercise" and "I don't like veggies" and "I could not give up my [fill in the blank]."

You may think of yourself as "ordinary." I am here to tell you that ordinary people are capable of extraordinary things. I am blessed to be able to witness this on a daily basis. I see people completely turn their lives around, starting with their weight. I see them going down a path where life is a long rut to be endured, and then they become somebody totally new, and totally exciting.

Do you want to be awed and inspired? If so, go out and watch an Ironman race or a marathon. In the early hours, the superhumans finish.

They are amazing, for sure. But if you want to be reminded of what we're all capable of, stick around and watch all the other people finishing and realizing their dreams. The mother who works a day job and cares for her kids, and still makes time to train. The father who works long hours and is still able to finish his first marathon. The gal who just dropped a hundred pounds and has gone from the couch to a triathlon finish line. It is inspiring to see people break through their self-imposed concepts of what is possible.

It's important to have role models to aspire to, but you should be one of them. Take time to constantly remind yourself of your own progress. Be your own inspiration. I find people to be so self-critical that they are actually keeping themselves down. Many of my patients lose lots of weight, yet are upset that they didn't lose more. We are always comparing ourselves to others, admiring them and denigrating ourselves. Instead, practice being impressed by what you accomplish. If you go from the couch to a 5K, don't think, *Well that was just a 5K; anybody can do it.* Be in awe that you were able to break out of that rut. Each milestone should motivate you to the next achievement, as your respect and admiration for yourself grow.

Also, remember it is not about the finish line. Life is a journey. Goals are important, but what is more important is that you are trying to be your best self daily. To me, each finish line is just the start of a new adventure. The race is the icing on the cake. The work, the training, the pushing myself beyond my comfort zone; that's what it is all about.

When I first started changing my life and getting healthy, I signed up for a triathlon, which seemed like an absolutely impossible task. My sister sent me a shirt that said IMPOSSIBLE IS A DARE. Well, I dare you.

Practice Aversion/Attraction Techniques

To further clarify your goals and align your thoughts, I suggest a visual reminder and thought provoker. I ask my patients to make a collage. First, take a picture of yourself that you do not like. You might be looking unhappy, or holding a bag of medications. Then surround that picture with the typical foods you eat: pizza, hamburger, ice cream, and so on. Next, find a picture that resonates with your goals. Maybe a picture of a healthy-looking person crossing a finish line. Now surround that picture with beautiful images of fruits and veggies. It is amazing how much prettier a salad is than a hamburger. Put these pictures up where you can see them. We know subconsciously that one set of choices leads to weight gain, ill health, and unhappiness, and another set of choices leads to a lean physique, radiant health, and joy. Let these pictures bring your subconscious knowing into the light of day. Let them be a visual reminder as to where your choices take you.

Keep a Journal

Probably one of the most important cognitive tools is journaling. We're so busy and distracted, most of us eat unconsciously. When I ask patients what they ate yesterday, they usually struggle to remember. Even breakfast is forgotten by lunchtime. I give my patients a journal to record what and when they eat. Just as important, I ask them to record how they feel after eating. The Okinawans practice purposely leaving the table only 80 percent full. We eat so unconsciously that we never stop to notice if we are full. We almost always leave the table stuffed and uncomfortable, but we forget this feeling by the time the next meal arrives. You may love hot dogs, but you quickly forget how they make you feel an hour later. I ask my patients to journal these feelings. Become cognizant of how the pizza makes you feel, as opposed to the kale salad.

Eat Consciously

Taking cognizance one step further, think about where your food came from before you start eating. Say grace, or at least give thanks to the people who made your food possible. When I first decided to get healthy, I signed up for a trip to a yoga resort. After I arrived, I discovered that it was a vegetarian establishment. At the time, I was a full-fledged meat eater. I had no choice but to give up the meat during my stay. The amazing thing to me was not just how delicious the food was but how wonderful it made me feel. In fact, the food ending up destroying my meditation and yoga: *OMMM, I wonder what's for dinner, OMMM, Stop thinking about the food, OMMM, That sesame dressing was amazing, OMMM...*

Eventually, I decided to find out from the chef how he made this food so nourishing on so many levels. I entered his kitchen, and it was like out of a movie. Birds were chirping, beautiful vegetables and fruits lay everywhere, and the chef was radiating joyful attention, chopping the food and whistling. I asked him why I felt so great eating his food, and his response changed my life: "Because I make it with love!"

This has stuck with me ever since. Every time I sit down to eat, I think about where my food came from. I visualize the love and caring that produced it and transported it and prepared it and served it to me. If it is a salad, I picture the beautiful scenery where it was harvested. This has completely changed my tastes. Now I crave salads. I want to fill my body with the love and nourishment.

I used to crave cheeseburgers, but now I imagine some poor cow, raised in a packed room, walking in feces, miserable and scared. I imagine the slaughter, and the chemicals given to the animal and used in processing the meat. I imagine the kid in the back of the fast-food joint preparing the burgers, sweating away at his minimum-wage job, his eyes lifeless, as he prepares my meal. Hardly an appetizing thought, and certainly devoid of love. In fact, I could not fathom ever eating a hamburger again. The whole scene disgusts me.

Stick to a Regimen

When it comes to actually eating, you need to train your body and mind in a regimen. I don't believe in counting calories, and Lord knows I don't want you counting grams of protein, carbs, and fat. I don't care how many beans you eat or how many whole fruits. That said, I prefer my patients to develop a pattern of eating. Three meals and one snack a day works well for many of them. I actually don't care how many times you eat, so long you develop a regimen that you adhere to and practice daily. One mistake I see in my patients is a tendency to graze: eating, unconsciously, whenever food happens to appear. Instead, train your body to eat food only at certain times. For instance, if you consistently eat at 6 A.M., noon, 3 P.M., and 6 P.M., your body will soon learn that those are the times you are supposed to eat. You'll lose the desire to eat in between, as your hunger patterns adapt to conform to your schedule.

Plan Your Meals

I can't stress enough the importance of planning your meals in advance. Don't go into lunch having to make a "game time decision" about what you are going to eat. If you have no plan and someone arrives with pizza, your knee-jerk reaction will be to reach for a slice. However, if you have planned your meal and brought a salad, or decided to go to a salad bar, it becomes far easier to resist the call of the junk food. Also, prepare for difficult situations where you know you will be tempted, and plan your responses. Write down what you are going to do if pizza is served at work, or how you are going to handle your craving for a hamburger as you drive home past the fast-food place. For instance, you can carry a little card that says, "When faced with a craving, I will drink water, eat an apple, and go for a walk."

When planning meals, keep it simple. I try and eat the same basic meals with a little variation. I find that the constant search for new and exciting meals can really throw people off. It is hard to prepare a gourmet meal every time you eat. I am not saying that your meals need to be boring, but they should be easy to shop for and prepare.

For breakfast, I like to stick with oatmeal. Steel-cut oats can take a while to cook, but if you soak them overnight they cook much faster. Rolled Quaker oats cook very easily and quickly. Sometimes I add organic almond butter and banana, other times I serve it with sliced almonds, berries, and ground flaxseed. I sweeten with honey or agave to taste. If I add lots of berries, I use less sweetener. I can have oatmeal every morning for a month and each time it will be a little bit different. I usually drink a cup of green tea with the meal.

Sometimes my breakfast consists of toasted whole-grain bread, such as Ezekiel brand, with almond butter, sliced banana, and sliced strawberry. Or I just pour a bowl of muesli, which is a mix of grains and nuts served like a cereal. I add soy or almond milk and top it off with berries.

For lunch, I always have a salad. I look for dark greens like spinach and kale, and then add all the veggies I can find. I add beans, and I finish it with vinegar dressing or low-fat vinaigrette. I usually include a side of sweet potato, or potato, or some lentil soup, depending on what is available.

For a snack during the day I look for whole fruits like an apple or banana and maybe a handful of walnuts or trail mix. I also love carrots or celery with hummus.

Dinner is where we have some variety. But you don't have to make it complicated. Jeff Novick has a series of *Fast Food* DVDs that reduce healthy cooking to its simplest, quickest form. My wife cooks up some delicious meals that I often photograph and feature on my Facebook page, but when she is not around I stick to Jeff's basics: a can of beans, a bag of frozen mixed veggies, spices, canned tomatoes, and a starch. If I am in the mood for Mexican food, for example, I put a can of black beans, a can of tomatoes, and a bag of frozen mixed veggies into a pot and warm on the stove. I add artichokes and Mexican seasoning and then serve it over brown basmati rice. If I want Italian food, then I throw a can of white cannellini beans, a can of chopped tomatoes, frozen mixed veggies, garlic, and Italian seasoning into a pot and serve it over whole-wheat pasta. Meals like this are quick, inexpensive, nutritious, and delicious.

Chapter 17 of this book includes several recipes that I give to my patients, which were created by Andy Bellati, RD.

I have even asked Dana McDonald RD, the Rebel Dietitian, to construct a sample meal plan that she would give to her clients. Dana has worked at our clinic and has the website https://rebeldietitian.us/. Dana really knows her stuff and puts together beautiful meal plans.

If you would like a more formal plan, I highly recommend signing up for the Physician's Committee for Responsible Medicine's 21-Day Vegan Kickstart at www.21daykisckstart.org. When I teach cooking classes in my office, I include the meals in this plan. My patients always comment how great they feel after completing the twenty-one days. They also tell me how surprised they are that the food is easy to make and actually tastes great.

Finding healthy options when eating out has become far easier over the years. Just about every restaurant menu includes a vegetarian option. Don't be afraid to ask the waiter if the restaurant has options without animal meat. Chefs love the variety of dishes they can make with veggies. When I go out to dinner with friends, they're always jealous of the beautiful dishes that I get served, simply because I asked. One very useful tactic is to look up the menu online and choose your dish before you even arrive at the restaurant, before you can be tempted by the smells and sights of dishes that don't support your big goals.

You will also find that restaurants offering ethnic foods cater well to a plant-based diet. Chinese restaurants serve lots of veggies. To avoid the oils, I order steamed veggies with tofu and eggplant, with garlic sauce on the side. At Mexican restaurants I ask for rice and beans and grilled peppers and onions. Japanese restaurants often make great veggie sushi. Middle Eastern restaurants and Greek restaurants have fantastic veggie dishes, just ask them to go easy on the olive oil. Ethiopian food hits the jackpot when it comes to delicious beans and veggies served curry style. I highly recommend it.

Surround Yourself with Positive People

One additional strategy that is crucial to success: surround yourself with people who share your goals and will celebrate your progress and your triumphs. As you know, I love the sport of triathlon. My best friend is also a triathlete, and we train together and compete against each other from time to time. So far, I'm sad to report, I have not beaten him. Not once. I haven't even scared him. But if that day ever comes, I know he would be happy for me.

All my good friends are very health conscious. I feel sorry for the waiters when we go out to dinner: "Can you put the oil on the side?" "Hold any cheese or dairy products." "Do you have a vegan plate?" (That last one is my line.) Collectively, we're like the restaurant scene from *When Harry Met Sally*. Our dinner conversations center around our exercise plans and the goals we're pursuing.

Now this may seem annoying. Why would I surround myself with people who trounce me in my sport and look better than me with our shirts off? Several years ago, I came across a fascinating article in the *New England Journal of Medicine* that showed that social groups or cliques tended to have similar weights (Christakis and Fowler 2007). In other words, we tend to mimic our peer groups' behaviors, and in so doing, share their successes and their failures.

I bring this up because when I see patients going through weight loss, their peer group often becomes a stumbling block. When my patients begin to lose weight, their friends and family may start to resent them. They are commonly told that they are losing too much weight, or that they look too skinny. Weight is an issue on everybody's mind and when spouses see their partners changing their lives, they become concerned about their own health and worth. Not only spouses, but also friends, neighbors, and coworkers may try to sabotage someone's healthy changes. Without consciously knowing it, they can feel threatened when somebody actually changes their life course and becomes healthy and happy.

The sad thing is this jealousy can actually lead to divorce or peer group isolation. I have had patients tell me some of their friends will take them to dinner and insist they eat a hamburger or some other junk food, purposely trying to sabotage their success. After all, the majority of people in this country are overweight, so your friends and family are likely to be overweight. If you lose weight, you are doing something they consider abnormal and therefore threatens their comfort zone.

> "Keep away from those who try to belittle your ambitions.
> Small people always do that, but the really great make you
> believe that you too can become great."
> —MARK TWAIN

I am not saying you have to leave your spouse or your friends, but you do need to have a discussion with them about the importance of this journey you are taking. You need to ask for their support and understanding and let them know that while your body and health may change, your feelings for them will not. Also, we're lucky to live in a time where we have so many ways to build new supportive peer groups. Facebook is filled with excellent group pages about exercise and plant-based eating. Joining a gym or a Zumba class can expose you to many new friends who share your goals. I personally joined a running group and am on several vegan web pages. I have made many new friends and built up a great support network.

My friends are a bit fanatical in their fitness, but that drives me. If my peer group drank beer and watched sports every weekend, I may have ended up the same despite my desire to get healthy. By putting together a social network that encourages and reinforces my goals, I've shifted the odds in my favor. My friends challenge me to become better and healthier, and I owe a lot of my success to their support.

Want a helping hand in changing your diet, getting healthy, and challenging all the "impossibles" in your life? We offer support, guidance, tips, recipes, and even coaching at Proteinaholic.com.

Meal Plan

Dana McDonald is a registered dietitian in Houston who has worked at my clinic. She goes by the name the "Rebel Dietitian" largely because she does not advocate the high-protein diets that her colleagues do from the moment they graduate. Dana also walks the talk. She is the picture of health and strength, all done on a diet filled with fruit and veggies. Like me, she doesn't advocate counting macronutrients, especially not protein. I have asked her to put together a typical weekly meal plan to help you see how easy and delicious it is once you break free of your obsession with protein.

This plan has more than enough protein. Do it for two weeks and you will feel strong and vibrant. You will be able to prove to yourself that you do not have to stuff your mouth with meat to be healthy. Actually, you will find quite the opposite to be true.

You can follow Dana at https://rebeldietitian.us or at Facebook.com/EatCleanTrainMeanLiveGreen.

General Information and Tips

You may be wondering why I chose to begin the meal plan on Saturday. Great question! I mean, who does that?

Rebel foodies! The reason I chose this layout for the book is to demonstrate weekly meal planning and preparation ("prepping"). By learning to

MEAL PLAN CHART

	Breakfast	Snack	Lunch	Snack	Dinner
Saturday (Prep for Sunday)	Carrot Cake Steel-Cut Oats	Strawberry Mint Fruit Salad	Sprouted Avocado Sandwich	Perfect Postworkout Smoothie	Hemp-Powered Green Machine Salad
Sunday (Official Prep Day)	Baked Apple Pie Steel-Cut Oats	Hit-the-Trail Mix Cup	Black Bean Soup Tip: Also create "refried" black beans.	Strawberry Patch Smoothie Tip: Dinner also uses collard greens.	Collard Green Wraps Tip: Calls for "refried" black beans.
Monday	Overnight Oats	Fresh Veggies with Dip	Black Bean Tacos Tip: Calls for black beans.	Coconut Lime Smoothie	Quinoa Power Bowl Tips: Calls for black beans; save some quinoa for breakfast!
Tuesday	Nutty Coconut Quinoa	Fresh Fruit and Nuts	Superfood Salad with Roasted Red Potatoes	Raw Banana "Ice Cream"	Baked Potatoes with Side Salad Tip: Prepare extra for lunch tomorrow.
Wednesday	Back-to-Nature Muesli	Fresh Veggies with Dip	Baked Potato with Side Salad	Mango Lime Sorbet	Cranberry Almond Wheat Berry Bowl Tip: Prepare extra for lunch tomorrow.
Thursday	Nutty Banana Wrap	Fresh Fruit and Nuts	Cranberry Almond Wheat Berry Bowl with Side Salad	Chocolate Protein Smoothie	Baked Sweet Potatoes with Side Salad Tip: Save 1½ cups sweet potato for tomorrow!
Friday	Whole-Grain Pancakes	Fresh Veggies with Dip	Berrylicious Salad	Pumpkin Pie Smoothie Tip: Calls for sweet potatoes.	Green Goddess Salad

plan and prep on Saturday and Sunday, you will be able to quickly prepare nutrient-dense meals for the rest of the week with little to no effort. Not to mention, you'll save yourself time and energy during the week. Examples of foods you may want to consider preparing on Sunday include black beans, quinoa, brown rice, and/or any other whole grains you'd like to use during the first half of the week. I list Saturday as the prep day for Sunday because that is when most people have extra time during the week.

Considering energy requirements vary from person-to-person based upon age, sex, and activity level, please feel free to adjust the portion sizes and/or quantity of snacks based upon your level of hunger. In general, raw fruits and vegetables are an ideal snack choice as these foods are naturally low in calories and high in fiber. For example, if you are still hungry after dinner, consider adding in either the "Fresh Veggies with Dip" or "Fresh Fruit and Nuts" snack option (described below). One of the great things about a plant-based lifestyle is the fact that it is a lifestyle of abundance, rather than restriction.

When it comes to storing your prepared food in the refrigerator, glass is generally your safest bet. While plastic storage containers may seem convenient, they are often a source of potentially harmful substances including endocrine-disrupting chemicals such as bisphenol A (BPA). The containers I use to store and transport my lunch in include glass and/or stainless steel containers. Stainless steel is a great choice for lunch because it less likely to break. As a reminder, be sure to wash all your produce well to remove any potentially harmful substances prior to eating it. Last, but not least, opt for local ingredients that are organic, free of genetically modified organisms (GMOs), and Fair Trade whenever possible.

Flexible Snack Options

Below are the instructions for the snacks found within your meal plan titled "Fresh Veggies with Dip" and "Fresh Fruit and Nuts." As always, the portion sizes described here are for your reference only. If you find they are not big enough, simply consume more raw fruits and vegetables. This is not intended to be a restrictive meal plan; rather, one that provides portion-size guidance for those who are interested in it.

Fresh Veggies with Dip

Within the menu, you will notice I've included "Fresh Veggies with Dip" as a snack on three separate occasions. The best part about this snack is, you get to eat as many raw vegetables as you like! Below I review how this snack option works.

Raw Vegetables

For your fresh vegetable option, you are free to choose from any of the following. If you'd like a combination of several veggies (e.g., cauliflower and broccoli florets), that works great too! Don't forget, for this snack, you are welcome to eat as much as you'd like!

- Bell peppers, sliced (green, red, yellow, orange or a combination)
- Broccoli florets
- Carrot sticks
- Cauliflower florets
- Celery sticks
- Cherry tomatoes
- Cucumber slices
- Eggplants
- Green onions
- Leafy greens
- Microgreens
- Mushrooms
- Purple onions
- Radishes
- Snap peas
- Zucchini

Vegetable Dip

For the dip, feel free to choose one of the following. Of course, you are always welcome to enjoy your vegetables without a dip. For your convenience, I am including the recipes for most of the dips described below within the recipe section; however, you are welcome to use your own recipe or purchase a low-fat minimally processed dip.

- Fresh salsa (enjoy as much fresh salsa as you'd like!)
- 3 tablespoons of fresh guacamole dip
- 3 tablespoons of "refried" bean dip

- 3 tablespoon of hummus

- 1 tablespoon of nut or seed butter (minimally processed; any type)

- 1 tablespoon of olive oil

- 1–2 tablespoons of low-fat salad dressing

- 1–2 tablespoons of low-fat veggie dip

Fresh Fruit and Nuts

Within the menu, you will notice I've included "Fresh Fruit and Nuts" as a snack on two separate occasions. Below I review how this snack option works.

Fresh Fruit

For the fresh fruit, you are free to choose one of the following. Of course, if you'd like to mix if up (e.g., half of a banana with half of an apple), that works great too!

- 1 medium apple (any variety)

- 1 medium banana

- 1 medium pomegranate

- 2 tangerines

- 2 oranges

- 2 small peaches

- 2 small nectarines

- 3 small figs

- 3 medium grapefruits

- 1 cup grapes (any type)

- 2 cups strawberries

- 1½ cups blackberries

- 1½ cups raspberries

- 1 cup blueberries
- 2 kiwi fruit
- 1 cup cherries (with pits)
- 1 cup mango, chopped
- 1 cup pineapple, chopped
- 2 cups watermelon, chopped
- 2 cups cantaloupe, chopped
- 2 cups papaya, chopped
- 2 Medjool dates
- 1 ounce raisins (or other naturally dried fruit)
- ½ avocado

Nuts/Nut Butter

For the nuts portion of the snack, feel free to choose one of the following. Of course, if you'd like to mix if up (e.g., 10 pecan halves with 10 walnut halves), that works great too.

- 15 almonds
- 15 hazelnuts
- 10 walnut halves
- 10 pecan halves
- 20 peanuts
- 25 pistachios
- 12 cashews
- 2½ tablespoons flaxseeds, whole
- 2 tablespoons sunflower seeds, whole
- 1½ tablespoons pumpkin seeds, whole
- 1½ tablespoons chia seeds, whole
- 1 tablespoon of nut or seed butter (minimally processed; any type)

Nut and/or Seed Allergies

For those of you with nut and/or seed allergies, please feel free to omit the nut and seed portion of the snack and consider one of the following options:

- Double the fruit portion
- Substitute raw vegetables

Whole Grains

Throughout the menu, you will notice I also include several recipes using whole grains to demonstrate how easy it is to incorporate different grains into your meals. If you are gluten intolerant, please feel free to make the necessary substitution.

Gluten-Free Grains

The gluten-free grains include sorghum, brown rice, corn, wild rice, buckwheat, amaranth, millet, teff, quinoa, oats,* and kañiwa.

*Oats are inherently gluten free, but they are frequently contaminated with wheat during growing or processing; however, there are several companies that sell oats that are guaranteed gluten free.

Edamame, Corn, and Green Peas

In general, when a recipe calls for edamame, corn, and/or green peas, I utilize frozen products that are certified organic and non-GMO. Simply cook these ingredients as directed on the package.

Herbs and Spices

Whenever possible, invest in quality food ingredients, including dried herbs and spices. As you will notice, I tend to use a lot of the same ingredients throughout this meal plan to keep the cost to a minimum.

Natural Sweeteners

Throughout this meal plan you will notice several recipes that include the option to add a natural sweetener. Please feel free to omit the sweetener or substitute it with the natural sweetener of your choice.

In general, natural sweeteners include the following:

- Raw honey*
- Pure maple syrup
- Granulated maple sugar
- Coconut palm sugar
- Dried fruit (e.g., Medjool dates)

Raw honey is not considered vegan.

Medjool Dates

If you prefer to substitute Medjool dates as your sweetener in any of the following recipes, consider the following:

- In general, substitute 1 chopped Medjool date for every 1 tablespoon of natural sweetener.

- In smoothie or raw food recipes, consider soaking your Medjool dates in filtered water for 1 to 2 hours prior to use. Soaking will soften the dates and enable a more even and consistent distribution of the sweetener.

- After soaking, be sure to rinse the dates with fresh water and remove the pits.

Black Beans

Welcome to Texas, y'all! No seriously, we love black beans in Texas. One of the great things about black beans is their versatility. For instance, black beans can easily be consumed as a soup or as "refried beans." If you are new to the border, have no fear—I provide tips on soaking and cooking beans just below and then, later in the chapter, provide a more detailed recipe, Black Bean Soup and "Refried" Beans, to use with your meal plan. Traditionally, to make refried beans, cooked black beans are literally refried using a pan and animal lard or vegetable oil. But using the simple blender method I describe in the later recipe, you'll see we've skipped the need for oil altogether. It's a simple way to make "refried" black beans to have on hand for veggie tacos and burritos—or even a dip!

General Tips on Cooking Black Beans

- Examine the beans and throw away any foreign particles or beans that are discolored or shriveled.

- Rinse the beans with water and then drain the water.

- Soak beans overnight prior to cooking them using one of the soak methods below. The benefits of soaking include:

- Significantly reduced cooking time

- Reduced concentrations of phytic acid levels (i.e., less gas and bloating)

- Improved nutrient bioavailability

- I recommend the "hot soak" method for 8 to 12 hours; see method below (start it Saturday night).

- Do not add salt to the soaking water.

- Add salt and any acids (e.g., lemon juice or vinegar) after cooking. The addition of salt or acid while cooking delays cooking time and results in a tough bean (that's no bueno!).

- Add tender herbs and spices near the end of the cooking process to prevent loss of flavor.

- Whatever you do, do not add baking soda to your beans at any time. Baking soda will rob your beans of flavor and important nutrients like vitamin B_1 (or thiamin).

- The exact cooking time will depend upon your altitude, water hardness, age of the beans, and soaking method.

- Generally, most beans cook within 45 to 90 minutes.

- To assess bean readiness, frequently sample your beans or take a fork and mash one of the beans against the side of the pot.

- When the beans are tender but firm, they're ready to eat!

- Oh, and don't be shocked if you happen to see a brownish-looking foam form at the top or around the edges during the cooking process. This is some of the protein from the beans coagulating and it is nothing to worry about. If it bothers you, you can skim it off.

- Have fun, foodies!

Bean-Soaking Methods

Hot Soak

- Reduces cooking time and phytic acid and produces tender beans (I prefer this method).

- Place beans in a pot and add 10 cups of water for every 2 cups of beans.

- Heat to boiling and boil for an additional 2 to 3 minutes.

- Remove beans from heat, cover, and let stand for 8 to 12 hours.

- Drain beans, discard soak water, and rinse with fresh, cool water.

Traditional Soak

- Pour cold water over the beans to cover.

- Soak beans for 8 hours or overnight.

- Drain beans, discard soak water, and rinse with fresh, cool water.

- Cold water starts the rehydration process slowly so beans will appear wrinkled after soaking.

Quick Soak

- Place beans in a large pot and add 10 cups of water for every 2 cups of beans.

- Bring to boil and boil for an additional 2 to 3 minutes.

- Drain beans, discard soak water, and rinse with fresh, cool water.

Back-to-Nature Muesli

Serves: 2 to 3

1 cup extra thick rolled oats
2 tablespoons hulled hemp seeds
2 tablespoons sunflower seeds
2 tablespoons almonds, chopped
2 tablespoons walnuts, chopped
2 tablespoons pistachios
2 tablespoons raisins, unsweetened
2 tablespoons unsweetened coconut flakes
½ teaspoon cinnamon, ground
1 tablespoon granulated maple sugar
1 cup nondairy milk
½ banana, sliced (optional)

1. In a medium bowl, gently toss extra thick rolled oats, hulled hemp seeds, sunflower seeds, almonds, walnuts, pistachios, raisins, cinnamon, granulated maple sugar, and unsweetened coconut flakes.

2. Serve with nondairy milk and fresh banana slices (optional).

3. Store muesli in an airtight container in the refrigerator.

Cinnamon Almond Muesli (Extra Recipe)

···

Serves: 2 to 3

    1 cup extra thick rolled oats
    2 tablespoons walnuts, chopped
    2 tablespoons almonds, chopped
    2 tablespoons unsweetened coconut flakes
    2 tablespoons raisins
    1 tablespoon granulated maple sugar
    1/4 teaspoon cinnamon, ground
    1 cup (8 ounces) nondairy milk
    1/3 cup fresh blueberries

1. In a medium bowl, gently toss extra thick rolled oats, walnuts, almonds, unsweetened coconut flakes, raisins, maple sugar, and cinnamon.

2. Serve muesli with nondairy milk and fresh blueberries.

3. Store muesli in an airtight container in the refrigerator.

Overnight Oats

···

Serves: 2 to 3

    1 cup extra thick rolled oats, uncooked
    1 cup of nondairy milk
    1 tablespoon sweetener of choice
    Your favorite toppings and/or other ingredients*

*Toppings/Optional Ingredients

- *Fresh fruit, chopped (e.g., fresh apple, baked cinnamon apples, strawberries, banana, blueberries, and kiwi)*
- *Nuts and/or seeds (e.g., almond butter, chia, flax, hulled hemp seeds, and almonds)*
- *Dried fruit (e.g., unsweetened coconut flakes, Medjool dates, goji berries, and raisins)*
- *Cacao (e.g., raw cacao nibs and raw cacao powder)*

- *Spices (e.g., cinnamon, vanilla, ginger, and nutmeg)*
- *Other (e.g., granola, muesli, and acai)*
- *Nondairy yogurt (e.g., coconut yogurt)*

1. Add 1 cup uncooked oats to a tall glass container with a lid (e.g., mason jar).

2. Add in 1–2 tablespoons each of your favorite ingredients (see above), optional.

3. Pour in nondairy milk and sweetener of choice.

4. Close lid and give the container a gentle shake.

5. Store oats in refrigerator overnight.

6. Wake up, grab your oats, and add any additional toppings.

7. Enjoy!

8. Store in an airtight container for up to 3 days (or freeze for up to 3 months).

Baked Apple Pie Steel-Cut Oats

Serves: 3 to 4

Steel-Cut Oats Ingredients

1 cup steel-cut oats, uncooked
1½ cups filtered water
1½ cups coconut milk, unsweetened
3 tablespoons shelled hemp seeds
¼ cup walnuts, chopped
1 teaspoon cinnamon, ground
¼ teaspoon ginger, ground
⅛ teaspoon nutmeg, ground
¾ teaspoon pure vanilla
2 tablespoons pure maple syrup
¼ teaspoon salt (optional)

Baked Apple Ingredients

1 large Granny Smith apple, peeled, cored, and evenly sliced
  (divided)
1–2 tablespoons of fresh lemon juice
1 tablespoon granulated maple sugar
1 tablespoon of cinnamon, ground

To Bake the Apple:

1. Preheat oven to 350°F and line a baking pan with parchment paper.

2. Peel, core, and evenly slice the apple.

3. In a medium bowl, toss apple slices with 1–2 tablespoons of
   lemon juice, 1 tablespoon of granulated maple sugar, and
   1 tablespoon of cinnamon until evenly coated.

4. Move the coated apples to the baking sheet lined with parchment
   paper.

5. Gently fold (or wrap) the apples within the parchment paper
   (to prevent moisture loss) and bake for 12 minutes.

6. Flip the folded apple mixture and bake for additional 10–12
   minutes, or until tender.

7. Set aside and allow to stand for 2 minutes.

8. Divide baked apples in half (half for steel-cut oats and half for
   garnish).

9. Set aside half of the baked apples for the garnish.

10. On a cutting board, gently dice up the other half of the apples and
    set aside (to be added to the steel-cut oats).

To Make the Steel-Cut Oats:

1. Add 1½ cups of filtered water and 1½ cups coconut milk to a medium
   pot and bring to boil.

2. Once boiling, add ¼ teaspoon salt (optional) and 1 cup of steel-
   cut oats.

3. Reduce heat to low and cook uncovered for 20 minutes, or until
   tender, stirring every few minutes.

4. When the oats are approximately 75 percent cooked, mix in ½ of the baked apples (diced), shelled hemp seeds, walnuts, cinnamon, ginger, nutmeg, vanilla, and maple syrup.

5. Cook for another 5 minutes, or until desired consistency.

6. Remove oats from heat and allow to stand for 2 minutes.

7. Garnish oats with remaining baked apples and serve.

8. Store in an airtight container for up to 3 days (or freeze for up to 3 months).

Carrot Cake Steel-Cut Oats

....

Serves: 3 to 4

1 cup steel-cut oats, uncooked
1½ cups filtered water
1½ cups coconut milk, unsweetened
⅓ cup unsweetened coconut flakes
1 cup finely grated carrots
1 teaspoon cinnamon, ground
¼ teaspoon ginger, ground
⅛ teaspoon nutmeg, ground
¾ teaspoon pure vanilla
2 tablespoons pure maple syrup
3 tablespoons shelled hemp seeds
¼ cup walnuts, chopped (plus a little extra for the garnish)
¼ cup raisins (plus a little extra for the garnish)
¼ teaspoon salt (optional)

1. Finely grate 3 or 4 medium-size carrots and set to the side (amount should equal 1 heaping cup).

2. Add 1½ cups of filtered water and 1½ cups coconut milk to a medium pot and bring to boil.

3. Reduce heat to low and add 1 cup of steel-cut oats, grated carrots, and ¼ teaspoon salt (optional).

4. Cook uncovered for 20 minutes, or until tender, stirring every few minutes.

5. When the oats are approximately 75 percent cooked, mix in unsweetened coconut flakes, raisins, shelled hemp seeds, walnuts, cinnamon, ginger, nutmeg, vanilla, and maple syrup. Mix well.

6. Cook for another 5 minutes, or until desired consistency.

7. Remove oats from heat and allow to stand for 2 minutes.

8. Garnish oats with walnuts and raisins (optional) and serve.

9. Store in an airtight container for up to 3 days (or freeze for up to 3 months).

Nutty Coconut Quinoa

Serves: 3 to 4

2 cups quinoa, cooked (1 cup dry quinoa yields about 3 cups cooked)
4 Medjool dates, chopped finely
½ teaspoon pure vanilla
1 teaspoon cinnamon, ground
2 tablespoons sunflower seeds
2 tablespoons almonds, chopped
2 tablespoons walnuts, chopped
2 tablespoons pistachio seeds
⅓ cup unsweetened coconut flakes
½–1 cup coconut milk, unsweetened

1. In a large bowl gently toss cooked quinoa with coconut milk, vanilla, chopped Medjool dates, and cinnamon.

2. Next, layer on chopped almonds, chopped walnuts, pistachios, and sunflower seeds.

3. Last, sprinkle on unsweetened coconut flakes.

4. Serve and enjoy!

Whole-Grain Pancakes

··

Serves: 2 to 3

> 1 cup Bob's Red Mill Organic 7 Grain Pancake and Waffle Mix*
> 2 tablespoons olive oil, plus a little extra to grease the pan
> ¾ cup (6 ounces) nondairy milk
> ½ cup pureed banana**
> ½ teaspoon pure vanilla extract
> Pure maple syrup

> *If gluten intolerant, substitute 1 cup of Bob's Red Mill Buckwheat
> Pancake Mix.*
> **If banana intolerant, substitute 1 flax egg (see recipe below).*

1. First, combine dry ingredients in a medium bowl and mix thoroughly.

2. Next, combine the wet ingredients in a separate bowl and mix well.

3. Now, add the wet ingredients to the dry ingredients and stir gently; overmixing results in tough pancakes.

4. Once mixed, preheat your griddle, heavy-bottomed stainless steel pan to 375°F (185°C) or until a drop of water skitters across the pan.

3. Lightly grease the hot pan with olive oil.*

4. Pour in an even amount of pancake batter into the center of the pan.

5. Do not press your pancake.

6. Flip the pancakes when edges begin to brown and bubbles show in the center.

7. Serve with maple syrup and fresh fruit, optional.

> *If you prefer, you can bake your pancakes in the oven using a baking
> sheet lined with parchment paper. Bake at 350°F for 20 to 25 minutes,
> or until golden brown.*

Flax Egg

1 tablespoon ground flaxseed
3 tablespoons filtered water

1. In a small bowl, mix ground flaxseed and water.
2. Set aside for 3 to 5 minutes until it thickens.

Nutty Banana Wrap

Serves: 1

1 Ezekiel 4:9 New Mexico Style Sprouted Grain Tortillas*
1 tablespoon fresh nut or seed butter
½ medium banana, sliced
1 teaspoon natural sweetener of choice

*If gluten intolerant, consider the black bean, brown rice, corn tortilla,
  or gluten-free bread of choice.*

1. Slice up the banana and set aside.
2. On a clean plate, lay out tortilla and apply nut butter.
3. Add banana slices and drizzle on natural sweetener.
4. Roll it up and enjoy!

Sprouted Avocado Sandwich

Serves: 1

2 slices sprouted whole-grain bread
½ cup sprouts (microgreens)
Romaine lettuce, whole leaves
Ripe tomato, thinly sliced
¼ avocado, sliced
Cucumber, thinly sliced

Salt and pepper, to taste
2 dill pickles
1 cup fresh fruit, chopped

1. Layer sprouts, lettuce, tomato, avocado, and cucumber between slices of bread. Salt and pepper to taste.

2. Serve with pickles and fresh fruit.

3. Enjoy!

SMOOTHIES

Strawberry Patch Smoothie

Serves: 1 to 2

2 large collard greens, stems removed
3 large basil leaves
3 strawberries, whole
1 mango, cut into chunks
1 kiwifruit, quartered*
1 tablespoon natural sweetener
1 to 1½ cups nondairy milk
1 cup ice

*Leave the kiwifruit peel for extra fiber and nutrition!

1. First, add ice, collard greens, and basil to high-speed blender.

2. Next, add strawberries, mango, and kiwi.

3. Last, pour in nondairy milk and natural sweetener.

4. Blend until creamy and smooth.

5. Enjoy!

Pumpkin Pie Smoothie

Serves: 2 to 3

1½ cups sweet potato, cooked*
1 banana, peeled, quartered, and frozen overnight
½ teaspoon cinnamon, ground
¼ teaspoon ginger, ground
¼ teaspoon nutmeg, ground
½ teaspoon pure vanilla
1 tablespoon pure maple syrup
1 to 1½ cups coconut milk, unsweetened
1 cup ice cubes

Include the sweet potato peel for extra fiber and nutrition!

1. First, add ice, cooked sweet potato, and frozen banana to high-speed blender.
2. Next, add dry spices (i.e., cinnamon, ginger, and nutmeg).
3. Last, add in vanilla, maple syrup, and coconut milk.
4. Blend until creamy and smooth.
5. Enjoy!

Perfect Postworkout Smoothie

Serves: 2 to 3

1 cup extra thick rolled oats, cooked
1 banana, peeled, quartered, and frozen overnight
3 tablespoons shelled hemp seeds
1 teaspoon cinnamon, ground
½ teaspoon pure vanilla
2 tablespoons Medjool dates, soaked
1½ cups nondairy milk
1 cup ice cubes

1. Prepare extra thick oats per instructions, allow to cool, and set to side.
2. First, add the ice, frozen banana, and cooked oats to high-speed blender.
3. Next, add in the soaked Medjool dates (or sweetener of choice), cinnamon, and shelled hemp seeds.
4. Last, add in pure vanilla and nondairy milk.
5. Blend until creamy and smooth.
6. Enjoy!

Chocolate Protein Smoothie

Serves: 2

2 bananas, quartered and frozen overnight
3 tablespoons shelled hemp seeds
1 to 2 teaspoons raw cacao powder
2 tablespoons raw cacao nibs, plus extra for garnish (optional)
½ teaspoon pure vanilla
1 tablespoon natural sweetener of choice
1 to 1½ cups nondairy milk
2 handfuls of ice

1. First, add ice, frozen bananas, and shelled hemp seeds to high-speed blender.
2. Next, add cacao nibs, cacao powder, and sweetener of choice.
3. Last, pour in vanilla and nondairy milk.
4. Blend until creamy and smooth.
5. Garnish smoothie with cacao nibs and enjoy!

Coconut Lime Smoothie

Serves: 2

2 cups baby spinach
2 cups coconut ice, frozen overnight*

½ teaspoon fresh lime zest
¼ cup fresh lime juice
1 cup coconut water
1 tablespoon natural sweetener of choice
Handful of unsweetened coconut flakes, for garnish

To make coconut ice, freeze pure coconut water in ice cube trays overnight. Enjoy!

1. First, add coconut ice and baby spinach to high-speed blender.

2. Next, add in lime zest and natural sweetener.

3. Last, pour in lime juice and coconut water.

4. Blend until creamy and smooth.

5. Garnish with unsweetened coconut flakes and enjoy!

Hemp-Powered Green Machine Salad

Serves: 3 to 4

4 cups of mixed leafy greens (e.g., baby kale, spinach, and romaine)
1 green bell pepper, sliced
½ cup broccoli florets, chopped
½ cup cauliflower florets, chopped
½ cup purple cabbage, shredded
½ cup green peas, cooked (frozen)
½ cup celery, sliced
¼ cup green olives
½ cup cashews
½ cup almonds
⅓ cup dried cranberries
⅓ cup shelled hemp seeds
Salad dressing of choice

1. Prepare green peas per package instructions and set to the side.

2. Thoroughly wash all produce and pat dry.

3. Prepare produce (e.g., chop, dice, or slice) and set to the side.

4. In a large bowl, add leafy greens, bell pepper, broccoli, cauliflower, cabbage, and celery.

5. Next add in the green peas, olives, cashews, almonds, and dried cranberries.

6. Last, sprinkle on shelled hemp seeds and serve with salad dressing of choice, and enjoy!

Green Goddess Salad

Serves: 3 to 4

> **4 cups of mixed leafy greens (e.g., baby kale, spinach, and romaine)**
> **1 cup sprouts (microgreens)**
> **½ cup broccoli florets, chopped**
> **1 green bell pepper, sliced**
> **½ cup green zucchini, shredded**
> **½ cup purple cabbage, shredded**
> **½ cup green peas, cooked (I purchase frozen)**
> **½ cup edamame, cooked (I purchase frozen)**
> **½ cup blueberries**
> **½ cup cashews**
> **½ cup almonds**
> **2 kiwis, quartered**
> **1 avocado, cubed**
> **Salad dressing of choice**

1. Prepare green peas and edamame per package instructions and set to the side.

2. Thoroughly wash all produce and pat dry.

3. Prepare produce (e.g., chop, dice, or slice) and set to the side.

4. In a large bowl, add leafy greens, sprouts, broccoli, bell pepper, and zucchini.

5. Next layer on the purple cabbage, green peas, edamame, and blueberries.

6. Next, sprinkle on your cashews and almonds.

7. Last, add in your avocado and kiwi.

8. Serve with salad dressing of choice and enjoy!

Berrylicious Salad

Serves: 1 to 2

> **2 cups of mixed leafy greens (e.g., baby kale, spinach, arugula, and romaine)**
> **½ cup carrots, diced**
> **½ cup green peas, cooked**
> **½ cup edamame, cooked**
> **½ cup blueberries**
> **½ cup strawberries, sliced**
> **¼ cup almonds**
> **¼ cup dried cranberries**
> **3 tablespoons shelled hemp seeds**
> **Salad dressing of choice**

1. Prepare green peas and edamame per package instructions, and set to the side.

2. Thoroughly wash all produce and pat dry.

3. Prepare produce (e.g. chop, dice, or slice) and set to the side.

4. In a large bowl, add leafy greens, carrots, green peas, edamame, blueberries, strawberries, and almonds.

5. Next, sprinkle on shelled hemp seeds and dried cranberries.

6. Serve with salad dressing of choice and enjoy!

Superfood Salad

Serves: 2 to 4

> **4 cups of mixed leafy greens (e.g., baby kale, spinach, arugula, and romaine)**
> **½ cup broccoli florets**

½ cup celery, chopped
⅓ cup carrots, shredded
⅓ cup purple cabbage, shredded
½ cup cherry tomatoes
½ cup red and green bell peppers, sliced
⅓ cup green peas, cooked
⅓ cup edamame, cooked
⅓ cup corn, cooked
⅓ cup blueberries
½ cup strawberries, sliced
⅓ cup cashews
⅓ cup almonds
3 tablespoons shelled hemp seeds
Salad dressing of choice

1. Prepare green peas, corn, and edamame per package instructions, and set to the side.

2. Thoroughly wash all produce and pat dry.

3. Prepare produce (e.g., chop, dice, or slice) and set to the side.

4. In a large bowl, add leafy greens, broccoli, cherry tomatoes, celery, carrots, purple cabbage, bell peppers, green peas, edamame, corn, blueberries, strawberries, cashews, almonds, and shelled hemp seeds.

5. Serve with salad dressing of choice and enjoy!

Quinoa Power Bowl

·····

Serves: 2 to 4

4 cups crisp romaine lettuce, shredded
2 cups quinoa, cooked (1 cup dry quinoa yields about 3 cups cooked)
1 cup black beans, cooked
1 cup tomatoes, diced
½ cup sweet onions, diced
1 cup corn, cooked
1 cup edamame, cooked

1 avocado, diced (or cubed)
Fresh lime juice, to taste
Salt and pepper, to taste

1. Prepare quinoa, black beans, corn, and edamame per instructions, and set aside.

2. Rinse and prepare produce (e.g., chop, slice, dice) and set aside.

3. In a large bowl, layer ingredients in the following order: romaine lettuce, quinoa, black beans, tomatoes, onions, corn, edamame, and diced avocado.

4. Serve with fresh lime juice and enjoy!

Optional: If you prefer, you can substitute pico de gallo for the diced tomatoes and onions and/or guacamole dip for the sliced avocado.

Collard Green Wraps

Serves: 2

2 large collard green leafs
½ to ¾ cup "refried" black beans
1 cup quinoa, cooked (1 cup dry quinoa yields about 3 cups cooked)
¼ cup shelled hemp seeds
1½ cup sprouts (microgreens)
½ cup purple cabbage, shredded
½ cup carrots, shredded
½ cup cucumber, thinly sliced
⅓ cup fresh guacamole dip
Fresh lime juice, to taste
Salt and pepper, to taste

1. Prepare quinoa, guacamole dip, and refried beans per instructions in the later recipes for them and set aside.

2. Rinse and prepare produce (e.g., chop, dice, and shred).

3. On a clean surface, lay collard greens flat and layer ingredients in the following order: "refried" black beans, quinoa, shelled hemp seeds, sprouts, cabbage, carrots, and cucumber.

4. Last, garnish with fresh guacamole dip.

5. Serve with fresh lime juice and enjoy!

Black Bean Tacos

Serves: 2

>2 Ezekiel 4:9 New Mexico Style Sprouted Grain Tortillas*
>½ to ¾ cup black beans
>¾ cup quinoa, cooked (1 cup dry quinoa yields about 3 cups
>   cooked)
>1 cup crisp romaine lettuce, shredded
>¼ cup Roma tomatoes, diced**
>¼ cup sweet onions, diced**
>½ Haas avocado, sliced (save the remaining avocado for dinner!)**
>Fresh lime juice, to taste
>Salt and pepper, to taste

1. On a clean plate, lay out whole-grain tortillas.

2. Add layer on the black beans, quinoa, lettuce, tomatoes, and onions.

3. Garnish with fresh guacamole and lime juice.

4. Enjoy!

>*If gluten intolerant, consider black bean tortillas, brown rice tortillas, corn tortillas, or 2 large collard green leaves.*
>**Optional: If you prefer, you can substitute pico de gallo for the diced tomatoes and onions and/or guacamole dip for the sliced avocado.*

Cranberry Almond Wheat Berry Bowl

Serves: 2 to 4

>1 cup wheat berries, uncooked*
>3⅓ cups filtered water
>¼ teaspoon salt, optional

¼ cup dried cranberries
¼ cup almonds, sliced
1 tablespoon fresh lemon juice, optional

1. Using a colander, rinse wheat berries.

2. In a medium pot, bring filtered water, wheat berries, and salt to a boil.

3. Reduce heat, cover, and simmer for 1 hour or until tender.

4. Remove from heat and let stand for 5 minutes.

5. In a medium bowl, gently toss the wheat berries, cranberries, almonds, and lemon juice (optional).

6. Enjoy!

If gluten intolerant, consider substituting quinoa or brown rice, or your favorite gluten-free grain.

Baked Sweet Potatoes

Serves: 4

4 medium sweet potatoes, scrubbed and patted dry
1 to 2 tablespoons coconut oil or nondairy butter
   (e.g., Earth Balance).
¼ cup raisins or dried cranberries
½ cup walnuts, chopped
1 teaspoon cinnamon, ground
1 tablespoon maple sugar, granulated (optional)

1. Line a baking sheet with parchment paper and set to the side.

2. Preheat oven to 400°F and place the lined baking sheet on the lowest rack (the baking sheet will be used to catch any sweet potato drippings).

3. Prick each sweet potato five or six times with a knife or a fork.

4. Lightly coat each sweet potato with coconut oil or nondairy butter.

5. Place the sweet potatoes inside the oven on the top rack.

6. Bake for 45 to 60 minutes, or until tender.

7. Remove from heat and let stand for 3 to 5 minutes.

8. Cut a slit in the top of each sweet potato and serve with cinnamon, raisins (or dried cranberries), walnuts, and maple sugar (optional).

Baked Potatoes

Serves: 4

4 medium russet potatoes, scrubbed and patted dry
1 to 2 tablespoons coconut oil or nondairy butter
1 to 2 tablespoons nondairy butter, optional
¼ cup shelled hemp seeds
¼ cup green onions, diced
Salt and pepper, to taste

1. Line a baking sheet with parchment paper and set to the side.

2. Preheat oven to 400°F and place the lined baking sheet on the lowest rack (the baking sheet will be used to catch any potato drippings).

3. Prick each potato five or six times with a knife or a fork.

4. Lightly coat each potato with coconut oil or nondairy butter.

5. Place the potatoes inside the oven on the top rack.

6. Bake for 45 to 60 minutes, or until tender.

7. Remove from heat and let stand for 3 to 5 minutes.

8. Cut a slit in the top of each potato and serve with 1 teaspoon nondairy butter, 1½ tablespoons shelled hemp seeds, 1 tablespoon green onions, and salt/pepper, to taste.

9. Enjoy!

Black Bean Soup and "Refried" Beans

....

Serves: 8 to 10

> 16 ounces (1 pound) black beans
> 10 cups filtered water (plus water for soaking)
> 1 bay leaf
> ½ teaspoon cumin, ground
> ¼ teaspoon dried oregano
> 4 cloves garlic, minced (divided)
> ½ cup cilantro, chopped finely
> 1 yellow onion, diced
> 1 green bell pepper, diced
> 1 teaspoon red wine vinegar
> 2 tablespoons olive oil
> 2 teaspoons salt, or to taste
> ½ avocado, sliced (optional)

1. Soak beans overnight (I prefer the hot soak I described earlier).

2. Add rinsed beans to a large pot with 10 cups of filtered water, bring to boil.

3. Reduce temperature to low, cover, and cook for 45 to 60 minutes or until tender, stir occasionally.

4. In a separate pan, heat the oil over medium heat and sauté the diced onion, bell pepper, and 2 cloves of minced garlic.

5. When beans are approximately 75 percent cooked, add bay leaf, cilantro, oregano, cumin, 2 cloves of garlic (minced), red wine vinegar, salt, and the sautéed ingredients (i.e., sautéed onion, bell pepper, and garlic), and stir.

6. Remove from heat and remove the bay leaf.

7. Serve with chopped cilantro and fresh avocado (optional).

8. Store black bean soup in an airtight container for up to 3 to 5 days in the refrigerator (or up to 3 months in the freezer).

9. Alternatively, you can add your bean soup to your blender to create "refried beans."

10. When making refried black beans, add 1 cup black beans and a small amount of bean broth to a high-speed blender, and blend well, or until desired consistency.

11. If refried beans are too watery, add in additional black beans without the broth, and mix.

12. If refried beans are too thick, add a small amount of additional broth, and mix.

13. Store refried black beans in an airtight container for up to 3 to 5 days in the refrigerator (or up to 3 months in the freezer).

Roasted Red Potatoes

Serves: 2 to 4

1 pound red new potatoes, cut in quarters
1 tablespoon of extra virgin olive oil
1 tablespoon fresh parsley, finely chopped
1 tablespoon fresh dill, finely chopped
2 garlic cloves, minced
Salt and pepper, to taste

1. Preheat oven to 400°F.

2. In a large bowl, toss quartered potatoes with extra virgin olive oil, fresh herbs, garlic, salt, and pepper.

3. Move potatoes to a large roasting pan and roast for 35 to 45 minutes, or until tender and golden brown.

4. Turn potatoes a few times while roasting to ensure they cook evenly.

5. Enjoy!

Guacamole Dip

Serves: 6 to 8

4 ripe Haas avocados
2 ripe Roma tomatoes, seeded and diced

½ cup sweet onion, diced
1 to 2 serrano chilies, seeded and minced
½ cup cilantro, finely chopped
1 clove garlic, minced
½ teaspoon cumin, ground
4 tablespoons fresh lime juice
¼ to ½ teaspoon salt, or to taste

1. Using a large spoon, remove the flesh from the avocados and place in a medium bowl or molcajete.

2. Gently mash the avocados with a fork, leaving some some larger chunks for texture.

3. Gently mix in remaining ingredients.

4. Immediately serve or refrigerate for 1 hour prior to serving (optional).

5. Store within an airtight container in the refrigerator.

6. Guacamole is best fresh (within one day of preparation).

Pico De Gallo

Serves: Yields ~3 cups

4 ripe Roma tomatoes, diced
1 small sweet onion, diced
⅓ cup fresh lime juice
2 to 3 serrano chilies, seeded and minced
¼ cup cilantro, finely chopped
2 teaspoons salt, or to taste

1. Combine the tomatoes, onion, lime juice, serranos, cilantro, and 2 teaspoons salt in a large bowl.

2. Gently toss all ingredients.

3. Enjoy!

Hummus

....

Serves: 8 to 10

> 2 cups chickpeas, cooked and drained
> 3 tablespoons extra virgin olive oil, unrefined and cold-pressed
> 3 tablespoons tahini
> 1½ tablespoons fresh lemon juice, or to taste
> 1 small clove of garlic, minced
> 1 teaspoon salt
> ½ teaspoon finely ground black pepper

1. Prepare, drain, and rinse chickpeas, and set aside.

2. For a smooth consistency, pinch the skins from each of the chickpeas.

3. Combine all ingredients in a food processor (or high-speed blender).

4. Blend until creamy and smooth.

5. If the hummus is too thick, add additional lemon juice (or a small amount of filtered water).

6. If the hummus is too thin, add additional rinsed chickpeas.

7. Transfer hummus to an airtight container and chill for 1 hour prior to serving (optional).

8. Enjoy!

Optional: To spice things up, consider adding in 1 to 3 teaspoons of cumin, sumac, harissa, or smoked paprika. For a vegetable-flavored hummus, blend in 1 cup of roasted eggplant, zucchini, bell pepper, or garlic.

Strawberry Mint Fruit Salad

Serves: 2 to 3

> 2 cups fresh strawberries, halved
> 1 cups fresh blackberries
> 1 to 2 teaspoons fresh lemon juice
> 1 tablespoon fresh mint, finely chopped
> 2 tablespoons maple syrup or sweetener of choice

1. In a large bowl, whisk maple syrup and lemon juice.
2. Add strawberries and blackberries and gently toss all ingredients, except mint.
3. Chill in the refrigerator for 30 to 60 minutes before serving.
4. Stir in mint just before serving.
5. Enjoy!

Raw Banana "Ice Cream"

Serves: 2

> 2 ripe bananas, peeled, chopped, and frozen overnight

1. Add frozen bananas to high-speed blender and blend.
2. Mix in optional ingredients.*
3. Blend until creamy.
4. Enjoy!

> *Optional Ingredients: Ready to take your raw banana ice cream to the next level? Consider mixing in one or more of the following ingredients:*
>
> - *Fresh fruit (e.g. strawberries)*
> - *1 tablespoon of raw cacao nibs*
> - *1 teaspoon of raw cacao powder*
> - *1 tablespoon nut butter*
> - *½ teaspoon cinnamon, ground*

- ¼ cup unsweetened coconut flakes
- ¼ teaspoon pure vanilla
- ½ teaspoon orange zest

Mango Lime Sorbet

Serves: 2

4 cups frozen mango, chunks
¼ cup fresh lime juice
¼ cup fresh lemon juice
1 tablespoon maple syrup (optional)

1. Add frozen mango, fresh lemon and lime juice, and maple syrup to blender and blend well.
2. Enjoy!

Hit-the-Trail Mix

Serves: 6 to 8

½ cup walnuts
½ cup almonds
½ cup pistachios
½ cup cashews
½ cup pecans
½ cup cranberries
½ cup raisins
½ cup unsweetened coconut flakes

1. In a large bowl, gently toss all ingredients.
2. Store in an airtight container in the refrigerator and enjoy!

SALAD DRESSINGS

When it comes to creating your own vinaigrettes with balsamic vinegar, quality matters. For a quality balsamic vinegar, look for either the D.O.P. or I.G.P. stamp. Balsamic vinegar without one of these stamps is likely poor quality (i.e., imitation).

Balsamic Vinegar Quality Assurance Stamps:

- Aceto Balsamico Tradizionale with the Denominazione di Origine Protetta (D.O.P.)
- Balsamic Vinegar of Modena Protected Geographic Identification (I.G.P.)

Blackberry Vinaigrette

Serves: 6 to 8

1 cup fresh blackberries, rinsed and chilled
6 tablespoons (90 mL) extra virgin olive oil, unrefined and cold-pressed
2 tablespoons (30 mL) Italian balsamic vinegar
1 tablespoon (15 mL) pure maple syrup

1. Add fresh blackberries to blender with olive oil, balsamic vinegar, and pure maple syrup.

2. Blend well (approximately 30 to 60 seconds).

3. Chill in the refrigerator for 1 hour prior to serving.

4. Store in an airtight container in the refrigerator for up to 3 days.

Raspberry Vinaigrette

Serves: 6 to 8

1 cup fresh raspberries, rinsed and chilled
6 tablespoons (90 mL) extra virgin olive oil, unrefined and cold-pressed
2 tablespoons (30 mL) Italian balsamic vinegar
1 tablespoon (15 mL) pure maple syrup

1. Add fresh raspberries to blender with olive oil, balsamic vinegar, and pure maple syrup.
2. Blend well (approximately 30 to 60 seconds).
3. Chill in the refrigerator for 1 hour prior to serving.
4. Store in an airtight container in the refrigerator for up to 3 days.

Alternatives to Salad Dressing

- Fresh salsa
- Balsamic vinegar (my favorite!)
- Fresh citrus juice
- Guacamole dip
- Hummus
- "Refried" black beans
- Pomegranate seeds

WHOLE GRAINS
COOKING INSTRUCTIONS

Quinoa

Serves: 4 to 6

1 cup quinoa, uncooked*
2 cups filtered water
¼ teaspoon salt (optional)

*Unless you are using a quinoa product that says the grain is prerinsed, it's a good idea before cooking quinoa to rinse it in a fine-mesh strainer to get rid of the natural, sometimes bitter or soapy-tasting coating.

1. Bring 2 cups filtered water to a boil.
2. Reduce heat to low, add 1 cup quinoa, and salt.

3. Cover with lid and cook for 15 minutes, or until tender.

4. Stir every few minutes.

5. Remove from heat and let stand for 5 minutes.

6. Fluff with fork and serve.

Wheat Berries

Serves: 4 to 6

> 1 cup wheat berries, uncooked
> 3⅓ cups filtered water
> ¼ teaspoon salt (optional)

1. Rinse wheat berries.

2. In a medium pot, bring filtered water, wheat berries, and salt to a boil.

3. Reduce heat, cover, and simmer for 1 hour, or until tender.

4. Stir every few minutes.

5. Remove from heat and let stand for 5 minutes.

6. Fluff with fork and serve.

Brown Rice

Serves: 4 to 6

> 1 cup brown rice, uncooked
> 1¾ cup filtered water
> ¼ teaspoon salt (optional)

1. In a medium pot, bring filtered water to a boil.

2. Reduce heat, add brown rice, and salt.

3. Cover with a lid and simmer for 25 to 30 minutes, or until tender.

4. Stir every few minutes.

5. Remove from heat and let stand for 5 minutes.

6. Fluff with fork and serve.

Steel-Cut Oats

Serves: 4 to 6

> 1 cup steel-cut oats, uncooked
> 3 cups filtered water
> ¼ teaspoon salt (optional)

1. In a medium pot, bring 3 cups of filtered water to a boil.
2. Reduce heat, add steel-cut oats, and salt.
3. Simmer for 20 minutes, or until tender.
4. Stir every few minutes.
5. Remove from heat and let stand for 2 minutes.
6. Fluff with a fork and serve.

Extra Thick Rolled Oats

Serves: 2 to 4

> 1 cup extra thick rolled oats, uncooked
> 3 cups filtered water
> ¼ teaspoon salt (optional)

1. In a medium pot, bring 2 cups filtered water and salt to a boil.
2. Reduce heat to low, add rolled oats, and simmer for 20 minutes, or until tender.
3. Stir every few minutes.
4. Remove from heat and let stand for 2 minutes.
5. Fluff with a fork and serve.

For more recipes, meal ideas, restaurant guides, cooking videos, and all around helpful stuff, go to Proteinaholic.com.

Acknowledgments

This book has been an absolute labor of love, not just for me, but also for my family. After long workweeks, I spent many long weekends in the library studying all this research, and that has taken me away from that which is so special to me. The other day my six-year-old daughter asked me when I would be done with the book so we could play together and talk together and be together. To my daughters, Avery and Dylan, I am done, and I love you for all the times I made you turn off the TV, and all the times I couldn't go roller-skating. I promise I will make it up to you.

To my beautiful wife, thank you so much for your patience. Thanks for being my sounding board, my psychiatrist, and my rock. Most of all, thank you for taking this journey with me.

I would also like to thank my father who has evolved from a parent to a teacher, to a partner, and to a friend. Thanks for always caring so much. I so appreciate you reviewing this book, and your simple words, *This book must be published,* meant so much to me.

I cannot give enough thanks to Gideon Weil, my editor. This book could never have been published by anybody else. When I brought the idea for the book to Gideon, it was simply a vague notion. Gideon was the one who asked me what I thought was the foremost problem in this country when it comes to nutrition. My answer was, of course, the fact that we are a country of proteinaholics, but it took his keen sense to make me realize it. I am not sure if Gideon has worked with a surgeon before, and I doubt he will again. Thank you so much for allowing me to miss so many deadlines and sticking with me for years before I could deliver to you exactly what I wanted to say.

Finally, I would like to thank my friend Howard Jacobson for helping me tie my thoughts together. If it were not for Howard, this book would never have been finished. Howard became my compass. He took what I had written and made it readable and logical. I cannot thank you enough.

Bibliography/References

Abelow, B. J., Holford, T. R., & Insogna, K. L. (1992). Cross-cultural association between dietary animal protein and hip fracture: a hypothesis. *Calcif Tissue Int, 50*(1), 14–18.

Acheson, K. J., Schutz, Y., Bessard, T., Anantharaman, K., Flatt, J. P., & Jéquier, E. (1988). Glycogen storage capacity and de novo lipogenesis during massive carbohydrate overfeeding in man. *Am J Clin Nutr, 48*(2), 240–247.

Adam, O., Beringer, C., Kless, T., Lemmen, C., Adam, A., Wiseman, M., . . . Forth, W. (2003). Anti-inflammatory effects of a low arachidonic acid diet and fish oil in patients with rheumatoid arthritis. *Rheumatol Int, 23*(1), 27–36. doi:10.1007/s00296-002-0234-7

Adam, T. C., Hasson, R. E., Ventura, E. E., Toledo-Corral, C., Le, K. A., Mahurkar, S., . . . Goran, M. I. (2010). Cortisol is negatively associated with insulin sensitivity in overweight Latino youth. *J Clin Endocrinol Metab, 95*(10), 4729–4735. doi:10.1210/jc.2010-0322

Adeva, M. M., & Souto, G. (2011). Diet-induced metabolic acidosis. *Clin Nutr, 30*(4), 416–421. doi:10.1016/j.clnu.2011.03.008

Ahmadi-Abhari, S., Luben, R. N., Powell, N., Bhaniani, A., Chowdhury, R., Wareham, N. J., . . . Khaw, K. T. (2014). Dietary intake of carbohydrates and risk of type 2 diabetes: the European Prospective Investigation into Cancer-Norfolk study. *Br J Nutr, 111*(2), 342–352. doi:10.1017/S0007114513002298

Akbaraly, T., Sabia, S., Hagger-Johnson, G., Tabak, A. G., Shipley, M. J., Jokela, M., . . . Kivimaki, M. (2013). Does overall diet in midlife predict future aging phenotypes? A cohort study. *Am J Med, 126*(5), 411–419. e413. doi:10.1016/j.amjmed.2012.10.028

Aldoori, W. H., Giovannucci, E. L., Stampfer, M. J., Rimm, E. B., Wing, A. L., & Willett, W. C. (1997). Prospective study of diet and the risk of duodenal ulcer in men. *Am J Epidemiol, 145*(1), 42–50.

Alford, B. B., Blankenship, A. C., & Hagen, R. D. (1990). The effects of variations in carbohydrate, protein, and fat content of the diet upon weight loss, blood values, and nutrient intake of adult obese women. *J Am Diet Assoc, 90*(4), 534–540.

Alhassan, S., Kim, S., Bersamin, A., King, A. C., & Gardner, C. D. (2008). Dietary adherence and weight loss success among overweight women: results from the A TO Z weight loss study. *Int J Obes (Lond), 32*(6), 985–991. doi:10.1038/ijo.2008.8

Allam, A. H., Thompson, R. C., Wann, L. S., Miyamoto, M. I., Nur El-Din, A. l.-H., El-Maksoud, G. A., . . . Thomas, G. S. (2011). Atherosclerosis in ancient Egyptian mummies: The Horus study. *JACC Cardiovasc Imaging, 4*(4), 315–327. doi:10.1016/j.jcmg.2011.02.002

Allen, N. E., Appleby, P. N., Davey, G. K., Kaaks, R., Rinaldi, S., & Key, T. J. (2002). The associations of diet with serum insulin-like growth factor I and its main binding proteins in 292 women meat-eaters, vegetarians, and vegans. *Cancer Epidemiol Biomarkers Prev, 11*(11), 1441–1448.

Allen, N. E., Appleby, P. N., Davey, G. K., & Key, T. J. (2000). Hormones and diet: low insulin-like growth factor-I but normal bioavailable androgens in vegan men. *Br J Cancer, 83*(1), 95–97. doi:10.1054/bjoc.2000.1152

Alpha-Tocopherol, Beta Carotene Cancer Prevention Study Group. The effect of vitamin E and beta carotene on the incidence of lung cancer and other cancers in male smokers. (1994). *N Engl J Med, 330*(15), 1029–1035. doi:10.1056/NEJM199404143301501

Alvarez-León, E. E., Román-Viñas, B., & Serra-Majem, L. (2006). Dairy products and health: a review of the epidemiological evidence. *Br J Nutr, 96*(1 Suppl), S94–S99.

Anderson, A. S., Haynie, K. R., McMillan, R. P., Osterberg, K. L., Boutagy, N. E., Frisard, M. I., . . . Hulver, M. W. (2015). Early skeletal muscle adaptations to short-term high-fat diet in humans before changes in insulin sensitivity. *Obesity (Silver Spring), 23*(4), 720–724. doi:10.1002/oby.21031

Anderson, J. W., Johnstone, B. M., & Cook-Newell, M. E. (1995). Meta-analysis of the effects of soy protein intake on serum lipids. *N Engl J Med, 333*(5), 276–282. doi:10.1056/NEJM199508033330502

Appel, L. J. (2008). Dietary patterns and longevity: Expanding the blue zones. *Circulation, 118*(3), 214–215. doi:10.1161/CIRCULATIONAHA.108.788497

Appel, L. J., Moore, T. J., Obarzanek, E., Vollmer, W. M., Svetkey, L. P., Sacks, F. M., . . . Karanja, N. (1997). A clinical trial of the effects of dietary patterns on blood pressure. DASH Collaborative Research Group. *N Engl J Med, 336*(16), 1117–1124. doi:10.1056/NEJM199704173361601

Appel, L. J., Sacks, F. M., Carey, V. J., Obarzanek, E., Swain, J. F., Miller, E. R., . . . OCR Group. (2005). Effects of protein, monounsaturated fat, and carbohydrate intake on blood pressure and serum lipids: Results of the OmniHeart randomized trial. *JAMA, 294*(19), 2455–2464. doi:10.1001/jama.294.19.2455

Appleby, P., Roddam, A., Allen, N., & Key, T. (2007). Comparative fracture risk in vegetarians and nonvegetarians in EPIC-Oxford. *Eur J Clin Nutr, 61*(12), 1400–1406. doi:10.1038/sj.ejcn.1602659

Appleby, P. N., Allen, N. E., & Key, T. J. (2011). Diet, vegetarianism, and cataract risk. *Am J Clin Nutr, 93*(5), 1128–1135. doi:10.3945/ajcn.110.004028

Appleby, P. N., Davey, G. K., & Key, T. J. (2002). Hypertension and blood pressure among meat eaters, fish eaters, vegetarians and vegans in EPIC-Oxford. *Public Health Nutr, 5*(5), 645–654. doi:10.1079/PHN2002332

Appleby, P. N., Key, T. J., Thorogood, M., Burr, M. L., & Mann, J. (2002). Mortality in British vegetarians. *Public Health Nutr, 5*(1), 29–36. doi:10.1079/PHN2001248

Appleby, P. N., Thorogood, M., Mann, J. I., & Key, T. J. (1999). The Oxford Vegetarian Study: an overview. *Am J Clin Nutr, 70*(3 Suppl), 525S–531S.

Appleby, P. N., Thorogood, M., McPherson, K., & Mann, J. (1995). Associations between plasma lipid concentrations and dietary, lifestyle and physical factors in the Oxford Vegetarian Study. *J Hum Nutri Diet, 8*(5), 305–314.

Arts, I. C., & Hollman, P. C. (2005). Polyphenols and disease risk in epidemiologic studies. *Am J Clin Nutr, 81*(1 Suppl), 317S–325S.

Arya, F., Egger, S., Colquhoun, D., Sullivan, D., Pal, S., & Egger, G. (2010). Differences in postprandial inflammatory responses to a "modern" v. traditional meat meal: A preliminary study. *Br J Nutr, 104*(5), 724–728. doi:10.1017/S0007114510001042

Association, A. D., & Canada, D. O. (2003). Position of the American Dietetic Association and Dietitians of Canada: Vegetarian diets. *J Am Diet Assoc, 103*(6), 748–765. doi:10.1053/jada.2003.50142

Astrup, A., Dyerberg, J., Elwood, P., Hermansen, K., Hu, F. B., Jakobsen, M. U., . . . Willett, W. C. (2011). The role of reducing intakes of saturated fat in the prevention of cardiovascular disease: Where does the evidence stand in 2010? *Am J Clin Nutr, 93*(4), 684–688. doi:10.3945/ajcn.110.004622

Astrup, A., Meinert Larsen, T., & Harper, A. (2004). Atkins and other low-carbohydrate diets: hoax or an effective tool for weight loss? *Lancet, 364*(9437), 897–899. doi:10.1016/S0140-6736(04)16986-9

Atherton, P. J., Etheridge, T., Watt, P. W., Wilkinson, D., Selby, A., Rankin, D., . . . Rennie, M. J. (2010). Muscle full effect after oral protein: Time-dependent concordance and discordance between human muscle protein synthesis and mTORC1 signaling. *Am J Clin Nutr, 92*(5), 1080–1088. doi:10.3945/ajcn.2010.29819

Aune, D., De Stefani, E., Ronco, A., Boffetta, P., Deneo-Pellegrini, H., Acosta, G., & Mendilaharsu, M. (2009). Meat consumption and cancer risk: A case-control study in Uruguay. *Asian Pac J Cancer Prev, 10*(3), 429–436.

Aune, D., Navarro Rosenblatt, D. A., Chan, D. S., Vieira, A. R., Vieira, R., Greenwood, D. C., . . . Norat, T. (2015). Dairy products, calcium, and prostate cancer risk: A systematic review and meta-analysis of cohort studies. *Am J Clin Nutr, 101*(1), 87–117. doi:10.3945/ajcn.113.067157

Aune, D., Ursin, G., & Veierød, M. B. (2009). Meat consumption and the risk of type 2 diabetes: A systematic review and meta-analysis of cohort studies. *Diabetologia, 52*(11), 2277–2287. doi:10.1007/s00125-009-1481-x

Azadbakht, L., & Esmaillzadeh, A. (2009). Soy-protein consumption and kidney-related biomarkers among type 2 diabetics: A crossover, randomized clinical trial. *J Ren Nutr, 19*(6), 479–486. doi:10.1053/j.jrn.2009.06.002

Baer, H. J., Glynn, R. J., Hu, F. B., Hankinson, S. E., Willett, W. C., Colditz, G. A., . . . Rosner, B. (2011). Risk factors for mortality in the nurses' health study: A competing risks analysis. *Am J Epidemiol, 173*(3), 319–329. doi:10.1093/aje/kwq368

Ball, M. J., & Bartlett, M. A. (1999). Dietary intake and iron status of Australian vegetarian women. *Am J Clin Nutr, 70*(3), 353–358.

Bandosz, P., O'Flaherty, M., Drygas, W., Rutkowski, M., Koziarek, J., Wyrzykowski, B., . . . Capewell, S. (2012). Decline in mortality from coronary heart disease in Poland after socioeconomic transformation: Modelling study. *BMJ, 344,* d8136.

Bao, W., Rong, Y., Rong, S., & Liu, L. (2012). Dietary iron intake, body iron stores, and the risk of type 2 diabetes: a systematic review and meta-analysis. *BMC Med, 10,* 119. doi:10.1186/1741-7015-10-119

Bao, Y., Han, J., Hu, F. B., Giovannucci, E. L., Stampfer, M. J., Willett, W. C., & Fuchs, C. S. (2013). Association of nut consumption with total and cause-specific mortality. *N Engl J Med, 369*(21), 2001–2011. doi:10.1056/NEJMoa1307352

Barbaresko, J., Koch, M., Schulze, M. B., & Nöthlings, U. (2013). Dietary pattern analysis and biomarkers of low-grade inflammation: A systematic literature review. *Nutr Rev, 71*(8), 511–527. doi:10.1111/nure.12035

Barnard, N. D., Cohen, J., Jenkins, D. J., Turner-McGrievy, G., Gloede, L., Green, A., & Ferdowsian, H. (2009). A low-fat vegan diet and a conventional diabetes diet in the treatment of type 2 diabetes: A randomized, controlled, 74-wk clinical trial. *Am J Clin Nutr, 89*(5), 1588S–1596S. doi:10.3945/ajcn.2009.26736H

Barnard, N. D., Cohen, J., Jenkins, D. J., Turner-McGrievy, G., Gloede, L., Jaster, B., . . . Talpers, S. (2006). A low-fat vegan diet improves glycemic control and cardiovascular risk factors in a randomized clinical trial in individuals with type 2 diabetes. *Diabetes Care, 29*(8), 1777–1783. doi:10.2337/dc06-0606

Barnard, R. J., Roberts, C. K., Varon, S. M., & Berger, J. J. (1998). Diet-induced insulin resistance precedes other aspects of the metabolic syndrome. *J Appl Physiol (1985), 84*(4), 1311–1315.

Barzel, U. S., & Massey, L. K. (1998). Excess dietary protein can adversely affect bone. *J Nutr, 128*(6), 1051–1053.

Basu, S., Yoffe, P., Hills, N., & Lustig, R. H. (2013). The relationship of sugar to population-level diabetes prevalence: An econometric analysis of repeated cross-sectional data. *PLoS One, 8*(2), e57873. doi:10.1371/journal.pone.0057873

Bauer, J., Biolo, G., Cederholm, T., Cesari, M., Cruz-Jentoft, A. J., Morley, J. E., . . . Boirie, Y. (2013). Evidence-based recommendations for optimal dietary protein intake in older people: A position paper from the PROT-AGE Study Group. *J Am Med Dir Assoc, 14*(8), 542–559. doi:10.1016/j.jamda.2013.05.021

Bautista-Castaño, I., & Serra-Majem, L. (2012). Relationship between bread consumption, body weight, and abdominal fat distribution: evidence from epidemiological studies. *Nutr Rev, 70*(4), 218–233. doi:10.1111/j.1753-4887.2012.00454.x

Bazzano, L. A., He, J., Ogden, L. G., Loria, C., Vupputuri, S., Myers, L., & Whelton, P. K. (2001). Legume consumption and risk of coronary heart disease in US men and women: NHANES I Epidemiologic Follow-up Study. *Arch Intern Med, 161*(21), 2573–2578.

Bazzano, L. A., He, J., Ogden, L. G., Loria, C. M., Vupputuri, S., Myers, L., & Whelton, P. K. (2002). Fruit and vegetable intake and risk of cardiovascular disease in US adults: The first National Health and Nutrition Examination Survey Epidemiologic Follow-up Study. *Am J Clin Nutr, 76*(1), 93–99.

Beasley, J. M., Newcomb, P. A., Trentham-Dietz, A., Hampton, J. M., Bersch, A. J., Passarelli, M. N., . . . Willett, W. C. (2011). Post-diagnosis dietary factors and survival after invasive breast cancer. *Breast Cancer Res Treat, 128*(1), 229–236. doi:10.1007/s10549-010-1323-z

Beeson, W. L., Mills, P. K., Phillips, R. L., Andress, M., & Fraser, G. E. (1989). Chronic disease among Seventh-day Adventists, a low-risk group: Rationale, methodology, and description of the population. *Cancer, 64*(3), 570–581.

Beezhold, B. L., & Johnston, C. S. (2012). Restriction of meat, fish, and poultry in omnivores improves mood: A pilot randomized controlled trial. *Nutr J, 11*, 9. doi:10.1186/1475-2891-11-9

Beier, K., Eppanapally, S., Bazick, H. S., Chang, D., Mahadevappa, K., Gibbons, F. K., & Christopher, K. B. (2011). Elevation of blood urea nitrogen is predictive of long-term mortality in critically ill patients independent of "normal" creatinine. *Crit Care Med, 39*(2), 305–313. doi:10.1097/CCM.0b013e3181ffe22a

Bell, R. A., Mayer-Davis, E. J., Jackson, Y., & Dresser, C. (1997). An epidemiologic review of dietary intake studies among American Indians and Alaska Natives: Implications for heart disease and cancer risk. *Ann Epidemiol, 7*(4), 229–240.

Benzie, I. F., & Wachtel-Galor, S. (2009). Biomarkers in long-term vegetarian diets. *Adv Clin Chem, 47*, 171–222.

Bergen, W. G., & Wu, G. (2009). Intestinal nitrogen recycling and utilization in health and disease. *J Nutr, 139*(5), 821–825. doi:10.3945/jn.109.104497

Berkemeyer, S. (2009). Acid-base balance and weight gain: Are there crucial links via protein and organic acids in understanding obesity? *Med Hypotheses, 73*(3), 347–356. doi:10.1016/j.mehy.2008.09.059

Berkow, S. E., Barnard, N., Eckart, J., & Katcher, H. (2010). Four therapeutic diets: Adherence and acceptability. *Can J Diet Pract Res, 71*(4), 199–204.

Bernstein, A. M., Sun, Q., Hu, F. B., Stampfer, M. J., Manson, J. E., & Willett, W. C. (2010). Major dietary protein sources and risk of coronary heart disease in women. *Circulation, 122*(9), 876–883. doi:10.1161/CIRCULATIONAHA.109.915165

Best, T. H., Franz, D. N., Gilbert, D. L., Nelson, D. P., & Epstein, M. R. (2000). Cardiac complications in pediatric patients on the ketogenic diet. *Neurology, 54*(12), 2328–2330.

Bidlack, W. R. (1996). Interrelationships of food, nutrition, diet and health: The National Association of State Universities and Land Grant Colleges White Paper. *J Am Coll Nutr, 15*(5), 422–433.

Biesiekierski, J. R., Muir, J. G., & Gibson, P. R. (2013). Is gluten a cause of gastrointestinal symptoms in people without celiac disease? *Curr Allergy Asthma Rep, 13*(6), 631–638. doi:10.1007/s11882-013-0386-4

Biesiekierski, J. R., Peters, S. L., Newnham, E. D., Rosella, O., Muir, J. G., & Gibson, P. R. (2013). No effects of gluten in patients with self-reported non-celiac gluten sensitivity after dietary reduction of fermentable, poorly absorbed, short-chain carbohydrates. *Gastroenterology, 145*(2), 320–328. e321-323. doi:10.1053/j.gastro.2013.04.051

Biet, S. S. (2014). The ratio of macronutrients, not caloric intake, dictates cardiometabolic health, aging, and longevity in ad libitum-fed mice. *Cell Metab, 19,* 4128–4430.

Bilsborough, S., & Mann, N. (2006). A review of issues of dietary protein intake in humans. *Int J Sport Nutr Exerc Metab, 16*(2), 129–152.

Bilsborough, S. A., & Crowe, T. C. (2003). Low-carbohydrate diets: What are the potential short- and long-term health implications? *Asia Pacific J Clin Nutr, 12*(4), 396–404.

Bingham, S. A. (1999). High-meat diets and cancer risk. *Proc Nutr Soc, 58*(2), 243–248.

Bingham, S. A., Day, N. E., Luben, R., Ferrari, P., Slimani, N., Norat, T., ... Nutrition, E. P. I. i. C. a. (2003). Dietary fibre in food and protection against colorectal cancer in the European Prospective Investigation into Cancer and Nutrition (EPIC): An observational study. *Lancet, 361*(9368), 1496–1501.

Bingham, S. A., Hughes, R., & Cross, A. J. (2002). Effect of white versus red meat on endogenous N-nitrosation in the human colon and further evidence of a dose response. *J Nutr, 132*(11 Suppl), 3522S–3525S.

Bingham, S. A., Pignatelli, B., Pollock, J. R., Ellul, A., Malaveille, C., Gross, G., ... O'Neill, I. K. (1996). Does increased endogenous formation of N-nitroso compounds in the human colon explain the association between red meat and colon cancer? *Carcinogenesis, 17*(3), 515–523.

Biolo, G., Ciocchi, B., Lebenstedt, M., Barazzoni, R., Zanetti, M., Platen, P., ... Guarnieri, G. (2004). Short-term bed rest impairs amino acid-induced protein anabolism in humans. *J Physiol, 558*(Pt 2), 381–388. doi:10.1113/jphysiol.2004.066365

Biritwum, R., Gyapong, J., & Mensah, G. (2005). The epidemiology of obesity in Ghana. *Ghana Med J, 39*(3), 82–85.

Bjerregaard, P., Young, T. K., & Hegele, R. A. (2003). Low incidence of cardiovascular disease among the Inuit—what is the evidence? *Atherosclerosis, 166*(2), 351–357.

Bjornsson, J. (1942). Arteriosclerosis: A Chemical and Statistical Study: CPH.

Blackburn, H. (2012). 20th-century "medical Marco Polos" in the origins of preventive cardiology and cardiovascular disease epidemiology. *Am J Cardiol, 109*(5), 756–767.

Bloomer, R. J., Kabir, M. M., Canale, R. E., Trepanowski, J. F., Marshall, K. E., Farney, T. M., & Hammond, K. G. (2010). Effect of a 21 day Daniel Fast on metabolic and cardiovascular disease risk factors in men and women. *Lipids Health Dis, 9*, 94. doi:10.1186/1476-511X-9-94

Blüher, M., Michael, M. D., Peroni, O. D., Ueki, K., Carter, N., Kahn, B. B., & Kahn, C. R. (2002). Adipose tissue selective insulin receptor knockout protects against obesity and obesity-related glucose intolerance. *Dev Cell, 3*(1), 25–38.

Boelsma, E., Brink, E. J., Stafleu, A., & Hendriks, H. F. (2010). Measures of postprandial wellness after single intake of two protein-carbohydrate meals. *Appetite, 54*(3), 456–464. doi:10.1016/j.appet.2009.12.014

Böger, R. H. (2003). Association of asymmetric dimethylarginine and endothelial dysfunction. *Clin Chem Lab Med, 41*(11), 1467–1472. doi:10.1515/CCLM.2003.225

Bowen, J., Noakes, M., & Clifton, P. M. (2006). Appetite regulatory hormone responses to various dietary proteins differ by body mass index status despite similar reductions in ad libitum energy intake. *J Clin Endocrinol Metab, 91*(8), 2913–2919. doi:10.1210/jc.2006-0609

Bowen, J., Noakes, M., Trenerry, C., & Clifton, P. M. (2006). Energy intake, ghrelin, and cholecystokinin after different carbohydrate and protein preloads in overweight men. *J Clin Endocrinol Metab, 91*(4), 1477–1483. doi:10.1210/jc.2005-1856

Bowman, S. A., & Spence, J. T. (2002). A comparison of low-carbohydrate vs. high-carbohydrate diets: energy restriction, nutrient quality and correlation to body mass index. *J Am Coll Nutr, 21*(3), 268–274.

Boyce, V. L., & Swinburn, B. A. (1993). The traditional Pima Indian diet. Composition and adaptation for use in a dietary intervention study. *Diabetes Care, 16*(1), 369–371.

Boyd, N. F., Stone, J., Vogt, K. N., Connelly, B. S., Martin, L. J., & Minkin, S. (2003). Dietary fat and breast cancer risk revisited: A meta-analysis of the published literature. *Br J Cancer, 89*(9), 1672–1685. doi:10.1038/sj.bjc.6601314

Brand-Miller, J., Hayne, S., Peťocz, P., & Colagiuri, S. (2003). Low-glycemic index diets in the management of diabetes: A meta-analysis of randomized controlled trials. *Diabetes Care, 26*(8), 2261–2267.

Brasky, T. M., Darke, A. K., Song, X., Tangen, C. M., Goodman, P. J., Thompson, I. M., . . . Kristal, A. R. (2013). Plasma phospholipid fatty acids and prostate cancer risk in the SELECT trial. *J Natl Cancer Inst, 105*(15), 1132–1141. doi:10.1093/jnci/djt174

Bravata, D. M., Sanders, L., Huang, J., Krumholz, H. M., Olkin, I., & Gardner, C. D. (2003). Efficacy and safety of low-carbohydrate diets: a systematic review. *JAMA, 289*(14), 1837–1850. doi:10.1001/jama.289.14.1837

Bray, G. A., & Popkin, B. M. (1998). Dietary fat intake does affect obesity! *Am J Clin Nutr, 68*(6), 1157–1173.

Bray, G. A., Smith, S. R., de Jonge, L., Xie, H., Rood, J., Martin, C. K., . . . Redman, L. M. (2012). Effect of dietary protein content on weight gain, energy expenditure, and body composition during overeating: A randomized controlled trial. *JAMA, 307*(1), 47–55. doi:10.1001/jama.2011.1918

Briel, M., Ferreira-Gonzalez, I., You, J. J., Karanicolas, P. J., Akl, E. A., Wu, P., . . . Guyatt, G. H. (2009). Association between change in high density lipoprotein cholesterol and cardiovascular disease morbidity and mortality: systematic review and meta-regression analysis. *BMJ, 338*, b92.

Brighenti, F., Benini, L., Del Rio, D., Casiraghi, C., Pellegrini, N., Scazzina, F., . . . Vantini, I. (2006). Colonic fermentation of indigestible carbohydrates contributes to the second-meal effect. *Am J Clin Nutr, 83*(4), 817–822.

Brinkworth, G. D., Buckley, J. D., Noakes, M., Clifton, P. M., & Wilson, C. J. (2009). Long-term effects of a very low-carbohydrate diet and a low-fat diet on mood and cognitive function. *Arch Intern Med, 169*(20), 1873–1880. doi:10.1001/archinternmed.2009.329

Brinton, E. A., Eisenberg, S., & Breslow, J. L. (1990). A low-fat diet decreases high density lipoprotein (HDL) cholesterol levels by decreasing HDL apolipoprotein transport rates. *J Clin Invest, 85*(1), 144–151. doi:10.1172/JCI114405

Brüning, J. C., Gautam, D., Burks, D. J., Gillette, J., Schubert, M., Orban, P. C., . . . Kahn, C. R. (2000). Role of brain insulin receptor in control of body weight and reproduction. *Science, 289*(5487), 2122–2125.

Brunzell, J. D., Lerner, R. L., Hazzard, W. R., Porte, D., & Bierman, E. L. (1971). Improved glucose tolerance with high carbohydrate feeding in mild diabetes. *N Engl J Med, 284*(10), 521–524. doi:10.1056/NEJM197103112841004

Büchner, F. L., Bueno-de-Mesquita, H. B., Ros, M. M., Overvad, K., Dahm, C. C., Hansen, L., . . . Riboli, E. (2010). Variety in fruit and vegetable consumption and the risk of lung cancer in the European prospective investigation into cancer and nutrition. *Cancer Epidemiol Biomarkers Prev, 19*(9), 2278–2286. doi:10.1158/1055-9965.EPI-10-0489

Buijsse, B., Feskens, E. J., Schulze, M. B., Forouhi, N. G., Wareham, N. J., Sharp, S., . . . Boeing, H. (2009). Fruit and vegetable intakes and subsequent changes in body weight in European populations: results from the project on Diet, Obesity, and Genes (DiOGenes). *Am J Clin Nutr, 90*(1), 202–209. doi:10.3945/ajcn.2008.27394

Bujnowski, D., Xun, P., Daviglus, M. L., Van Horn, L., He, K., & Stamler, J. (2011). Longitudinal association between animal and vegetable protein intake and obesity among men in the United States: The Chicago Western Electric Study. *J Am Diet Assoc, 111*(8), 1150–1155. e1151. doi:10.1016/j.jada.2011.05.002

Burkert, N. T., Muckenhuber, J., Großschädl, F., Rásky, E., & Freidl, W. (2014). Nutrition and health—the association between eating behavior and various health parameters: a matched sample study. *PLoS One, 9*(2), e88278. doi:10.1371/journal.pone.0088278

Burkitt, D. (1991). An approach to the reduction of the most common Western cancers. The failure of therapy to reduce disease. *Arch Surg, 126*(3), 345–347.

Burkitt, D. P. (1971). Epidemiology of cancer of the colon and rectum. *Cancer, 28*(1), 3–13.

Burkitt, D. P. (1981). *Western diseases: Their emergence and prevention.* Cambridge, MA: Harvard University Press.

Butler, L. M., Sinha, R., Millikan, R. C., Martin, C. F., Newman, B., Gammon, M. D., . . . Sandler, R. S. (2003). Heterocyclic amines, meat intake, and association with colon cancer in a population-based study. *Am J Epidemiol, 157*(5), 434–445.

Cai, H., Shu, X. O., Gao, Y. T., Li, H., Yang, G., & Zheng, W. (2007). A prospective study of dietary patterns and mortality in Chinese women. *Epidemiology, 18*(3), 393–401. doi:10.1097/01.ede.0000259967.21114.45

Calloway, D. H. (1975). Nitrogen balance of men with marginal intakes of protein and energy. *J Nutr, 105*(7), 914–923.

Campbell, W. W., Johnson, C. A., McCabe, G. P., & Carnell, N. S. (2008). Dietary protein requirements of younger and older adults. *Am J Clin Nutr, 88*(5), 1322–1329.

Campbell, W. W., & Leidy, H. J. (2007). Dietary protein and resistance training effects on muscle and body composition in older persons. *J Am Coll Nutr, 26*(6), 696S–703S.

Campbell, W. W., Trappe, T. A., Jozsi, A. C., Kruskall, L. J., Wolfe, R. R., & Evans, W. J. (2002). Dietary protein adequacy and lower body versus whole body resistive training in older humans. *J Physiol, 542*(Pt 2), 631–642.

Capewell, S., & Ford, E. S. (2011). Why have total cholesterol levels declined in most developed countries? *BMC Public Health, 11*, 641. doi:10.1186/1471-2458-11-641

Carlson, M. G., & Campbell, P. J. (1993). Intensive insulin therapy and weight gain in IDDM. *Diabetes, 42*(12), 1700–1707.

Casas-Agustench, P., Bulló, M., Ros, E., Basora, J., Salas-Salvadó, J., & investigators, N.-P. (2011). Cross-sectional association of nut intake with adiposity in a Mediterranean population. *Nutr Metab Cardiovasc Dis, 21*(7), 518–525. doi:10.1016/j.numecd.2009.11.010

Cellarier, E., Durando, X., Vasson, M. P., Farges, M. C., Demiden, A., Maurizis, J. C., . . . Chollet, P. (2003). Methionine dependency and cancer treatment. *Cancer Treat Rev, 29*(6), 489–499.

Cermak, N. M., Res, P. T., de Groot, L. C., Saris, W. H., & van Loon, L. J. (2012). Protein supplementation augments the adaptive response of skeletal muscle to resistance-type exercise training: a meta-analysis. *Am J Clin Nutr, 96*(6), 1454–1464. doi:10.3945/ajcn.112.037556

Cerqueira, M. T., Fry, M. M., & Connor, W. E. (1979). The food and nutrient intakes of the Tarahumara Indians of Mexico. *Am J Clin Nutr, 32*(4), 905–915.

Chagas, P., Caramori, P., Galdino, T. P., Barcellos, C. a. S., Gomes, I., & Schwanke, C. H. (2013). Egg consumption and coronary atherosclerotic burden. *Atherosclerosis, 229*(2), 381–384. doi:10.1016/j.atherosclerosis.2013.05.008

Chan, D. S., Lau, R., Aune, D., Vieira, R., Greenwood, D. C., Kampman, E., & Norat, T. (2011). Red and processed meat and colorectal cancer incidence: Meta-analysis of prospective studies. *PLoS One, 6*(6), e20456. doi:10.1371/journal.pone.0020456

Chan, J., Jaceldo-Siegl, K., & Fraser, G. E. (2009). Serum 25-hydroxyvitamin D status of vegetarians, partial vegetarians, and nonvegetarians: The Adventist Health Study-2. *Am J Clin Nutr, 89*(5), 1686S–1692S. doi:10.3945/ajcn.2009.26736X

Chan, J. M., Stampfer, M. J., Giovannucci, E., Gann, P. H., Ma, J., Wilkinson, P., . . . Pollak, M. (1998). Plasma insulin-like growth factor-I and prostate cancer risk: A prospective study. *Science, 279*(5350), 563–566.

Chandalia, M., Garg, A., Lutjohann, D., von Bergmann, K., Grundy, S. M., & Brinkley, L. J. (2000). Beneficial effects of high dietary fiber intake in patients with type 2 diabetes mellitus. *N Engl J Med, 342*(19), 1392–1398. doi:10.1056/NEJM200005113421903

Chang, W. C., Wahlqvist, M. L., Chang, H. Y., Hsu, C. C., Lee, M. S., Wang, W. S., & Hsiung, C. A. (2012). A bean-free diet increases the risk of all-cause mortality among Taiwanese women: The role of the metabolic syndrome. *Public Health Nutr, 15*(4), 663–672. doi:10.1017/S1368980011002151

Chang-Claude, J., Frentzel-Beyme, R., & Eilber, U. (1992). Mortality pattern of German vegetarians after 11 years of follow-up. *Epidemiology, 3*(5), 395–401.

Chavarro, J. E., Rich-Edwards, J. W., Rosner, B. A., & Willett, W. C. (2008). Protein intake and ovulatory infertility. *Am J Obstet Gynecol, 198*(2), 210. e211-217. doi:10.1016/j.ajog.2007.06.057

Chen, H. M., Yu, Y. N., Wang, J. L., Lin, Y. W., Kong, X., Yang, C. Q., . . . Fang, J. Y. (2013). Decreased dietary fiber intake and structural alteration of gut microbiota in patients with advanced colorectal adenoma. *Am J Clin Nutr, 97*(5), 1044–1052. doi:10.3945/ajcn.112.046607

Chen, M., Pan, A., Malik, V. S., & Hu, F. B. (2012). Effects of dairy intake on body weight and fat: A meta-analysis of randomized controlled trials. *Am J Clin Nutr, 96*(4), 735–747. doi:10.3945/ajcn.112.037119

Cheng, G., Buyken, A. E., Shi, L., Karaolis-Danckert, N., Kroke, A., Wudy, S. A., . . . Remer, T. (2012). Beyond overweight: Nutrition as an important lifestyle factor influencing timing of puberty. *Nutr Rev, 70*(3), 133–152. doi:10.1111/j.1753-4887.2011.00461.x

Cheng, G., Remer, T., Prinz-Langenohl, R., Blaszkewicz, M., Degen, G. H., & Buyken, A. E. (2010). Relation of isoflavones and fiber intake in childhood to the timing of puberty. *Am J Clin Nutr, 92*(3), 556–564. doi:10.3945/ajcn.2010.29394

Cheuvront, S. N. (2003). The Zone Diet phenomenon: A closer look at the science behind the claims. *J Am Coll Nutr, 22*(1), 9–17.

Chiba, M., Abe, T., Tsuda, H., Sugawara, T., Tsuda, S., Tozawa, H., . . . Imai, H. (2010). Lifestyle-related disease in Crohn's disease: Relapse prevention by a semi-vegetarian diet. *World J Gastroenterol, 16*(20), 2484–2495.

Chiu, T. H., Huang, H. Y., Chiu, Y. F., Pan, W. H., Kao, H. Y., Chiu, J. P., . . . Lin, C. L. (2014). Taiwanese vegetarians and omnivores: Dietary composition, prevalence of diabetes and IFG. *PLoS One, 9*(2), e88547. doi:10.1371/journal.pone.0088547

Chlebowski, R. T., Blackburn, G. L., Thomson, C. A., Nixon, D. W., Shapiro, A., Hoy, M. K., . . . Elashoff, R. M. (2006). Dietary fat reduction and breast cancer outcome: Interim efficacy results from the Women's Intervention Nutrition Study. *J Natl Cancer Inst, 98*(24), 1767–1776. doi:10.1093/jnci/djj494

Choi, H. K., Atkinson, K., Karlson, E. W., Willett, W., & Curhan, G. (2004). Purine-rich foods, dairy and protein intake, and the risk of gout in men. *N Engl J Med, 350*(11), 1093–1103. doi:10.1056/NEJMoa035700

Choinière, R. (1992). Mortality among the Baffin Inuit in the mid-80s. *Arctic Med Res, 51*(2), 87–93.

Chowdhury, R., Warnakula, S., Kunutsor, S., Crowe, F., Ward, H. A., Johnson, L., . . . Di Angelantonio, E. (2014). Association of dietary, circulating, and supplement fatty acids with coronary risk: a systematic review and meta-analysis. *Ann Intern Med, 160*(6), 398–406. doi:10.7326/M13-1788

Christakis, N. A., & Fowler, J. H. (2007). The spread of obesity in a large social network over 32 years. *N Engl J Med, 357*(4), 370–379. doi:10.1056/NEJMsa066082

Christensen, A. S., Viggers, L., Hasselström, K., & Gregersen, S. (2013). Effect of fruit restriction on glycemic control in patients with type 2 diabetes—a randomized trial. *Nutr J, 12*, 29. doi:10.1186/1475-2891-12-29

Chuang, S. C., Norat, T., Murphy, N., Olsen, A., Tjønneland, A., Overvad, K., . . . Vineis, P. (2012). Fiber intake and total and cause-specific mortality in the European Prospective Investigation into Cancer and Nutrition cohort. *Am J Clin Nutr, 96*(1), 164–174. doi:10.3945/ajcn.111.028415

Clarke, R., Frost, C., Collins, R., Appleby, P., & Peto, R. (1997). Dietary lipids and blood cholesterol: Quantitative meta-analysis of metabolic ward studies. *BMJ, 314*(7074), 112–117.

Clifton, P. M., & Keogh, J. (2007). Metabolic effects of high-protein diets. *Curr Atheroscler Rep, 9*(6), 472–478.

Cohen, M. N. (2012). History, diet, and hunter-gatherers. In K. Kiple & K. C. Ornelas (Eds.), *Cambridge World History of Food.* Cambridge, UK: Cambridge University Press.

Cohen, P., Peehl, D. M., & Rosenfeld, R. G. (1994). The IGF axis in the prostate. *Horm Metab Res, 26*(2), 81–84. doi:10.1055/s-2007-1000777

Coletta, D. K., & Mandarino, L. J. (2011). Mitochondrial dysfunction and insulin resistance from the outside in: extracellular matrix, the cytoskeleton, and mitochondria. *Am J Physiol Endocrinol Metab, 301*(5), E749–E755. doi:10.1152/ajpendo.00363.2011

Connor, W. E., Cerqueira, M. T., Connor, R. W., Wallace, R. B., Malinow, M. R., & Casdorph, H. R. (1978). The plasma lipids, lipoproteins, and diet of the Tarahumara indians of Mexico. *Am J Clin Nutr, 31*(7), 1131–1142.

Connor, W. E., & Connor, S. L. (1972). The key role of nutritional factors in the prevention of coronary heart disease. *Prev Med, 1*(1), 49–83.

Connor, W. E., & Connor, S. L. (1997). Should a low-fat, high-carbohydrate diet be recommended for everyone? The case for a low-fat, high-carbohydrate diet. *N Engl J Med, 337*(8), 562–563; discussion 566–567. doi:10.1056/NEJM199708213370811

Consortium, I. (2013). Association between dietary meat consumption and incident type 2 diabetes: The EPIC-InterAct study. *Diabetologia, 56*(1), 47–59. doi:10.1007/s00125-012-2718-7

Consortium, I. (2014). Adherence to predefined dietary patterns and incident type 2 diabetes in European populations: EPIC-InterAct Study. *Diabetologia, 57*(2), 321–333. doi:10.1007/s00125-013-3092-9

Cooper, A. J., Sharp, S. J., Lentjes, M. A., Luben, R. N., Khaw, K. T., Wareham, N. J., & Forouhi, N. G. (2012). A prospective study of the association between quantity and variety of fruit and vegetable intake and incident type 2 diabetes. *Diabetes Care, 35*(6), 1293–1300. doi:10.2337/dc11-2388

Corti, M. C., Guralnik, J. M., Salive, M. E., Harris, T., Ferrucci, L., Glynn, R. J., & Havlik, R. J. (1997). Clarifying the direct relation between total cholesterol levels and death from coronary heart disease in older persons. *Ann Intern Med, 126*(10), 753–760.

Cozma, A. I., Sievenpiper, J. L., de Souza, R. J., Chiavaroli, L., Ha, V., Wang, D. D., . . . Jenkins, D. J. (2012). Effect of fructose on glycemic control in diabetes: A systematic review and meta-analysis of controlled feeding trials. *Diabetes Care, 35*(7), 1611–1620. doi:10.2337/dc12-0073

Craig, W. J., Mangels, A. R., & Association, A. D. (2009). Position of the American Dietetic Association: Vegetarian diets. *J Am Diet Assoc, 109*(7), 1266–1282.

Cross, A. J., Leitzmann, M. F., Gail, M. H., Hollenbeck, A. R., Schatzkin, A., & Sinha, R. (2007). A prospective study of red and processed meat intake in relation to cancer risk. *PLoS Med, 4*(12), e325. doi:10.1371/journal.pmed.0040325

Cross, A. J., Peters, U., Kirsh, V. A., Andriole, G. L., Reding, D., Hayes, R. B., & Sinha, R. (2005). A prospective study of meat and meat mutagens and prostate cancer risk. *Cancer Res, 65*(24), 11779–11784. doi:10.1158/0008-5472.CAN-05-2191

Cross, A. J., Pollock, J. R., & Bingham, S. A. (2003). Haem, not protein or inorganic iron, is responsible for endogenous intestinal N-nitrosation arising from red meat. *Cancer Res, 63*(10), 2358–2360.

Crowe, F. L., Appleby, P. N., Allen, N. E., & Key, T. J. (2011). Diet and risk of diverticular disease in Oxford cohort of European Prospective Investigation into Cancer and Nutrition (EPIC): Prospective study of British vegetarians and non-vegetarians. *BMJ, 343*, d4131.

Crowe, F. L., Appleby, P. N., Travis, R. C., & Key, T. J. (2013). Risk of hospitalization or death from ischemic heart disease among British vegetarians and nonvegetarians: Results from the EPIC-Oxford cohort study. *Am J Clin Nutr, 97*(3), 597–603. doi:10.3945/ajcn.112.044073

Cruz-Jentoft, A. J., Landi, F., Schneider, S. M., Zúñiga, C., Arai, H., Boirie, Y., . . . Cederholm, T. (2014). Prevalence of and interventions for sarcopenia in ageing adults: a systematic review. Report of the International Sarcopenia Initiative (EWGSOP and IWGS). *Age Ageing, 43*(6), 748–759. doi:10.1093/ageing/afu115

Cuadrado, C., Hajos, G., Burbano, C., Pedrosa, M., Ayet, G., Muzquiz, M., . . . Gelencser, E. (2002). The effects of natural fermentation of the lectin in lentils measured by immunolgic methods. *Food Agric Immunol, 14*, 41–49.

Dancause, K. N., Vilar, M., Wilson, M., Soloway, L. E., DeHuff, C., Chan, C., . . . Garruto, R. M. (2013). Behavioral risk factors for obesity during health transition in Vanuatu, South Pacific. *Obesity (Silver Spring), 21*(1), E98–E104. doi:10.1002/oby.20082

Daniel, C. R., Cross, A. J., Graubard, B. I., Hollenbeck, A. R., Park, Y., & Sinha, R. (2011). Prospective investigation of poultry and fish intake in relation to cancer risk. *Cancer Prev Res (Phila),* 4(11), 1903–1911. doi:10.1158/1940-6207.CAPR-11-0241

Daniel, C. R., Cross, A. J., Graubard, B. I., Park, Y., Ward, M. H., Rothman, N., . . . Sinha, R. (2012). Large prospective investigation of meat intake, related mutagens, and risk of renal cell carcinoma. *Am J Clin Nutr,* 95(1), 155–162. doi:10.3945/ajcn.111.019364

Daniel, C. R., Park, Y., Chow, W. H., Graubard, B. I., Hollenbeck, A. R., & Sinha, R. (2013). Intake of fiber and fiber-rich plant foods is associated with a lower risk of renal cell carcinoma in a large US cohort. *Am J Clin Nutr,* 97(5), 1036–1043. doi:10.3945/ajcn.112.045351

Danilo, C., & Frank, P. G. (2012). Cholesterol and breast cancer development. *Curr Opin Pharmacol,* 12(6), 677–682. doi:10.1016/j.coph.2012.07.009

Dansinger, M. L., Gleason, J. A., Griffith, J. L., Selker, H. P., & Schaefer, E. J. (2005). Comparison of the Atkins, Ornish, Weight Watchers, and Zone diets for weight loss and heart disease risk reduction: a randomized trial. *JAMA,* 293(1), 43–53. doi:10.1001/jama.293.1.43

Dar, B., Dar, N. & Bashir, S. (2012). Calorie restriction: The fountain of youth. *Food Nutr Sci,* 3(11), 1522–1526.

Darmadi-Blackberry, I., Wahlqvist, M. L., Kouris-Blazos, A., Steen, B., Lukito, W., Horie, Y., & Horie, K. (2004). Legumes: The most important dietary predictor of survival in older people of different ethnicities. *Asia Pacific J Clin Nutr,* 13(2), 217–220.

Dauchet, L., Ferrières, J., Arveiler, D., Yarnell, J. W., Gey, F., Ducimetière, P., . . . Dallongeville, J. (2004). Frequency of fruit and vegetable consumption and coronary heart disease in France and Northern Ireland: the PRIME study. *Br J Nutr,* 92(6), 963–972.

Davey, G. K., Spencer, E. A., Appleby, P. N., Allen, N. E., Knox, K. H., & Key, T. J. (2003). EPIC-Oxford: Lifestyle characteristics and nutrient intakes in a cohort of 33,883 meat-eaters and 31,546 non meat-eaters in the UK. *Public Health Nutr,* 6(3), 259–269. doi:10.1079/PHN2002430

David, L. A., Maurice, C. F., Carmody, R. N., Gootenberg, D. B., Button, J. E., Wolfe, B. E., . . . Turnbaugh, P. J. (2013). Diet rapidly and reproducibly alters the human gut microbiome. *Nature.* doi:10.1038/nature12820

David, L. A., Maurice, C. F., Carmody, R. N., Gootenberg, D. B., Button, J. E., Wolfe, B. E., . . . Turnbaugh, P. J. (2014). Diet rapidly and reproducibly alters the human gut microbiome. *Nature,* 505(7484), 559–563. doi:10.1038/nature12820

Daviglus, M. L., Stamler, J., Orencia, A. J., Dyer, A. R., Liu, K., Greenland, P., . . . Shekelle, R. B. (1997). Fish consumption and the 30-year risk of fatal myocardial infarction. *N Engl J Med,* 336(15), 1046–1053. doi:10.1056/NEJM199704103361502

Dawson-Hughes, B., Harris, S. S., & Ceglia, L. (2008). Alkaline diets favor lean tissue mass in older adults. *Am J Clin Nutr,* 87(3), 662–665.

de Carvalho, A. M., César, C. L., Fisberg, R. M., & Marchioni, D. M. (2013). Excessive meat consumption in Brazil: Diet quality and environmental impacts. *Public Health Nutr,* 16(10), 1893–1899. doi:10.1017/S1368980012003916

de Castro, J. M. (1987). Macronutrient relationships with meal patterns and mood in the spontaneous feeding behavior of humans. *Physiol Behav,* 39(5), 561–569.

de Koning, L., Malik, V. S., Kellogg, M. D., Rimm, E. B., Willett, W. C., & Hu, F. B. (2012).

Sweetened beverage consumption, incident coronary heart disease, and biomarkers of risk in men. *Circulation, 125*(14), 1735–1741, S1731. doi:10.1161/CIRCULATIONAHA.111.067017

de Lorgeril, M., Salen, P., Martin, J. L., Monjaud, I., Delaye, J., & Mamelle, N. (1999). Mediterranean diet, traditional risk factors, and the rate of cardiovascular complications after myocardial infarction: Final report of the Lyon Diet Heart Study. *Circulation, 99*(6), 779–785.

de Nadai, T. R., de Nadai, M. N., Albuquerque, A. A., de Carvalho, M. T., Celotto, A. C., & Evora, P. R. (2013). Metabolic acidosis treatment as part of a strategy to curb inflammation. *Int J Inflam, 2013,* 601424. doi:10.1155/2013/601424

de Silva, P. S., Olsen, A., Christensen, J., Schmidt, E. B., Overvaad, K., Tjonneland, A., & Hart, A. R. (2010). An association between dietary arachidonic acid, measured in adipose tissue, and ulcerative colitis. *Gastroenterology, 139*(6), 1912–1917. doi:10.1053/j.gastro.2010.07.065

de Souza, R. J., Bray, G. A., Carey, V. J., Hall, K. D., LeBoff, M. S., Loria, C. M., . . . Smith, S. R. (2012). Effects of 4 weight-loss diets differing in fat, protein, and carbohydrate on fat mass, lean mass, visceral adipose tissue, and hepatic fat: Results from the POUNDS LOST trial. *Am J Clin Nutr, 95*(3), 614–625. doi:10.3945/ajcn.111.026328

Deapen, D., Liu, L., Perkins, C., Bernstein, L., & Ross, R. K. (2002). Rapidly rising breast cancer incidence rates among Asian-American women. *Int J Cancer, 99*(5), 747–750. doi:10.1002/ijc.10415

Deopurkar, R., Ghanim, H., Friedman, J., Abuaysheh, S., Sia, C. L., Mohanty, P., . . . Dandona, P. (2010). Differential effects of cream, glucose, and orange juice on inflammation, endotoxin, and the expression of Toll-like receptor-4 and suppressor of cytokine signaling-3. *Diabetes Care, 33*(5), 991–997. doi:10.2337/dc09-1630

Dewailly, E., Blanchet, C., Lemieux, S., Sauvé, L., Gingras, S., Ayotte, P., & Holub, B. J. (2001). n-3 Fatty acids and cardiovascular disease risk factors among the Inuit of Nunavik. *Am J Clin Nutr, 74*(4), 464–473.

Dewell, A., Weidner, G., Sumner, M. D., Chi, C. S., & Ornish, D. (2008). A very-low-fat vegan diet increases intake of protective dietary factors and decreases intake of pathogenic dietary factors. *J Am Diet Assoc, 108*(2), 347–356. doi:10.1016/j.jada.2007.10.044

Dideriksen, K., Reitelseder, S., & Holm, L. (2013). Influence of amino acids, dietary protein, and physical activity on muscle mass development in humans. *Nutrients, 5*(3), 852–876. doi:10.3390/nu5030852

Diethelm, P., & McKee, M. (2009). Denialism: What is it and how should scientists respond? *Eur J Public Health, 19*(1), 2–4. doi:10.1093/eurpub/ckn139

Djoussé, L., & Gaziano, J. M. (2008). Egg consumption in relation to cardiovascular disease and mortality: the Physicians' Health Study. *Am J Clin Nutr, 87*(4), 964–969.

Du, H., van der A, D. L., Boshuizen, H. C., Forouhi, N. G., Wareham, N. J., Halkjaer, J., . . . Feskens, E. J. (2010). Dietary fiber and subsequent changes in body weight and waist circumference in European men and women. *Am J Clin Nutr, 91*(2), 329–336. doi:10.3945/ajcn.2009.28191

Ducimetiere, P. (2008). The French paradox: Fact or fiction. *Dialogues Cardio Med,* 13, 193.

Duncan, S. H., Belenguer, A., Holtrop, G., Johnstone, A. M., Flint, H. J., & Lobley, G. E. (2007). Reduced dietary intake of carbohydrates by obese subjects results in decreased concentrations of butyrate and butyrate-producing bacteria in feces. *Appl Environ Microbiol, 73*(4), 1073–1078. doi:10.1128/AEM.02340-06

Dwyer, J. T. (1988). Health aspects of vegetarian diets. *Am J Clin Nutr, 48*(3 Suppl), 712–738.

Eaton, S. B., & Konner, M. (1985). Paleolithic nutrition. A consideration of its nature and current implications. *N Engl J Med, 312*(5), 283–289. doi:10.1056/NEJM198501313120505

Ebbeling, C. B., Swain, J. F., Feldman, H. A., Wong, W. W., Hachey, D. L., Garcia-Lago, E., & Ludwig, D. S. (2012). Effects of dietary composition on energy expenditure during weight-loss maintenance. *JAMA, 307*(24), 2627–2634. doi:10.1001/jama.2012.6607

Eckel, R. H., Grundy, S. M., & Zimmet, P. Z. (2005). The metabolic syndrome. *Lancet, 365*(9468), 1415–1428. doi:10.1016/S0140-6736(05)66378-7

Edenharder, R., Sager, J. W., Glatt, H., Muckel, E., & Platt, K. L. (2002). Protection by beverages, fruits, vegetables, herbs, and flavonoids against genotoxicity of 2-acetylaminofluorene and 2-amino-1-methyl-6-phenylimidazo[4,5-b]pyridine (PhIP) in metabolically competent V79 cells. *Mutat Res, 521*(1-2), 57–72.

El, S. N., & Karakaya, S. (2004). Radical scavenging and iron-chelating activities of some greens used as traditional dishes in Mediterranean diet. *Int J Food Sci Nutr, 55*(1), 67–74. doi:10.1080/09637480310001642501

el-Khoury, A. E., Forslund, A., Olsson, R., Branth, S., Sjödin, A., Andersson, A., . . . Young, V. R. (1997). Moderate exercise at energy balance does not affect 24-h leucine oxidation or nitrogen retention in healthy men. *Am J Physiol, 273*(2 Pt 1), E394–E407.

Elango, R., Humayun, M. A., Ball, R. O., & Pencharz, P. B. (2010). Evidence that protein requirements have been significantly underestimated. *Curr Opin Clin Nutr Metab Care, 13*(1), 52–57. doi:10.1097/MCO.0b013e328332f9b7

Elango, R., Humayun, M. A., Ball, R. O., & Pencharz, P. B. (2011). Protein requirement of healthy school-age children determined by the indicator amino acid oxidation method. *Am J Clin Nutr, 94*(6), 1545–1552. doi:10.3945/ajcn.111.012815

Elkan, A. C., Sjöberg, B., Kolsrud, B., Ringertz, B., Hafström, I., & Frostegård, J. (2008). Gluten-free vegan diet induces decreased LDL and oxidized LDL levels and raised atheroprotective natural antibodies against phosphorylcholine in patients with rheumatoid arthritis: A randomized study. *Arthritis Res Ther, 10*(2), R34. doi:10.1186/ar2388

Elliott, P., Stamler, J., Dyer, A. R., Appel, L., Dennis, B., Kesteloot, H., . . . Zhou, B. (2006). Association between protein intake and blood pressure: The INTERMAP Study. *Arch Intern Med, 166*(1), 79–87. doi:10.1001/archinte.166.1.79

Ello-Martin, J. A., Ledikwe, J. H., & Rolls, B. J. (2005). The influence of food portion size and energy density on energy intake: implications for weight management. *Am J Clin Nutr, 82*(1 Suppl), 236S–241S.

Elmadfa, I., & Singer, I. (2009). Vitamin B-12 and homocysteine status among vegetarians: a global perspective. *Am J Clin Nutr, 89*(5), 1693S–1698S. doi:10.3945/ajcn.2009.26736Y

English, D. R., MacInnis, R. J., Hodge, A. M., Hopper, J. L., Haydon, A. M., & Giles, G. G. (2004). Red meat, chicken, and fish consumption and risk of colorectal cancer. *Cancer Epidemiol Biomarkers Prev, 13*(9), 1509–1514.

Epner, D. E. (2001). Can dietary methionine restriction increase the effectiveness of chemotherapy in treatment of advanced cancer? *J Am Coll Nutr, 20*(5 Suppl), 443S–449S; discussion 473S-475S.

Epstein, S. S. (2001). Re: Role of the insulin-like growth factors in cancer development and progression. *J Natl Cancer Inst, 93*(3), 238.

Ericson, U., Hellstrand, S., Brunkwall, L., Schulz, C. A., Sonestedt, E., Wallström, P., . . . Orho-Melander, M. (2015). Food sources of fat may clarify the inconsistent role of dietary fat intake for incidence of type 2 diabetes. *Am J Clin Nutr.* doi:10.3945/ajcn.114.103010

Erridge, C., Attina, T., Spickett, C. M., & Webb, D. J. (2007). A high-fat meal induces low-grade endotoxemia: Evidence of a novel mechanism of postprandial inflammation. *Am J Clin Nutr, 86*(5), 1286–1292.

Esmarck, B., Andersen, J. L., Olsen, S., Richter, E. A., Mizuno, M., & Kjaer, M. (2001). Timing of postexercise protein intake is important for muscle hypertrophy with resistance training in elderly humans. *J Physiol, 535*(Pt 1), 301–311.

Esposito, K., & Giugliano, D. (2006). Diet and inflammation: A link to metabolic and cardiovascular diseases. *Eur Heart J, 27*(1), 15–20. doi:10.1093/eurheartj/ehi605

Esposito, K., Nappo, F., Giugliano, F., Di Palo, C., Ciotola, M., Barbieri, M., . . . Giugliano, D. (2003). Meal modulation of circulating interleukin 18 and adiponectin concentrations in healthy subjects and in patients with type 2 diabetes mellitus. *Am J Clin Nutr, 78*(6), 1135–1140.

Esposito, K., Nappo, F., Giugliano, F., Giugliano, G., Marfella, R., & Giugliano, D. (2003). Effect of dietary antioxidants on postprandial endothelial dysfunction induced by a high-fat meal in healthy subjects. *Am J Clin Nutr, 77*(1), 139–143.

Esselstyn, C. B. (1999). Updating a 12-year experience with arrest and reversal therapy for coronary heart disease (an overdue requiem for palliative cardiology). *Am J Cardiol, 84*(3), 339-341, A338.

Esselstyn, C. B., Ellis, S. G., Medendorp, S. V., & Crowe, T. D. (1995). A strategy to arrest and reverse coronary artery disease: A 5-year longitudinal study of a single physician's practice. *J Fam Pract, 41*(6), 560–568.

Esselstyn, C. B., Gendy, G., Doyle, J., Golubic, M., & Roizen, M. F. (2014). A way to reverse CAD? *J Fam Pract, 63*(7), 356–364b.

Fagherazzi, G., Vilier, A., Bonnet, F., Lajous, M., Balkau, B., Boutron-Ruault, M. C., & Clavel-Chapelon, F. (2013). Dietary acid load and risk of type 2 diabetes: The E3N-EPIC cohort study. *Diabetologia.* doi:10.1007/s00125-013-3100-0

Faramawi, M. F., Johnson, E., Fry, M. W., Sall, M., Zhou, Y., & Yi, Z. (2007). Consumption of different types of meat and the risk of renal cancer: Meta-analysis of case-control studies. *Cancer Causes Control, 18*(2), 125–133. doi:10.1007/s10552-006-0104-9

Farmer, B., Larson, B. T., Fulgoni, V. L., Rainville, A. J., & Liepa, G. U. (2011). A vegetarian dietary pattern as a nutrient-dense approach to weight management: An analysis of the national health and nutrition examination survey 1999–2004. *J Am Diet Assoc, 111*(6), 819–827. doi:10.1016/j.jada.2011.03.012

Farvid, M. S., Ding, M., Pan, A., Sun, Q., Chiuve, S. E., Steffen, L. M., . . . Hu, F. B. (2014). Dietary linoleic acid and risk of coronary heart disease: A systematic review and meta-analysis of prospective cohort studies. *Circulation.* doi:10.1161/CIRCULATIONAHA.114.010236

Fedewa, S. A., Etzioni, R., Flanders, W. D., Jemal, A., & Ward, E. M. (2010). Association of insurance and race/ethnicity with disease severity among men diagnosed with prostate cancer, National Cancer Database 2004–2006. *Cancer Epidemiol Biomarkers Prev, 19*(10), 2437–2444. doi:10.1158/1055-9965.EPI-10-0299

Ferrari, P., Rinaldi, S., Jenab, M., Lukanova, A., Olsen, A., Tjønneland, A., . . . Romieu, I. (2013). Dietary fiber intake and risk of hormonal receptor-defined breast cancer in the European Prospective Investigation into Cancer and Nutrition study. *Am J Clin Nutr, 97*(2), 344–353. doi:10.3945/ajcn.112.034025

Feskanich, D., Willett, W. C., Stampfer, M. J., & Colditz, G. A. (1996). Protein consumption and bone fractures in women. *Am J Epidemiol, 143*(5), 472–479.

Feskens, E. J., & Kromhout, D. (1993). Epidemiologic studies on Eskimos and fish intake. *Ann N Y Acad Sci, 683*, 9–15.

Flanagan, A. M., Brown, J. L., Santiago, C. A., Aad, P. Y., Spicer, L. J., & Spicer, M. T. (2008). High-fat diets promote insulin resistance through cytokine gene expression in growing female rats. *J Nutr Biochem, 19*(8), 505–513. doi:10.1016/j.jnutbio.2007.06.005

Fleming, R. M. (2000). The effect of high-protein diets on coronary blood flow. *Angiology, 51*(10), 817–826.

Flores-Mateo, G., Rojas-Rueda, D., Basora, J., Ros, E., & Salas-Salvadó, J. (2013). Nut intake and adiposity: Meta-analysis of clinical trials. *Am J Clin Nutr, 97*(6), 1346–1355. doi:10.3945/ajcn.111.031484

Fodor, J. G., Helis, E., Yazdekhasti, N. & Vohnout, B. (2014). "Fishing" for the origins of the "Eskimos and heart disease" story: Facts or wishful thinking? *Can J Cardiol, 30* (8), 864–868. doi:10.1016/j.cjca.2014.04.007

Fontana, L., Weiss, E. P., Villareal, D. T., Klein, S., & Holloszy, J. O. (2008). Long-term effects of calorie or protein restriction on serum IGF-1 and IGFBP-3 concentration in humans. *Aging Cell, 7*(5), 681–687.

Fontana L, A. V., Atella, V., & Kammen DM. (2013). Energy efficiency as a unifying principle for human, environmental, and global health. *F1000 Research, 2*, 101. doi:10.12688/f1000research.2-101.v1

Ford, E. S., & Mokdad, A. H. (2001). Fruit and vegetable consumption and diabetes mellitus incidence among U.S. adults. *Prev Med, 32*(1), 33–39. doi:10.1006/pmed.2000.0772

Forslund, A. H., Hambraeus, L., Olsson, R. M., El-Khoury, A. E., Yu, Y. M., & Young, V. R. (1998). The 24-h whole body leucine and urea kinetics at normal and high protein intakes with exercise in healthy adults. *Am J Physiol, 275*(2 Pt 1), E310–E320.

Foster, G. D., Wadden, T. A., Vogt, R. A., & Brewer, G. (1997). What is a reasonable weight loss? Patients' expectations and evaluations of obesity treatment outcomes. *J Consult Clin Psychol, 65*(1), 79–85.

Foster, G. D., Wyatt, H. R., Hill, J. O., McGuckin, B. G., Brill, C., Mohammed, B. S., . . . Klein, S. (2003). A randomized trial of a low-carbohydrate diet for obesity. *N Engl J Med, 348*(21), 2082–2090. doi:10.1056/NEJMoa022207

Frandsen, H. (2008). Biomonitoring of urinary metabolites of 2-amino-1-methyl-6-phenylim idazo[4,5-b]pyridine (PhIP) following human consumption of cooked chicken. *Food Chem Toxicol, 46*(9), 3200–3205. doi:10.1016/j.fct.2008.07.008

Fraser, G. E. (1999). Associations between diet and cancer, ischemic heart disease, and all-cause mortality in non-Hispanic white California Seventh-day Adventists. *Am J Clin Nutr, 70*(3 Suppl), 532S–538S.

Fraser, G. E. (2005). A comparison of first event coronary heart disease rates in two contrasting California populations. *J Nutr Health Aging, 9*(1), 53–58.

Fraser, G. E. (2009). Vegetarian diets: What do we know of their effects on common chronic diseases? *Am J Clin Nutr, 89*(5), 1607S–1612S. doi:10.3945/ajcn.2009.26736K

Fraser, G. E., & Shavlik, D. J. (2001). Ten years of life: Is it a matter of choice? *Arch Intern Med, 161*(13), 1645–1652.

Frassetto, L., Morris, R. C., Sellmeyer, D. E., Todd, K., & Sebastian, A. (2001). Diet, evolution and aging—the pathophysiologic effects of the post-agricultural inversion of the potassium-to-sodium and base-to-chloride ratios in the human diet. *Eur J Nutr, 40*(5), 200–213.

Freedman, M. R., King, J., & Kennedy, E. (2001). Popular diets: A scientific review. *Obes Res, 9*(Suppl 1), 1S–40S. doi:10.1038/oby.2001.113

French, S. A., Jeffery, R. W., Forster, J. L., McGovern, P. G., Kelder, S. H., & Baxter, J. E. (1994). Predictors of weight change over two years among a population of working adults: the Healthy Worker Project. *Int J Obes Relat Metab Disord, 18*(3), 145–154.

Freudenberg, N. (2014). *Lethal but legal: Corporations, consumption, and protecting public health.* New York: Oxford University Press.

Freudenheim, J. L., Marshall, J. R., Vena, J. E., Laughlin, R., Brasure, J. R., Swanson, M. K., ... Graham, S. (1996). Premenopausal breast cancer risk and intake of vegetables, fruits, and related nutrients. *J Natl Cancer Inst, 88*(6), 340–348.

Friborg, J. T., & Melbye, M. (2008). Cancer patterns in Inuit populations. *Lancet Oncol, 9*(9), 892–900. doi:10.1016/S1470-2045(08)70231-6

Fung, T. T., Schulze, M., Manson, J. E., Willett, W. C., & Hu, F. B. (2004). Dietary patterns, meat intake, and the risk of type 2 diabetes in women. *Arch Intern Med, 164*(20), 2235–2240. doi:10.1001/archinte.164.20.2235

Fung, T. T., van Dam, R. M., Hankinson, S. E., Stampfer, M., Willett, W. C., & Hu, F. B. (2010). Low-carbohydrate diets and all-cause and cause-specific mortality: Two cohort studies. *Ann Intern Med, 153*(5), 289–298. doi:10.1059/0003-4819-153-5-201009070-00003

Fung, T. T., Willett, W. C., Stampfer, M. J., Manson, J. E., & Hu, F. B. (2001). Dietary patterns and the risk of coronary heart disease in women. *Arch Intern Med, 161*(15), 1857–1862.

Galland, L. (2010). Diet and inflammation. *Nutr Clin Pract, 25*(6), 634–640. doi:10.1177/0884533610385703

Gallinetti, J., Harputlugil, E., & Mitchell, J. R. (2013). Amino acid sensing in dietary-restriction-mediated longevity: Roles of signal-transducing kinases GCN2 and TOR. *Biochem J, 449*(1), 1–10. doi:10.1042/BJ20121098

Gao, X., Bermudez, O. I., & Tucker, K. L. (2004). Plasma C-reactive protein and homocysteine concentrations are related to frequent fruit and vegetable intake in Hispanic and non-Hispanic white elders. *J Nutr, 134*(4), 913–918.

García-Unciti, M., Martinez, J. A., Izquierdo, M., Gorostiaga, E. M., Grijalba, A., & Ibañez, J. (2012). Effect of resistance training and hypocaloric diets with different protein content on body composition and lipid profile in hypercholesterolemic obese women. *Nutr Hosp, 27*(5), 1511–1520. doi:10.3305/nh.2012.27.5.5921

Gardner, C. D., Coulston, A., Chatterjee, L., Rigby, A., Spiller, G., & Farquhar, J. W. (2005). The effect of a plant-based diet on plasma lipids in hypercholesterolemic adults: A randomized trial. *Ann Intern Med, 142*(9), 725–733.

Gardner, C. D., Kiazand, A., Alhassan, S., Kim, S., Stafford, R. S., Balise, R. R., . . . King, A. C. (2007). Comparison of the Atkins, Zone, Ornish, and LEARN diets for change in weight and related risk factors among overweight premenopausal women: The A TO Z Weight Loss Study: A randomized trial. *JAMA, 297*(9), 969–977. doi:10.1001/jama.297.9.969

Garlick, P. J., McNurlan, M. A., & Patlak, C. S. (1999). Adaptation of protein metabolism in relation to limits to high dietary protein intake. *Eur J Clin Nutr, 53*(1 Suppl), S34–S43.

Gear, J. S., Ware, A., Fursdon, P., Mann, J. I., Nolan, D. J., Brodribb, A. J., & Vessey, M. P. (1979). Symptomless diverticular disease and intake of dietary fibre. *Lancet, 1*(8115), 511–514.

Geppert, J., Kraft, V., Demmelmair, H., & Koletzko, B. (2005). Docosahexaenoic acid supplementation in vegetarians effectively increases omega-3 index: A randomized trial. *Lipids, 40*(8), 807–814.

Ghanim, H., Abuaysheh, S., Sia, C. L., Korzeniewski, K., Chaudhuri, A., Fernandez-Real, J. M., & Dandona, P. (2009). Increase in plasma endotoxin concentrations and the expression of Toll-like receptors and suppressor of cytokine signaling-3 in mononuclear cells after a high-fat, high-carbohydrate meal: implications for insulin resistance. *Diabetes Care, 32*(12), 2281–2287. doi:10.2337/dc09-0979

Giem, P., Beeson, W. L., & Fraser, G. E. (1993). The incidence of dementia and intake of animal products: Preliminary findings from the Adventist Health Study. *Neuroepidemiology, 12*(1), 28–36.

Gil, A., Ortega, R. M., & Maldonado, J. (2011). Wholegrain cereals and bread: A duet of the Mediterranean diet for the prevention of chronic diseases. *Public Health Nutr, 14*(12A), 2316–2322. doi:10.1017/S1368980011002576

Gilbert, J. A., Bendsen, N. T., Tremblay, A., & Astrup, A. (2011). Effect of proteins from different sources on body composition. *Nutr Metab Cardiovasc Dis, 21*(2 Suppl), B16–B31. doi:10.1016/j.numecd.2010.12.008

Gimeno, S. G., Ferreira, S. R., Franco, L. J., Hirai, A. T., Matsumura, L., & Moisés, R. S. (2002). Prevalence and 7-year incidence of type II diabetes mellitus in a Japanese-Brazilian population: An alarming public health problem. *Diabetologia, 45*(12), 1635–1638. doi:10.1007/s00125-002-0963-x

Giovannucci, E., Rimm, E. B., Stampfer, M. J., Colditz, G. A., Ascherio, A., & Willett, W. C. (1994). Intake of fat, meat, and fiber in relation to risk of colon cancer in men. *Cancer Res, 54*(9), 2390–2397.

Goff, L. M., Bell, J. D., So, P. W., Dornhorst, A., & Frost, G. S. (2005). Veganism and its relationship with insulin resistance and intramyocellular lipid. *Eur J Clin Nutr, 59*(2), 291–298. doi:10.1038/sj.ejcn.1602076

Golay, A., Allaz, A. F., Morel, Y., de Tonnac, N., Tankova, S., & Reaven, G. (1996). Similar weight loss with low- or high-carbohydrate diets. *Am J Clin Nutr, 63*(2), 174–178.

Goldman, L., & Cook, E. F. (1984). The decline in ischemic heart disease mortality rates. An analysis of the comparative effects of medical interventions and changes in lifestyle. *Ann Intern Med, 101*(6), 825–836.

González, C. A. (2006a). The European Prospective Investigation into Cancer and Nutrition (EPIC). *Public Health Nutr, 9*(1A), 124–126.

González, C. A. (2006b). Nutrition and cancer: The current epidemiological evidence. *Br J Nutr, 96*(1 Suppl), S42–S45.

González, C. A., Jakszyn, P., Pera, G., Agudo, A., Bingham, S., Palli, D., . . . Riboli, E. (2006). Meat intake and risk of stomach and esophageal adenocarcinoma within the European Prospective Investigation into Cancer and Nutrition (EPIC). *J Natl Cancer Inst, 98*(5), 345–354. doi:10.1093/jnci/djj071

Grant, W. (2014). A multicountry ecological study of cancer incidence rates in 2008 with respect to various risk-modifying factors. *Nutrients, 6*(1), 163–189. doi:10.339/nu6010163

Greco, A. V., Mingrone, G., Giancaterini, A., Manco, M., Morroni, M., Cinti, S., . . . Ferrannini, E. (2002). Insulin resistance in morbid obesity: reversal with intramyocellular fat depletion. *Diabetes, 51*(1), 144–151.

Groen, J. J., Balogh, M., Levy, M., & Yaron, E., Zemach, R., & Benaderet, S. (1964). Nutrition of the Bedouins in the Negev Desert. *Am J Clin Nutr, 14*(1), 37–46.

Grün, F., & Blumberg, B. (2006). Environmental obesogens: organotins and endocrine disruption via nuclear receptor signaling. *Endocrinology, 147*(6 Suppl), S50–S55. doi: 10.1210/en.2005-1129

Günther, A. L., Karaolis-Danckert, N., Kroke, A., Remer, T., & Buyken, A. E. (2010). Dietary protein intake throughout childhood is associated with the timing of puberty. *J Nutr, 140*(3), 565–571. doi:10.3945/jn.109.114934

Haddad, E. H., Berk, L. S., Kettering, J. D., Hubbard, R. W., & Peters, W. R. (1999). Dietary intake and biochemical, hematologic, and immune status of vegans compared with non-vegetarians. *Am J Clin Nutr, 70*(3 Suppl), S86S–593S.

Haddad, E. H., & Tanzman, J. S. (2003). What do vegetarians in the United States eat? *Am J Clin Nutr, 78*(3 Suppl), 626S–632S.

Halkjær, J., Olsen, A., Overvad, K., Jakobsen, M. U., Boeing, H., Buijsse, B., . . . Tjønneland, A. (2011). Intake of total, animal and plant protein and subsequent changes in weight or waist circumference in European men and women: The Diogenes project. *Int J Obes (Lond), 35*(8), 1104–1113. doi:10.1038/ijo.2010.254

Halton, T. L., Willett, W. C., Liu, S., Manson, J. E., Albert, C. M., Rexrode, K., & Hu, F. B. (2006). Low-carbohydrate-diet score and the risk of coronary heart disease in women. *N Engl J Med, 355*(19), 1991–2002. doi:10.1056/NEJMoa055317

Hankinson, S. E., Willett, W. C., Colditz, G. A., Hunter, D. J., Michaud, D. S., Deroo, B., . . . Pollak, M. (1998). Circulating concentrations of insulin-like growth factor-I and risk of breast cancer. *Lancet, 351*(9113), 1393–1396. doi:10.1016/S0140-6736(97)10384-1

Harland, J. I., & Haffner, T. A. (2008). Systematic review, meta-analysis and regression of randomised controlled trials reporting an association between an intake of circa 25 g soya protein per day and blood cholesterol. *Atherosclerosis, 200*(1), 13–27. doi:10.1016/j.atherosclerosis.2008.04.006

Havel, P. J., Townsend, R., Chaump, L., & Teff, K. (1999). High-fat meals reduce 24-h circulating leptin concentrations in women. *Diabetes, 48*(2), 334–341.

Hawkes, C. (2006). Uneven dietary development: Linking the policies and processes of globalization with the nutrition transition, obesity and diet-related chronic diseases. *Global Health, 2,* 4. doi:10.1186/1744-8603-2-4

He, F. J., Nowson, C. A., Lucas, M., & MacGregor, G. A. (2007). Increased consumption of fruit and vegetables is related to a reduced risk of coronary heart disease: Meta-analysis of cohort studies. *J Hum Hypertens, 21*(9), 717–728. doi:10.1038/sj.jhh.1002212

He, J., Gu, D., Wu, X., Chen, J., Duan, X., & Whelton, P. K. (2005). Effect of soybean protein on blood pressure: A randomized, controlled trial. *Ann Intern Med, 143*(1), 1–9.

Heidemann, C., Schulze, M. B., Franco, O. H., van Dam, R. M., Mantzoros, C. S., & Hu, F. B. (2008). Dietary patterns and risk of mortality from cardiovascular disease, cancer, and all causes in a prospective cohort of women. *Circulation, 118*(3), 230–237. doi:10.1161/CIRCULATIONAHA.108.771881

Hellerstein, M. K. (1999). De novo lipogenesis in humans: Metabolic and regulatory aspects. *Eur J Clin Nutr, 53*(1 Suppl), S53–S65.

Henry, A. G., Brooks, A. S., & Piperno, D. R. (2011). Microfossils in calculus demonstrate consumption of plants and cooked foods in Neanderthal diets (Shanidar III, Iraq; Spy I and II, Belgium). *Proc Natl Acad Sci U S A, 108*(2), 486–491. doi:10.1073/pnas.1016868108

Henry, A. G., Ungar, P. S., Passey, B. H., Sponheimer, M., Rossouw, L., Bamford, M., . . . Berger, L. (2012). The diet of Australopithecus sediba. *Nature, 487*(7405), 90–93. doi:10.1038/nature11185

Hernández-Alonso, P., Salas-Salvadó, J., Ruiz-Canela, M., Corella, D., Estruch, R., Fitó, M., . . . Bulló, M. (2015). High dietary protein intake is associated with an increased body weight and total death risk. *Clin Nutr.* doi:10.1016/j.clnu.2015.03.016

Heys, M., Jiang, C., Cheng, K. K., Zhang, W., Lam, T. H., Leung, G. M., & Schooling, C. M. (2011). Does childhood meat eating contribute to sex differences in risk factors for ischaemic heart disease in a developing population? *J Epidemiol Community Health, 65*(6), 522–528. doi:10.1136/jech.2009.099143

Hill, J. O., Drougas, H., & Peters, J. C. (1993). Obesity treatment: Can diet composition play a role? *Ann Intern Med, 119*(7 Pt 2), 694–697.

Ho-Pham, L. T., Nguyen, N. D., & Nguyen, T. V. (2009). Effect of vegetarian diets on bone mineral density: A Bayesian meta-analysis. *Am J Clin Nutr, 90*(4), 943–950. doi:10.3945/ajcn.2009.27521

Ho-Pham, L. T., Nguyen, P. L., Le, T. T., Doan, T. A., Tran, N. T., Le, T. A., & Nguyen, T. V. (2009). Veganism, bone mineral density, and body composition: A study in Buddhist nuns. *Osteoporos Int, 20*(12), 2087–2093. doi:10.1007/s00198-009-0916-z

Holt, E. M., Steffen, L. M., Moran, A., Basu, S., Steinberger, J., Ross, J. A., . . . Sinaiko, A. R. (2009). Fruit and vegetable consumption and its relation to markers of inflammation and oxidative stress in adolescents. *J Am Diet Assoc, 109*(3), 414–421. doi:10.1016/j.jada.2008.11.036

Holt, H. B., Wild, S. H., Postle, A. D., Zhang, J., Koster, G., Umpleby, M., . . . Byrne, C. D. (2007). Cortisol clearance and associations with insulin sensitivity, body fat and fatty liver in middle-aged men. *Diabetologia, 50*(5), 1024–1032. doi:10.1007/s00125-007-0629-9

Holt, S. H., Miller, J. C., & Petocz, P. (1997). An insulin index of foods: The insulin demand generated by 1000-kJ portions of common foods. *Am J Clin Nutr, 66*(5), 1264–1276.

Holt, S. H., Miller, J. C., Petocz, P., & Farmakalidis, E. (1995). A satiety index of common foods. *Eur J Clin Nutr, 49*(9), 675–690.

Hooper, L., Summerbell, C. D., Thompson, R., Sills, D., Roberts, F. G., Moore, H., & Davey

Smith, G. (2011). Reduced or modified dietary fat for preventing cardiovascular disease. *Cochrane Database Syst Rev*(7), CD002137. doi:10.1002/14651858.CD002137.pub2

Horton, T. J., Drougas, H., Brachey, A., Reed, G. W., Peters, J. C., & Hill, J. O. (1995). Fat and carbohydrate overfeeding in humans: different effects on energy storage. *Am J Clin Nutr, 62*(1), 19–29.

Howard, B. V., Manson, J. E., Stefanick, M. L., Beresford, S. A., Frank, G., Jones, B., . . . Prentice, R. (2006). Low-fat dietary pattern and weight change over 7 years: The Women's Health Initiative Dietary Modification Trial. *JAMA, 295*(1), 39–49. doi:10.1001/jama.295.1.39

Howie, B. J., & Shultz, T. D. (1985). Dietary and hormonal interrelationships among vegetarian Seventh-Day Adventists and nonvegetarian men. *Am J Clin Nutr, 42*(1), 127–134.

Hu, F. B. (2003). Plant-based foods and prevention of cardiovascular disease: An overview. *Am J Clin Nutr, 78*(3 Suppl), 544S–551S.

Hu, F. B. (2005). Protein, body weight, and cardiovascular health. *Am J Clin Nutr, 82*(1 Suppl), 242S–247S.

Hu, F. B., Rimm, E. B., Stampfer, M. J., Ascherio, A., Spiegelman, D., & Willett, W. C. (2000). Prospective study of major dietary patterns and risk of coronary heart disease in men. *Am J Clin Nutr, 72*(4), 912–921.

Hu, F. B., Stampfer, M. J., Manson, J. E., Ascherio, A., Colditz, G. A., Speizer, F. E., . . . Willett, W. C. (1999). Dietary saturated fats and their food sources in relation to the risk of coronary heart disease in women. *Am J Clin Nutr, 70*(6), 1001–1008.

Hu, F. B., Stampfer, M. J., Manson, J. E., Rimm, E., Colditz, G. A., Rosner, B. A., . . . Willett, W. C. (1997). Dietary fat intake and the risk of coronary heart disease in women. *N Engl J Med, 337*(21), 1491–1499. doi:10.1056/NEJM199711203372102

Hu, F. B., Stampfer, M. J., Manson, J. E., Rimm, E., Colditz, G. A., Speizer, F. E., . . . Willett, W. C. (1999). Dietary protein and risk of ischemic heart disease in women. *Am J Clin Nutr, 70*(2), 221–227.

Hu, F. B., Stampfer, M. J., Rimm, E. B., Manson, J. E., Ascherio, A., Colditz, G. A., . . . Willett, W. C. (1999). A prospective study of egg consumption and risk of cardiovascular disease in men and women. *JAMA, 281*(15), 1387–1394.

Hu, F. B., & Willett, W. C. (2002). Optimal diets for prevention of coronary heart disease. *JAMA, 288*(20), 2569–2578.

Hu, T., Mills, K. T., Yao, L., Demanelis, K., Eloustaz, M., Yancy, W. S., . . . Bazzano, L. A. (2012). Effects of low-carbohydrate diets versus low-fat diets on metabolic risk factors: a meta-analysis of randomized controlled clinical trials. *Am J Epidemiol, 176*(7 Suppl), S44–S54. doi:10.1093/aje/kws264

Hua, N. W., Stoohs, R. A., & Facchini, F. S. (2001). Low iron status and enhanced insulin sensitivity in lacto-ovo vegetarians. *Br J Nutr, 86*(4), 515–519.

Huang, T., Yang, B., Zheng, J., Li, G., Wahlqvist, M. L., & Li, D. (2012). Cardiovascular disease mortality and cancer incidence in vegetarians: A meta-analysis and systematic review. *Ann Nutr Metab, 60*(4), 233–240. doi:10.1159/000337301

Hubbard, J. D., Inkeles, S., & Barnard, R. J. (1985). Nathan Pritikin's heart. *N Engl J Med, 313*(1), 52. doi:10.1056/NEJM198507043130118

Hughes, R., Cross, A. J., Pollock, J. R., & Bingham, S. (2001). Dose-dependent effect of dietary meat on endogenous colonic N-nitrosation. *Carcinogenesis, 22*(1), 199–202.

Hulston, C. J., Wolsk, E., Grøndahl, T. S., Yfanti, C., & Van Hall, G. (2011). Protein intake does not increase vastus lateralis muscle protein synthesis during cycling. *Med Sci Sports Exerc, 43*(9), 1635–1642. doi:10.1249/MSS.0b013e31821661ab

Humayun, M. A., Elango, R., Ball, R. O., & Pencharz, P. B. (2007). Reevaluation of the protein requirement in young men with the indicator amino acid oxidation technique. *Am J Clin Nutr, 86*(4), 995–1002.

Hunt, J. R. (2003). Bioavailability of iron, zinc, and other trace minerals from vegetarian diets. *Am J Clin Nutr, 78*(3 Suppl), 633S–639S.

Hutson, S. M., Sweatt, A. J., & Lanoue, K. F. (2005). Branched-chain [corrected] amino acid metabolism: Implications for establishing safe intakes. *J Nutr, 135*(6 Suppl), 1557S–1564S.

Huxley, R. R., & Neil, H. A. (2003). The relation between dietary flavonol intake and coronary heart disease mortality: A meta-analysis of prospective cohort studies. *Eur J Clin Nutr, 57*(8), 904–908. doi:10.1038/sj.ejcn.1601624

Iburg, K. M., Brønnum-Hansen, H., & Bjerregaard, P. (2001). Health expectancy in Greenland. *Scand J Public Health, 29*(1), 5–12.

Iglay, H. B., Apolzan, J. W., Gerrard, D. E., Eash, J. K., Anderson, J. C., & Campbell, W. W. (2009). Moderately increased protein intake predominately from egg sources does not influence whole body, regional, or muscle composition responses to resistance training in older people. *J Nutr Health Aging, 13*(2), 108–114.

Institute of Medicine. (2005). *Dietary reference intakes for energy, carbohydrate, fiber, fat, cholesterol, protein, and amino acids.* Washington, DC: National Academies Press.

Jacob, S., Machann, J., Rett, K., Brechtel, K., Volk, A., Renn, W., . . . Häring, H. U. (1999). Association of increased intramyocellular lipid content with insulin resistance in lean non-diabetic offspring of type 2 diabetic subjects. *Diabetes, 48*(5), 1113–1119.

Jacobs, D. R., Anderson, J. T., & Blackburn, H. (1979). Diet and serum cholesterol: Do zero correlations negate the relationship? *Am J Epidemiol, 110*(1), 77–87.

Jacobs, D. R., & Steffen, L. M. (2003). Nutrients, foods, and dietary patterns as exposures in research: A framework for food synergy. *Am J Clin Nutr, 78*(3 Suppl), 508S–513S.

Jakobsen, M. U., Due, K. M., Dethlefsen, C., Halkjaer, J., Holst, C., Forouhi, N. G., . . . Overvad, K. (2012). Fish consumption does not prevent increase in waist circumference in European women and men. *Br J Nutr, 108*(5), 924–931. doi:10.1017/S0007114511006039

JAMA. Book review of Weston Price's *Nutrition and physical degeneration: A comparison of primitive and modern diets and their effects.* (1940). *JAMA, 114*(26), 2589. doi:10.1001/jama.1940.02810260075024.

JAMA. The effects of nonpharmacologic interventions on blood pressure of persons with high normal levels. Results of the Trials of Hypertension Prevention, Phase I. (1992). *JAMA, 267*(9), 1213–1220.

Janket, S. J., Manson, J. E., Sesso, H., Buring, J. E., & Liu, S. (2003). A prospective study of sugar intake and risk of type 2 diabetes in women. *Diabetes Care, 26*(4), 1008–1015.

Jantchou, P., Morois, S., Clavel-Chapelon, F., Boutron-Ruault, M. C., & Carbonnel, F. (2010). Animal protein intake and risk of inflammatory bowel disease: The E3N prospective study. *Am J Gastroenterol, 105*(10), 2195–2201. doi:10.1038/ajg.2010.192

Järvisalo, M. J., Harmoinen, A., Hakanen, M., Paakkunainen, U., Viikari, J., Hartiala, J., . . . Raitakari, O. T. (2002). Elevated serum C-reactive protein levels and early arterial changes in healthy children. *Arterioscler Thromb Vasc Biol, 22*(8), 1323–1328.

Jemal, A., Center, M. M., DeSantis, C., & Ward, E. M. (2010). Global patterns of cancer incidence and mortality rates and trends. *Cancer Epidemiol Biomarkers Prev, 19*(8), 1893–1907. doi:10.1158/1055-9965.EPI-10-0437

Jenkins, D. J., Kendall, C. W., Faulkner, D., Vidgen, E., Trautwein, E. A., Parker, T. L., . . . Connelly, P. W. (2002). A dietary portfolio approach to cholesterol reduction: Combined effects of plant sterols, vegetable proteins, and viscous fibers in hypercholesterolemia. *Metabolism, 51*(12), 1596–1604. doi:10.1053/meta.2002.35578

Jenkins, D. J., Kendall, C. W., Marchie, A., Faulkner, D. A., Wong, J. M., de Souza, R., . . . Connelly, P. W. (2003). Effects of a dietary portfolio of cholesterol-lowering foods vs lovastatin on serum lipids and C-reactive protein. *JAMA, 290*(4), 502–510. doi:10.1001/jama.290.4.502

Jenkins, D. J., Kendall, C. W., Marchie, A., Jenkins, A. L., Augustin, L. S., Ludwig, D. S., . . . Anderson, J. W. (2003). Type 2 diabetes and the vegetarian diet. *Am J Clin Nutr, 78*(3 Suppl), 610S–616S.

Jenkins, P. J. (2006). Cancers associated with acromegaly. *Neuroendocrinology, 83*(3-4), 218–223. doi:10.1159/000095531

Jiang, R., Manson, J. E., Meigs, J. B., Ma, J., Rifai, N., & Hu, F. B. (2004). Body iron stores in relation to risk of type 2 diabetes in apparently healthy women. *JAMA, 291*(6), 711–717. doi:10.1001/jama.291.6.711

Jiao, L., Kramer, J. R., Rugge, M., Parente, P., Verstovsek, G., Alsarraj, A., & El-Serag, H. B. (2013). Dietary intake of vegetables, folate, and antioxidants and the risk of Barrett's esophagus. *Cancer Causes Control, 24*(5), 1005–1014. doi:10.1007/s10552-013-0175-3

Jibani, M. M., Bloodworth, L. L., Foden, E., Griffiths, K. D., & Galpin, O. P. (1991). Predominantly vegetarian diet in patients with incipient and early clinical diabetic nephropathy: Effects on albumin excretion rate and nutritional status. *Diabet Med, 8*(10), 949–953.

Jimenez-Cruz, A., Bacardi-Gascon, M., Turnbull, W. H., Rosales-Garay, P., & Severino-Lugo, I. (2003). A flexible, low-glycemic index mexican-style diet in overweight and obese subjects with type 2 diabetes improves metabolic parameters during a 6-week treatment period. *Diabetes Care, 26*(7), 1967–1970.

Johansson, I., Nilsson, L. M., Stegmayr, B., Boman, K., Hallmans, G., & Winkvist, A. (2012). Associations among 25-year trends in diet, cholesterol and BMI from 140,000 observations in men and women in Northern Sweden. *Nutr J, 11*, 40. doi:10.1186/1475-2891-11-40

John, J. H., Ziebland, S., Yudkin, P., Roe, L. S., Neil, H. A., & OFAVS Group. (2002). Effects of fruit and vegetable consumption on plasma antioxidant concentrations and blood pressure: a randomised controlled trial. *Lancet, 359*(9322), 1969–1974.

Johnson, E. S., Ndetan, H., & Lo, K. M. (2010). Cancer mortality in poultry slaughtering/processing plant workers belonging to a union pension fund. *Environ Res, 110*(6), 588–594. doi:10.1016/j.envres.2010.05.010

Johnson, S. C., Rabinovitch, P. S., & Kaeberlein, M. (2013). mTOR is a key modulator of ageing and age-related disease. *Nature, 493*(7432), 338–345. doi:10.1038/nature11861

Joosen, A. M., Kuhnle, G. G., Aspinall, S. M., Barrow, T. M., Lecommandeur, E., Azqueta, A.,

... Bingham, S. A. (2009). Effect of processed and red meat on endogenous nitrosation and DNA damage. *Carcinogenesis, 30*(8), 1402–1407. doi:10.1093/carcin/bgp130

Joosen, A. M., Lecommandeur, E., Kuhnle, G. G., Aspinall, S. M., Kap, L., & Rodwell, S. A. (2010). Effect of dietary meat and fish on endogenous nitrosation, inflammation and genotoxicity of faecal water. *Mutagenesis, 25*(3), 243–247. doi:10.1093/mutage/gep070

Jornayvaz, F. R., Jurczak, M. J., Lee, H. Y., Birkenfeld, A. L., Frederick, D. W., Zhang, D., ... Shulman, G. I. (2010). A high-fat, ketogenic diet causes hepatic insulin resistance in mice, despite increasing energy expenditure and preventing weight gain. *Am J Physiol Endocrinol Metab, 299*(5), E808–E815. doi:10.1152/ajpendo.00361.2010

Kahn, H. S., Tatham, L. M., Rodriguez, C., Calle, E. E., Thun, M. J., & Heath, C. W. (1997). Stable behaviors associated with adults' 10-year change in body mass index and likelihood of gain at the waist. *Am J Public Health, 87*(5), 747–754.

Kaluza, J., Wolk, A., & Larsson, S. C. (2012). Red meat consumption and risk of stroke: A meta-analysis of prospective studies. *Stroke, 43*(10), 2556–2560. doi:10.1161/STROKEAHA.112.663286

Kaluza, J., Wolk, A., & Larsson, S. C. (2013). Heme iron intake and risk of stroke: A prospective study of men. *Stroke, 44*(2), 334–339. doi:10.1161/STROKEAHA.112.679662

Kannel, W. B. (1995). Clinical misconceptions dispelled by epidemiological research. *Circulation, 92*(11), 3350–3360.

Kant, A. K., Schatzkin, A., Graubard, B. I., & Schairer, C. (2000). A prospective study of diet quality and mortality in women. *JAMA, 283*(16), 2109–2115.

Kato, H., Tillotson, J., Nichaman, M. Z., Rhoads, G. G., & Hamilton, H. B. (1973). Epidemiologic studies of coronary heart disease and stroke in Japanese men living in Japan, Hawaii and California. *Am J Epidemiol, 97*(6), 372–385.

Keim, N. L., Stern, J. S., & Havel, P. J. (1998). Relation between circulating leptin concentrations and appetite during a prolonged, moderate energy deficit in women. *Am J Clin Nutr, 68*(4), 794–801.

Kelemen, L. E., Kushi, L. H., Jacobs, D. R., & Cerhan, J. R. (2005). Associations of dietary protein with disease and mortality in a prospective study of postmenopausal women. *Am J Epidemiol, 161*(3), 239–249. doi:10.1093/aje/kwi038

Kelsey, J. L., & Horn-Ross, P. L. (1993). Breast cancer: Magnitude of the problem and descriptive epidemiology. *Epidemiol Rev, 15*(1), 7–16.

Kennedy, E. T., Bowman, S. A., Spence, J. T., Freedman, M., & King, J. (2001). Popular diets: Correlation to health, nutrition, and obesity. *J Am Diet Assoc, 101*(4), 411–420. doi:10.1016/S0002-8223(01)00108-0

Keogh, J. B., Grieger, J. A., Noakes, M., & Clifton, P. M. (2005). Flow-mediated dilatation is impaired by a high-saturated fat diet but not by a high-carbohydrate diet. *Arterioscler Thromb Vasc Biol, 25*(6), 1274–1279. doi:10.1161/01.ATV.0000163185.28245.a1

Key, T., & Davey, G. (1996). Prevalence of obesity is low in people who do not eat meat. *BMJ, 313*(7060), 816–817.

Key, T. J., Allen, N., Appleby, P., Overvad, K., Tjønneland, A., Miller, A., ... European Prospective Investigation into Cancer and Nutrition (EPIC). (2004). Fruits and vegetables and prostate cancer: no association among 1104 cases in a prospective study of 130544 men in the European Prospective Investigation into Cancer and Nutrition (EPIC). *Int J Cancer, 109*(1), 119–124. doi:10.1002/ijc.11671

Key, T. J., Appleby, P. N., Crowe, F. L., Bradbury, K. E., Schmidt, J. A., & Travis, R. C. (2014). Cancer in British vegetarians: Updated analyses of 4998 incident cancers in a cohort of 32,491 meat eaters, 8612 fish eaters, 18,298 vegetarians, and 2246 vegans. *Am J Clin Nutr, 100*(1 Suppl), 378S–385S. doi:10.3945/ajcn.113.071266

Key, T. J., Appleby, P. N., Davey, G. K., Allen, N. E., Spencer, E. A., & Travis, R. C. (2003). Mortality in British vegetarians: Review and preliminary results from EPIC-Oxford. *Am J Clin Nutr, 78*(3 Suppl), 533S–538S.

Key, T. J., Appleby, P. N., Reeves, G. K., Roddam, A. W., & Endogenous Hormones and Breast Cancer Collaborative Group. (2010). Insulin-like growth factor 1 (IGF1), IGF binding protein 3 (IGFBP3), and breast cancer risk: Pooled individual data analysis of 17 prospective studies. *Lancet Oncol, 11*(6), 530–542. doi:10.1016/S1470-2045(10)70095-4

Key, T. J., Appleby, P. N., & Rosell, M. S. (2006). Health effects of vegetarian and vegan diets. *Proc Nutr Soc, 65*(1), 35–41.

Key, T. J., Appleby, P. N., Spencer, E. A., Travis, R. C., Allen, N. E., Thorogood, M., & Mann, J. I. (2009a). Cancer incidence in British vegetarians. *Br J Cancer, 101*(1), 192–197. doi:10.1038/sj.bjc.6605098

Key, T. J., Appleby, P. N., Spencer, E. A., Travis, R. C., Roddam, A. W., & Allen, N. E. (2009b). Mortality in British vegetarians: Results from the European Prospective Investigation into Cancer and Nutrition (EPIC-Oxford). *Am J Clin Nutr, 89*(5), 1613S–1619S. doi:10.3945/ajcn.2009.26736L

Key, T. J., Appleby, P. N., Spencer, E. A., Travis, R. C., Roddam, A. W., & Allen, N. E. (2009). Cancer incidence in vegetarians: Results from the European Prospective Investigation into Cancer and Nutrition (EPIC-Oxford). *Am J Clin Nutr, 89*(5), 1620S–1626S. doi:10.3945/ajcn.2009.26736M

Key, T. J., Fraser, G. E., Thorogood, M., Appleby, P. N., Beral, V., Reeves, G., . . . McPherson, K. (1999). Mortality in vegetarians and nonvegetarians: detailed findings from a collaborative analysis of 5 prospective studies. *Am J Clin Nutr, 70*(3 Suppl), 516S–524S.

Key, T. J., Schatzkin, A., Willett, W. C., Allen, N. E., Spencer, E. A., & Travis, R. C. (2004). Diet, nutrition and the prevention of cancer. *Public Health Nutr, 7*(1A), 187–200.

Key, T. J., Thorogood, M., Appleby, P. N., & Burr, M. L. (1996). Dietary habits and mortality in 11,000 vegetarians and health conscious people: Results of a 17 year follow up. *BMJ, 313*(7060), 775–779.

Khor, G. L. (1997). Nutrition and cardiovascular disease: An Asia Pacific perspective. *Asia Pacific J Clin Nutr, 6*(2), 122–142.

Kim, J., Park, S., & Nam, B. H. (2011). The risk of colorectal cancer is associated with the frequency of meat consumption in a population-based cohort in Korea. *Asian Pac J Cancer Prev, 12*(9), 2371–2376.

Kirkmeyer, S. V., & Mattes, R. D. (2000). Effects of food attributes on hunger and food intake. *Int J Obes Relat Metab Disord, 24*(9), 1167–1175.

Kjeldsen-Kragh, J., Haugen, M., Førre, O., Laache, H., & Malt, U. F. (1994). Vegetarian diet for patients with rheumatoid arthritis: Can the clinical effects be explained by the psychological characteristics of the patients? *Br J Rheumatol, 33*(6), 569–575.

Knekt, P., Steineck, G., Järvinen, R., Hakulinen, T., & Aromaa, A. (1994). Intake of fried meat and risk of cancer: a follow-up study in Finland. *Int J Cancer, 59*(6), 756–760.

Knowler, W. C., Saad, M. F., Pettitt, D. J., Nelson, R. G., & Bennett, P. H. (1993). Determinants of diabetes mellitus in the Pima Indians. *Diabetes Care, 16*(1), 216–227.

Koeth, R. A., Wang, Z., Levison, B. S., Buffa, J. A., Org, E., Sheehy, B. T., . . . Hazen, S. L. (2013). Intestinal microbiota metabolism of L-carnitine, a nutrient in red meat, promotes atherosclerosis. *Nat Med, 19*(5), 576–585. doi:10.1038/nm.3145

Koh-Banerjee, P., Franz, M., Sampson, L., Liu, S., Jacobs, D. R., Spiegelman, D., . . . Rimm, E. (2004). Changes in whole-grain, bran, and cereal fiber consumption in relation to 8-y weight gain among men. *Am J Clin Nutr, 80*(5), 1237–1245.

Korzenik, J. R. (2006). Case closed? Diverticulitis: epidemiology and fiber. *J Clin Gastroenterol, 40, Suppl 3*, S112–S116. doi:10.1097/01.mcg.0000225503.59923.6c

Kraschnewski, J. L., Boan, J., Esposito, J., Sherwood, N. E., Lehman, E. B., Kephart, D. K., & Sciamanna, C. N. (2010). Long-term weight loss maintenance in the United States. *Int J Obes (Lond), 34*(11), 1644–1654. doi:10.1038/ijo.2010.94

Krebs, J. D., Elley, C. R., Parry-Strong, A., Lunt, H., Drury, P. L., Bell, D. A., . . . Mann, J. I. (2012). The Diabetes Excess Weight Loss (DEWL) Trial: A randomised controlled trial of high-protein versus high-carbohydrate diets over 2 years in type 2 diabetes. *Diabetologia, 55*(4), 905–914. doi:10.1007/s00125-012-2461-0

Kromhout, D., Bloemberg, B., Feskens, E., Menotti, A., & Nissinen, A. (2000). Saturated fat, vitamin C and smoking predict long-term population all-cause mortality rates in the Seven Countries Study. *Int J Epidemiol, 29*(2), 260–265.

Kromhout, D., Geleijnse, J. M., Menotti, A., & Jacobs, D. R. (2011). The confusion about dietary fatty acids recommendations for CHD prevention. *Br J Nutr, 106*(5), 627–632. doi:10.1017/S0007114511002236

Krssak, M., Falk Petersen, K., Dresner, A., DiPietro, L., Vogel, S. M., Rothman, D. L., . . . Shulman, G. I. (1999). Intramyocellular lipid concentrations are correlated with insulin sensitivity in humans: A 1H NMR spectroscopy study. *Diabetologia, 42*(1), 113–116. doi:10.1007/s001250051123

Kumagai, S., Shibata, H., Watanabe, S., Suzuki, T., & Haga, H. (1999). Effect of food intake pattern on all-cause mortality in the community elderly: A 7-year longitudinal study. *J Nutr Health Aging, 3*(1), 29–33.

Kwak, S. M., Myung, S. K., Lee, Y. J., Seo, H. G., & Korean Meta-analysis Study Group. (2012). Efficacy of omega-3 fatty acid supplements (eicosapentaenoic acid and docosahexaenoic acid) in the secondary prevention of cardiovascular disease: A meta-analysis of randomized, double-blind, placebo-controlled trials. *Arch Intern Med, 172*(9), 686–694. doi:10.1001/archinternmed.2012.262

Kwiterovich, P. O., Vining, E. P., Pyzik, P., Skolasky, R., & Freeman, J. M. (2003). Effect of a high-fat ketogenic diet on plasma levels of lipids, lipoproteins, and apolipoproteins in children. *JAMA, 290*(7), 912–920. doi:10.1001/jama.290.7.912

Laatikainen, T., Critchley, J., Vartiainen, E., Salomaa, V., Ketonen, M., & Capewell, S. (2005). Explaining the decline in coronary heart disease mortality in Finland between 1982 and 1997. *Am J Epidemiol, 162*(8), 764–773. doi:10.1093/aje/kwi274

Lagiou, P., Sandin, S., Lof, M., Trichopoulos, D., Adami, H. O., & Weiderpass, E. (2012).

Low carbohydrate-high protein diet and incidence of cardiovascular diseases in Swedish women: Prospective cohort study. *BMJ, 344,* e4026.

Lagiou, P., Sandin, S., Weiderpass, E., Lagiou, A., Mucci, L., Trichopoulos, D., & Adami, H. O. (2007). Low carbohydrate-high protein diet and mortality in a cohort of Swedish women. *J Intern Med, 261*(4), 366–374. doi:10.1111/j.1365-2796.2007.01774.x

Lampe, J. W. (1999). Health effects of vegetables and fruit: assessing mechanisms of action in human experimental studies. *Am J Clin Nutr, 70*(3 Suppl), 475S–490S.

Lappe, F. M. (1985). *Diet for a Small Planet.* New York: Ballantine Books.

Lara-Castro, C., & Garvey, W. T. (2004). Diet, insulin resistance, and obesity: Zoning in on data for Atkins dieters living in South Beach. *J Clin Endocrinol Metab, 89*(9), 4197–4205. doi:10.1210/jc.2004-0683

Lara-Castro, C., & Garvey, W. T. (2008). Intracellular lipid accumulation in liver and muscle and the insulin resistance syndrome. *Endocrinol Metab Clin North Am, 37*(4), 841–856. doi:10.1016/j.ecl.2008.09.002

Larsson, S. C., Kumlin, M., Ingelman-Sundberg, M., & Wolk, A. (2004). Dietary long-chain n-3 fatty acids for the prevention of cancer: a review of potential mechanisms. *Am J Clin Nutr, 79*(6), 935–945.

Larsson, S. C., & Orsini, N. (2013). Red meat and processed meat consumption and all-cause mortality: A meta-analysis. *Am J Epidemiol.* doi:10.1093/aje/kwt261

Lauber, S. N., & Gooderham, N. J. (2011). The cooked meat-derived mammary carcinogen 2-amino-1-methyl-6-phenylimidazo[4,5-b]pyridine promotes invasive behaviour of breast cancer cells. *Toxicology, 279*(1-3), 139–145. doi:10.1016/j.tox.2010.10.004

Laville, M., & Nazare, J. A. (2009). Diabetes, insulin resistance and sugars. *Obes Rev, 10*(1 Suppl), 24–33. doi:10.1111/j.1467-789X.2008.00562.x

Lee, J. E., Giovannucci, E., Smith-Warner, S. A., Spiegelman, D., Willett, W. C., & Curhan, G. C. (2006). Intakes of fruits, vegetables, vitamins A, C, and E, and carotenoids and risk of renal cell cancer. *Cancer Epidemiol Biomarkers Prev, 15*(12), 2445–2452. doi:10.1158/1055-9965.EPI-06-0553

Leenders, M., Sluijs, I., Ros, M. M., Boshuizen, H. C., Siersema, P. D., Ferrari, P., . . . Bueno-de-Mesquita, H. B. (2013). Fruit and vegetable consumption and mortality: European prospective investigation into cancer and nutrition. *Am J Epidemiol, 178*(4), 590–602. doi:10.1093/aje/kwt006

Leidy, H. J., Bossingham, M. J., Mattes, R. D., & Campbell, W. W. (2009). Increased dietary protein consumed at breakfast leads to an initial and sustained feeling of fullness during energy restriction compared to other meal times. *Br J Nutr, 101*(6), 798–803.

Leidy, H. J., Ortinau, L. C., Douglas, S. M., & Hoertel, H. A. (2013). Beneficial effects of a higher-protein breakfast on the appetitive, hormonal, and neural signals controlling energy intake regulation in overweight/obese, "breakfast-skipping," late-adolescent girls. *Am J Clin Nutr, 97*(4), 677–688. doi:10.3945/ajcn.112.053116

Lennerz, B. S., Alsop, D. C., Holsen, L. M., Stern, E., Rojas, R., Ebbeling, C. B., . . . Ludwig, D. S. (2013). Effects of dietary glycemic index on brain regions related to reward and craving in men. *Am J Clin Nutr, 98*(3), 641–647. doi:10.3945/ajcn.113.064113

Lesser, L. I., Ebbeling, C. B., Goozner, M., Wypij, D., & Ludwig, D. S. (2007). Relationship between funding source and conclusion among nutrition-related scientific articles. *PLoS Med, 4*(1), e5. doi:10.1371/journal.pmed.0040005

Levine, M. E., Suarez, J. A., Brandhorst, S., Balasubramanian, P., Cheng, C. W., Madia, F., ... Longo, V. D. (2014). Low protein intake is associated with a major reduction in IGF-1, cancer, and overall mortality in the 65 and younger but not older population. *Cell Metab, 19*(3), 407–417. doi:10.1016/j.cmet.2014.02.006

Ley, S. H., Sun, Q., Willett, W. C., Eliassen, A. H., Wu, K., Pan, A., ... Hu, F. B. (2014). Associations between red meat intake and biomarkers of inflammation and glucose metabolism in women. *Am J Clin Nutr, 99*(2), 352–360. doi:10.3945/ajcn.113.075663

Li, S., Chiuve, S. E., Flint, A., Pai, J. K., Forman, J. P., Hu, F. B., ... Rimm, E. B. (2013). Better diet quality and decreased mortality among myocardial infarction survivors. *JAMA Intern Med, 173*(19), 1808–1818. doi:10.1001/jamainternmed.2013.9768

Li, S., Flint, A., Pai, J. K., Forman, J. P., Hu, F. B., Willett, W. C., ... Rimm, E. B. (2014). Low carbohydrate diet from plant or animal sources and mortality among myocardial infarction survivors. *J Am Heart Assoc, 3*(5), e001169. doi:10.1161/JAHA.114.001169

Li, Y., Zhou, C., Zhou, X., & Li, L. (2013). Egg consumption and risk of cardiovascular diseases and diabetes: A meta-analysis. *Atherosclerosis.* doi:10.1016/j.atherosclerosis.2013.04.003

Li, Z., & Heber, D. (2012). Overeating and overweight: extra calories increase fat mass while protein increases lean mass. *JAMA, 307*(1), 86–87. doi:10.1001/jama.2011.1959

Lin, P.-H., Miwa, S., Li, Y., Wang, Y., Levy, E., Lastor, K., & Champagne, C. (2010). Influencing dietary protein sources in the PREMIER trial population. *J Am Diet Assoc, 110,* 291–295. doi:10.1016/j.jada.2009.10.041.

Lin, Y., Bolca, S., Vandevijvere, S., De Vriese, S., Mouratidou, T., De Neve, M., ... Huybrechts, I. (2011). Plant and animal protein intake and its association with overweight and obesity among the Belgian population. *Br J Nutr, 105*(7), 1106–1116. doi:10.1017/S0007114510004642

Liu, S., Stampfer, M. J., Hu, F. B., Giovannucci, E., Rimm, E., Manson, J. E., ... Willett, W. C. (1999). Whole-grain consumption and risk of coronary heart disease: Results from the Nurses' Health Study. *Am J Clin Nutr, 70*(3), 412–419.

Liu, S., Willett, W. C., Manson, J. E., Hu, F. B., Rosner, B., & Colditz, G. (2003). Relation between changes in intakes of dietary fiber and grain products and changes in weight and development of obesity among middle-aged women. *Am J Clin Nutr, 78*(5), 920–927.

Loh, Y. H., Jakszyn, P., Luben, R. N., Mulligan, A. A., Mitrou, P. N., & Khaw, K. T. (2011). N-nitroso compounds and cancer incidence: The European Prospective Investigation into Cancer and Nutrition (EPIC)-Norfolk Study. *Am J Clin Nutr, 93*(5), 1053–1061. doi:10.3945/ajcn.111.012377

López-Torres, M., & Barja, G. (2008). Lowered methionine ingestion as responsible for the decrease in rodent mitochondrial oxidative stress in protein and dietary restriction possible implications for humans. *Biochim Biophys Acta, 1780*(11), 1337–1347. doi:10.1016/j.bbagen.2008.01.007

Loria Kohen, V., Gómez Candela, C., Fernández Fernández, C., Pérez Torres, A., Villarino Sanz, M., & Bermejo, L. M. (2011). Impact of two low-calorie meals with and without bread on the sensation of hunger, satiety and amount of food consumed. *Nutr Hosp, 26*(5), 1155–1160. doi:10.1590/S0212-16112011000500035

Lowndes, J., Kawiecki, D., Pardo, S., Nguyen, V., Melanson, K. J., Yu, Z., & Rippe, J. M. (2012). The effects of four hypocaloric diets containing different levels of sucrose or high fructose corn syrup on weight loss and related parameters. *Nutr J, 11*, 55. doi:10.1186/1475-2891-11-55

Lu, S. C., Wu, W. H., Lee, C. A., Chou, H. F., Lee, H. R., & Huang, P. C. (2000). LDL of Taiwanese vegetarians are less oxidizable than those of omnivores. *J Nutr, 130*(6), 1591–1596.

Mann, G. V., Spoerry, A., Gray, M., & Jarashow, D. (1972). Atherosclerosis in the Masai. *Am J Epidemiol, 95*(1), 26–37.

Margetts, B. M., Beilin, L. J., Vandongen, R., & Armstrong, B. K. (1986). Vegetarian diet in mild hypertension: A randomised controlled trial. *Br Med J (Clin Res Ed), 293*(6560), 1468–1471.

Margetts, B. M., & Jackson, A. A. (1993). Vegetarians and longevity. *Epidemiology, 4*(3), 278–279.

Marmot, M. G., Syme, S. L., Kagan, A., Kato, H., Cohen, J. B., & Belsky, J. (1975). Epidemiologic studies of coronary heart disease and stroke in Japanese men living in Japan, Hawaii and California: Prevalence of coronary and hypertensive heart disease and associated risk factors. *Am J Epidemiol, 102*(6), 514–525.

Martens, E. A., Lemmens, S. G., & Westerterp-Plantenga, M. S. (2013). Protein leverage affects energy intake of high-protein diets in humans. *Am J Clin Nutr, 97*(1), 86–93. doi:10.3945/ajcn.112.046540

Martin, L. J., Li, Q., Melnichouk, O., Greenberg, C., Minkin, S., Hislop, G., & Boyd, N. F. (2011). A randomized trial of dietary intervention for breast cancer prevention. *Cancer Res, 71*(1), 123-133. doi:10.1158/0008-5472.CAN-10-1436

Mattei, J., Hu, F. B., & Campos, H. (2011). A higher ratio of beans to white rice is associated with lower cardiometabolic risk factors in Costa Rican adults. *Am J Clin Nutr, 94*(3), 869–876. doi:10.3945/ajcn.111.013219

McCarty, M. F. (1999). Vegan proteins may reduce risk of cancer, obesity, and cardiovascular disease by promoting increased glucagon activity. *Med Hypotheses, 53*(6), 459–485. doi:10.1054/mehy.1999.0784

McCarty, M. F., Barroso-Aranda, J., & Contreras, F. (2009). The low-methionine content of vegan diets may make methionine restriction feasible as a life extension strategy. *Med Hypotheses, 72*(2), 125–128. doi:10.1016/j.mehy.2008.07.044

McDougall, J., Bruce, B., Spiller, G., Westerdahl, J., & McDougall, M. (2002). Effects of a very low-fat, vegan diet in subjects with rheumatoid arthritis. *J Altern Complement Med, 8*(1), 71–75. doi:10.1089/107555302753507195

McGee, D. L., Reed, D. M., Yano, K., Kagan, A., & Tillotson, J. (1984). Ten-year incidence of coronary heart disease in the Honolulu Heart Program. Relationship to nutrient intake. *Am J Epidemiol, 119*(5), 667–676.

McGinnis, J. M., & Foege, W. H. (1993). Actual causes of death in the United States. *JAMA, 270*(18), 2207–2212.

McLaughlin, J., Middaugh, J., Boudreau, D., Malcom, G., Parry, S., Tracy, R., & Newman, W. (2005). Adipose tissue triglyceride fatty acids and atherosclerosis in Alaska Natives and non-Natives. *Atherosclerosis, 181*(2), 353–362. doi:10.1016/j.atherosclerosis.2005.01.019

Meigs, J. B., Hu, F. B., Rifai, N., & Manson, J. E. (2004). Biomarkers of endothelial dysfunction and risk of type 2 diabetes mellitus. *JAMA, 291*(16), 1978–1986. doi:10.1001/jama.291.16.1978

Mellen, P. B., Walsh, T. F., & Herrington, D. M. (2008). Whole grain intake and cardiovascular disease: A meta-analysis. *Nutr Metab Cardiovasc Dis, 18*(4), 283–290. doi:10.1016/j.numecd.2006.12.008

Menotti, A., Kromhout, D., Blackburn, H., Fidanza, F., Buzina, R., & Nissinen, A. (1999). Food intake patterns and 25-year mortality from coronary heart disease: cross-cultural correlations in the Seven Countries Study. The Seven Countries Study Research Group. *Eur J Epidemiol, 15*(6), 507–515.

Meredith, C. N., Zackin, M. J., Frontera, W. R., & Evans, W. J. (1989). Dietary protein requirements and body protein metabolism in endurance-trained men. *J Appl Physiol, 66*(6), 2850–2856.

Merino, J., Kones, R., Ferré, R., Plana, N., Girona, J., Aragonés, G., . . . Masana, L. (2013). Negative effect of a low-carbohydrate, high-protein, high-fat diet on small peripheral artery reactivity in patients with increased cardiovascular risk. *Br J Nutr, 109*(7), 1241–1247. doi:10.1017/S0007114512003091

Micha, R., Wallace, S. K., & Mozaffarian, D. (2010). Red and processed meat consumption and risk of incident coronary heart disease, stroke, and diabetes mellitus: A systematic review and meta-analysis. *Circulation, 121*(21), 2271–2283. doi:10.1161/CIRCULATIONAHA.109.924977

Michaud, D. S., Spiegelman, D., Clinton, S. K., Rimm, E. B., Willett, W. C., & Giovannucci, E. L. (1999). Fruit and vegetable intake and incidence of bladder cancer in a male prospective cohort. *J Natl Cancer Inst, 91*(7), 605–613.

Mikkelsen, P. B., Toubro, S., & Astrup, A. (2000). Effect of fat-reduced diets on 24-h energy expenditure: comparisons between animal protein, vegetable protein, and carbohydrate. *Am J Clin Nutr, 72*(5), 1135–1141.

Miller, E. R., Erlinger, T. P., Sacks, F. M., Svetkey, L. P., Charleston, J., Lin, P. H., & Appel, L. J. (2005). A dietary pattern that lowers oxidative stress increases antibodies to oxidized LDL: results from a randomized controlled feeding study. *Atherosclerosis, 183*(1), 175–182. doi:10.1016/j.atherosclerosis.2005.04.001

Miller, E. R., Pastor-Barriuso, R., Dalal, D., Riemersma, R. A., Appel, L. J., & Guallar, E. (2005). Meta-analysis: High-dosage vitamin E supplementation may increase all-cause mortality. *Ann Intern Med, 142*(1), 37–46.

Miller, M., Beach, V., Sorkin, J. D., Mangano, C., Dobmeier, C., Novacic, D., . . . Vogel, R. A. (2009). Comparative effects of three popular diets on lipids, endothelial function, and C-reactive protein during weight maintenance. *J Am Diet Assoc, 109*(4), 713–717. doi:10.1016/j.jada.2008.12.023

Millward, D. J. (1999a). Meat or wheat for the next millennium? Proceedings of a symposium. Guildford, United Kingdom, 29 June–2 July 1998. *Proc Nutr Soc, 58*(2), 209–275.

Millward, D. J. (1999b). The nutritional value of plant-based diets in relation to human amino acid and protein requirements. *Proc Nutr Soc, 58*(2), 249–260.

Milton, K. (2000). Hunter-gatherer diets—a different perspective. *Am J Clin Nutr, 71*(3), 665–667.

Mollard, R. C., Zykus, A., Luhovyy, B. L., Nunez, M. F., Wong, C. L., & Anderson, G. H.

(2012). The acute effects of a pulse-containing meal on glycaemic responses and measures of satiety and satiation within and at a later meal. *Br J Nutr, 108*(3), 509–517. doi:10.1017/S0007114511005836

Montonen, J., Boeing, H., Fritsche, A., Schleicher, E., Joost, H. G., Schulze, M. B., . . . Pischon, T. (2013). Consumption of red meat and whole-grain bread in relation to biomarkers of obesity, inflammation, glucose metabolism and oxidative stress. *Eur J Nutr, 52*(1), 337–345. doi:10.1007/s00394-012-0340-6

Moore, D. R., Robinson, M. J., Fry, J. L., Tang, J. E., Glover, E. I., Wilkinson, S. B., . . . Phillips, S. M. (2009). Ingested protein dose response of muscle and albumin protein synthesis after resistance exercise in young men. *Am J Clin Nutr, 89*(1), 161–168. doi:10.3945/ajcn.2008.26401

Morimoto, A. (2010). Trends in the epidemiology of patients with diabetes in Japan. *JMAJ, 53,* 36–40.

Mozaffarian, D., Hao, T., Rimm, E. B., Willett, W. C., & Hu, F. B. (2011). Changes in diet and lifestyle and long-term weight gain in women and men. *N Engl J Med, 364*(25), 2392–2404. doi:10.1056/NEJMoa1014296

Mozaffarian, D., Micha, R., & Wallace, S. (2010). Effects on coronary heart disease of increasing polyunsaturated fat in place of saturated fat: A systematic review and meta-analysis of randomized controlled trials. *PLoS Med, 7*(3), e1000252. doi:10.1371/journal.pmed.1000252

Mozaffarian, D., & Rimm, E. B. (2006). Fish intake, contaminants, and human health: evaluating the risks and the benefits. *JAMA, 296*(15), 1885–1899. doi:10.1001/jama.296.15.1885

Mozaffarian, D., Rimm, E. B., & Herrington, D. M. (2004). Dietary fats, carbohydrate, and progression of coronary atherosclerosis in postmenopausal women. *Am J Clin Nutr, 80*(5), 1175–1184.

Müller, H., de Toledo, F. W., & Resch, K. L. (2001). Fasting followed by vegetarian diet in patients with rheumatoid arthritis: a systematic review. *Scand J Rheumatol, 30*(1), 1–10.

Murad, M. H., & Montori, V. M. (2013). Synthesizing evidence: Shifting the focus from individual studies to the body of evidence. *JAMA, 309*(21), 2217–2218. doi:10.1001/jama.2013.5616

Murad, M. H., Montori, V. M., Ioannidis, J. P., Jaeschke, R., Devereaux, P. J., Prasad, K., . . . Guyatt, G. (2014). How to read a systematic review and meta-analysis and apply the results to patient care: Users' guides to the medical literature. *JAMA, 312*(2), 171–179. doi:10.1001/jama.2014.5559

Muraki, I., Imamura, F., Manson, J. E., Hu, F. B., Willett, W. C., van Dam, R. M., & Sun, Q. (2013). Fruit consumption and risk of type 2 diabetes: Results from three prospective longitudinal cohort studies. *BMJ, 347,* f5001.

Murphy, N., Norat, T., Ferrari, P., Jenab, M., Bueno-de-Mesquita, B., Skeie, G., . . . Riboli, E. (2012). Dietary fibre intake and risks of cancers of the colon and rectum in the European prospective investigation into cancer and nutrition (EPIC). *PLoS One, 7*(6), e39361. doi:10.1371/journal.pone.0039361

Nagura, J., Iso, H., Watanabe, Y., Maruyama, K., Date, C., Toyoshima, H., . . . JACC Study Group. (2009). Fruit, vegetable and bean intake and mortality from cardiovascular disease among Japanese men and women: the JACC Study. *Br J Nutr, 102*(2), 285–292. doi:10.1017/S0007114508143586

Nakagawa, S., Lagisz, M., Hector, K. L., & Spencer, H. G. (2012). Comparative and meta-analytic insights into life extension via dietary restriction. *Aging Cell, 11*(3), 401–409. doi:10.1111/j.1474-9726.2012.00798.x

Nakamura, Y., Okamura, T., Tamaki, S., Kadowaki, T., Hayakawa, T., Kita, Y., . . . NIPPON Data Research Group. (2004). Egg consumption, serum cholesterol, and cause-specific and all-cause mortality: the National Integrated Project for Prospective Observation of Non-communicable Disease and Its Trends in the Aged, 1980 (NIPPON DATA80). *Am J Clin Nutr, 80*(1), 58–63.

Nanri, A., Moore, M. A., & Kono, S. (2007). Impact of C-reactive protein on disease risk and its relation to dietary factors. *Asian Pac J Cancer Prev, 8*(2), 167–177.

National Center for Health Statistics. (2005). *National Health and Nutrition Examination Survey, 2005–2006.* Hyattsville, MD: Author.

Nechuta, S. J., Caan, B. J., Chen, W. Y., Lu, W., Chen, Z., Kwan, M. L., . . . Shu, X. O. (2012). Soy food intake after diagnosis of breast cancer and survival: An in-depth analysis of combined evidence from cohort studies of US and Chinese women. *Am J Clin Nutr, 96*(1), 123–132. doi:10.3945/ajcn.112.035972

Nestle, M. (1995). Mediterranean diets: Historical and research overview. *Am J Clin Nutr, 61*(6 Suppl), 1313S–1320S.

Nestle, M. (1999). Animal v. plant foods in human diets and health: Is the historical record unequivocal? *Proc Nutr Soc, 58*(2), 211–218.

Nettleton, J. A., Diez-Roux, A., Jenny, N. S., Fitzpatrick, A. L., & Jacobs, D. R. (2008). Dietary patterns, food groups, and telomere length in the Multi-Ethnic Study of Atherosclerosis (MESA). *Am J Clin Nutr, 88*(5), 1405–1412.

New, S. A. (2004). Do vegetarians have a normal bone mass? *Osteoporos Int, 15*(9), 679–688. doi:10.1007/s00198-004-1647-9

New, S. A., Bolton-Smith, C., Grubb, D. A., & Reid, D. M. (1997). Nutritional influences on bone mineral density: A cross-sectional study in premenopausal women. *Am J Clin Nutr, 65*(6), 1831–1839.

Newby, P. K., Muller, D., Hallfrisch, J., Qiao, N., Andres, R., & Tucker, K. L. (2003). Dietary patterns and changes in body mass index and waist circumference in adults. *Am J Clin Nutr, 77*(6), 1417–1425.

Newby, P. K., Tucker, K. L., & Wolk, A. (2005). Risk of overweight and obesity among semi-vegetarian, lactovegetarian, and vegan women. *Am J Clin Nutr, 81*(6), 1267–1274.

Nicholls, S. J., Lundman, P., Harmer, J. A., Cutri, B., Griffiths, K. A., Rye, K. A., . . . Celermajer, D. S. (2006). Consumption of saturated fat impairs the anti-inflammatory properties of high-density lipoproteins and endothelial function. *J Am Coll Cardiol, 48*(4), 715–720. doi:10.1016/j.jacc.2006.04.080

Nicholson, A. S., Sklar, M., Barnard, N. D., Gore, S., Sullivan, R., & Browning, S. (1999). Toward improved management of NIDDM: A randomized, controlled, pilot intervention using a lowfat, vegetarian diet. *Prev Med, 29*(2), 87–91. doi:10.1006/pmed.1999.0529

Norat, T., Bingham, S., Ferrari, P., Slimani, N., Jenab, M., Mazuir, M., . . . Riboli, E. (2005). Meat, fish, and colorectal cancer risk: The European Prospective Investigation into cancer and nutrition. *J Natl Cancer Inst, 97*(12), 906–916. doi:10.1093/jnci/dji164

Norat, T., Lukanova, A., Ferrari, P., & Riboli, E. (2002). Meat consumption and colorectal cancer risk: Dose-response meta-analysis of epidemiological studies. *Int J Cancer, 98*(2), 241–256.

Nordmann, A. J., Nordmann, A., Briel, M., Keller, U., Yancy, W. S., Brehm, B. J., & Bucher, H. C. (2006). Effects of low-carbohydrate vs low-fat diets on weight loss and cardiovascular risk factors: A meta-analysis of randomized controlled trials. *Arch Intern Med, 166*(3), 285–293. doi:10.1001/archinte.166.3.285

Nöthlings, U., Wilkens, L. R., Murphy, S. P., Hankin, J. H., Henderson, B. E., & Kolonel, L. N. (2005). Meat and fat intake as risk factors for pancreatic cancer: The multiethnic cohort study. *J Natl Cancer Inst, 97*(19), 1458–1465. doi:10.1093/jnci/dji292

Noto, H., Goto, A., Tsujimoto, T., & Noda, M. (2013). Low-carbohydrate diets and all-cause mortality: A systematic review and meta-analysis of observational studies. *PLoS One, 8*(1), e55030. doi:10.1371/journal.pone.0055030

O'Keefe, S. J., Kidd, M., Espitalier-Noel, G., & Owira, P. (1999). Rarity of colon cancer in Africans is associated with low animal product consumption, not fiber. *Am J Gastroenterol, 94*(5), 1373–1380. doi:10.1111/j.1572-0241.1999.01089.x

Ogden, C. L., Carroll, M. D., Curtin, L. R., McDowell, M. A., Tabak, C. J., & Flegal, K. M. (2006). Prevalence of overweight and obesity in the United States, 1999–2004. *JAMA, 295*(13), 1549–1555. doi:10.1001/jama.295.13.1549

Orlich, M. J., Singh, P. N., Sabaté, J., Jaceldo-Siegl, K., Fan, J., Knutsen, S., . . . Fraser, G. E. (2013). Vegetarian dietary patterns and mortality in adventist health study 2. *JAMA Intern Med, 173*(13), 1230–1238. doi:10.1001/jamainternmed.2013.6473

Ornish, D., Lin, J., Chan, J., Epel, E., Kemp, C., Weidner, G., Marlin, R., . . . Blackburn, E. (2013). Effect of comprehensive lifestyle changes on telomerase activity and telomere length in men with biopsy-proven low-risk prostate cancer: 5-year follow-up of a descriptive pilot study. *Lancet Oncol, 14*(11), 1112–1120.

Ornish, D., Lin, J., Daubenmier, J., Weidner, G., Epel, E., Kemp, C., . . . Blackburn, E. H. (2008). Increased telomerase activity and comprehensive lifestyle changes: A pilot study. *Lancet Oncol, 9*(11), 1048–1057. doi:10.1016/S1470-2045(08)70234-1

Ornish, D., Scherwitz, L. W., Billings, J. H., Brown, S. E., Gould, K. L., Merritt, T. A., . . . Brand, R. J. (1998). Intensive lifestyle changes for reversal of coronary heart disease. *JAMA, 280*(23), 2001–2007.

Ornish, D., Weidner, G., Fair, W. R., Marlin, R., Pettengill, E. B., Raisin, C. J., . . . Carroll, P. R. (2005). Intensive lifestyle changes may affect the progression of prostate cancer. *J Urol, 174*(3), 1065–1069; discussion 1069–1070. doi:10.1097/01.ju.0000169487.49018.73

Osler, M., Heitmann, B. L., Gerdes, L. U., Jørgensen, L. M., & Schroll, M. (2001). Dietary patterns and mortality in Danish men and women: a prospective observational study. *Br J Nutr, 85*(2), 219–225.

Otten, J., Hellwig, J., & Meyers, L. (Eds.). (2006). *Dietary reference intakes:The essential guide to nutrient requirements.* Washington, DC: National Academies Press.

Padler-Karavani, V., Yu, H., Cao, H., Chokhawala, H., Karp, F., Varki, N., . . . Varki, A. (2008). Diversity in specificity, abundance, and composition of anti-Neu5Gc antibodies in normal humans: Potential implications for disease. *Glycobiology, 18*(10), 818–830. doi:10.1093/glycob/cwn072

Paltoo, D. N., & Chu, K. C. (2004). Patterns in cancer incidence among American Indians/Alaska Natives, United States, 1992–1999. *Public Health Rep, 119*(4), 443–451. doi:10.1016/j.phr.2004.05.009

Pan, A., Sun, Q., Bernstein, A. M., Manson, J. E., Willett, W. C., & Hu, F. B. (2013). Changes in red meat consumption and subsequent risk of type 2 diabetes mellitus: Three cohorts of US men and women. *JAMA Intern Med*, 1–8. doi:10.1001/jamainternmed.2013.6633

Pan, A., Sun, Q., Bernstein, A. M., Schulze, M. B., Manson, J. E., Stampfer, M. J., . . . Hu, F. B. (2012). Red meat consumption and mortality: Results from 2 prospective cohort studies. *Arch Intern Med, 172*(7), 555–563. doi:10.1001/archinternmed.2011.2287

Pan, A., Sun, Q., Bernstein, A. M., Schulze, M. B., Manson, J. E., Willett, W. C., & Hu, F. B. (2011). Red meat consumption and risk of type 2 diabetes: 3 cohorts of US adults and an updated meta-analysis. *Am J Clin Nutr, 94*(4), 1088–1096. doi:10.3945/ajcn.111 .018978

Park, Y., Hunter, D. J., Spiegelman, D., Bergkvist, L., Berrino, F., van den Brandt, P. A., . . . Smith-Warner, S. A. (2005). Dietary fiber intake and risk of colorectal cancer: A pooled analysis of prospective cohort studies. *JAMA, 294*(22), 2849–2857. doi:10.1001/ jama.294.22.2849

Park, Y., Subar, A. F., Hollenbeck, A., & Schatzkin, A. (2011). Dietary fiber intake and mortality in the NIH-AARP diet and health study. *Arch Intern Med, 171*(12), 1061–1068. doi:10.1001/archinternmed.2011.18

Patel, J. V., Vyas, A., Cruickshank, J. K., Prabhakaran, D., Hughes, E., Reddy, K. S., . . . Durrington, P. N. (2006). Impact of migration on coronary heart disease risk factors: Comparison of Gujaratis in Britain and their contemporaries in villages of origin in India. *Atherosclerosis, 185*(2), 297–306. doi:10.1016/j.atherosclerosis.2005.06.005

Pedersen, J. I., James, P. T., Brouwer, I. A., Clarke, R., Elmadfa, I., Katan, M. B., . . . Uusitupa, M. (2011). The importance of reducing SFA to limit CHD. *Br J Nutr, 106*(7), 961–963. doi:10.1017/S000711451100506X

Pettersen, B. J., Anousheh, R., Fan, J., Jaceldo-Siegl, K., & Fraser, G. E. (2012). Vegetarian diets and blood pressure among white subjects: Results from the Adventist Health Study-2 (AHS-2). *Public Health Nutr, 15*(10), 1909–1916. doi:10.1017/S1368980011003454

Pickup, J. C. (2004). Inflammation and activated innate immunity in the pathogenesis of type 2 diabetes. *Diabetes Care, 27*(3), 813–823.

Pierce, J. P., Natarajan, L., Caan, B. J., Parker, B. A., Greenberg, E. R., Flatt, S. W., . . . Stefanick, M. L. (2007). Influence of a diet very high in vegetables, fruit, and fiber and low in fat on prognosis following treatment for breast cancer: The Women's Healthy Eating and Living (WHEL) randomized trial. *JAMA, 298*(3), 289–298. doi:10.1001/ jama.298.3.289

Pimentel, D., & Pimentel, M. (2003). Sustainability of meat-based and plant-based diets and the environment. *Am J Clin Nutr, 78*(3 Suppl), 660S–663S.

Pirro, M., Schillaci, G., Savarese, G., Gemelli, F., Mannarino, M. R., Siepi, D., . . . Mannarino, E. (2004). Attenuation of inflammation with short-term dietary intervention is associated with a reduction of arterial stiffness in subjects with hypercholesterolaemia. *Eur J Cardiovasc Prev Rehabil, 11*(6), 497–502.

Pixley, F., Wilson, D., McPherson, K., & Mann, J. (1985). Effect of vegetarianism on development of gall stones in women. *Br Med J (Clin Res Ed), 291*(6487), 11–12.

Poddar, K., Kolge, S., Bezman, L., Mullin, G. E., & Cheskin, L. J. (2011). Nutraceutical supplements for weight loss: A systematic review. *Nutr Clin Pract, 26*(5), 539–552. doi:10.1177/0884533611419859

Pollak, M. N. (1998). Endocrine effects of IGF-I on normal and transformed breast epithelial cells: Potential relevance to strategies for breast cancer treatment and prevention. *Breast Cancer Res Treat, 47*(3), 209–217.

Poulain, M., Pes, G. M., Grasland, C., Carru, C., Ferrucci, L., Baggio, G., . . . Deiana, L. (2004). Identification of a geographic area characterized by extreme longevity in the Sardinia island: The AKEA study. *Exp Gerontol, 39*(9), 1423–1429. doi:10.1016/j.exger.2004.06.016

Powell, J. J., Tucker, L., Fisher, A. G., & Wilcox, K. (1994). The effects of different percentages of dietary fat intake, exercise, and calorie restriction on body composition and body weight in obese females. *Am J Health Promot, 8*(6), 442–448.

Preis, S. R., Stampfer, M. J., Spiegelman, D., Willett, W. C., & Rimm, E. B. (2010). Lack of association between dietary protein intake and risk of stroke among middle-aged men. *Am J Clin Nutr, 91*(1), 39–45. doi:10.3945/ajcn.2009.28060

Preis, S. R., Stampfer, M. J., Spiegelman, D., Willett, W. C., & Rimm, E. B. (2010). Dietary protein and risk of ischemic heart disease in middle-aged men. *Am J Clin Nutr, 92*(5), 1265–1272. doi:10.3945/ajcn.2010.29626

Qiao, L., & Feng, Y. (2013). Intakes of heme iron and zinc and colorectal cancer incidence: A meta-analysis of prospective studies. *Cancer Causes Control, 24*(6), 1175–1183. doi:10.1007/s10552-013-0197-x

Rafii, M., Chapman, K., Owens, J., Elango, R., Campbell, W. W., Ball, R. O., . . . Courtney-Martin, G. (2015). Dietary protein requirement of female adults >65 years determined by the indicator amino acid oxidation technique is higher than current recommendations. *J Nutr, 145*(1), 18–24. doi:10.3945/jn.114.197517

Rajaram, S. (2003). The effect of vegetarian diet, plant foods, and phytochemicals on hemostasis and thrombosis. *Am J Clin Nutr, 78*(3 Suppl), 552S–558S.

Rand, W. M., Pellett, P. L., & Young, V. R. (2003). Meta-analysis of nitrogen balance studies for estimating protein requirements in healthy adults. *Am J Clin Nutr, 77*(1), 109–127.

Rankin, J. W., & Turpyn, A. D. (2007). Low carbohydrate, high fat diet increases C-reactive protein during weight loss. *J Am Coll Nutr, 26*(2), 163–169.

Rasmussen-Torvik, L. J., Shay, C. M., Abramson, J. G., Friedrich, C. A., Nettleton, J. A., Prizment, A. E., & Folsom, A. R. (2013). Ideal cardiovascular health is inversely associated with incident cancer: The atherosclerosis risk in communities study. *Circulation, 127*(12), 1270–1275. doi:10.1161/CIRCULATIONAHA.112.001183

Ravussin, E., Valencia, M. E., Esparza, J., Bennett, P. H., & Schulz, L. O. (1994). Effects of a traditional lifestyle on obesity in Pima Indians. *Diabetes Care, 17*(9), 1067–1074.

Ray, K., Wainwright, N. W., Visser, L., Witteman, J., Breteler, M., Ambegaonkar, B., . . . Sandhu, M. (2012). Changes in HDL cholesterol and cardiovascular outcomes after lipid modification therapy. *Heart, 98*(10), 780–785. doi:10.1136/heartjnl-2011-301405

Reddy, S. T., Wang, C. Y., Sakhaee, K., Brinkley, L., & Pak, C. Y. (2002). Effect of low-carbohydrate high-protein diets on acid-base balance, stone-forming propensity, and calcium metabolism. *Am J Kidney Dis, 40*(2), 265–274. doi:10.1053/ajkd.2002.34504

Reif, D. W. (1992). Ferritin as a source of iron for oxidative damage. *Free Radic Biol Med, 12*(5), 417–427.

Riboli, E., & Norat, T. (2003). Epidemiologic evidence of the protective effect of fruit and vegetables on cancer risk. *Am J Clin Nutr, 78*(3 Suppl), 559S–569S.

Richman, E. L., Kenfield, S. A., Stampfer, M. J., Giovannucci, E. L., & Chan, J. M. (2011). Egg, red meat, and poultry intake and risk of lethal prostate cancer in the prostate-specific antigen-era: Incidence and survival. *Cancer Prev Res (Phila), 4*(12), 2110–2121. doi:10.1158/1940-6207.CAPR-11-0354

Richman, E. L., Kenfield, S. A., Stampfer, M. J., Giovannucci, E. L., Zeisel, S. H., Willett, W. C., & Chan, J. M. (2012). Choline intake and risk of lethal prostate cancer: Incidence and survival. *Am J Clin Nutr, 96*(4), 855–863. doi:10.3945/ajcn.112.039784

Richman, E. L., Stampfer, M. J., Paciorek, A., Broering, J. M., Carroll, P. R., & Chan, J. M. (2010). Intakes of meat, fish, poultry, and eggs and risk of prostate cancer progression. *Am J Clin Nutr, 91*(3), 712–721. doi:10.3945/ajcn.2009.28474

Rizos, E. C., Ntzani, E. E., Bika, E., Kostapanos, M. S., & Elisaf, M. S. (2012). Association between omega-3 fatty acid supplementation and risk of major cardiovascular disease events: a systematic review and meta-analysis. *JAMA, 308*(10), 1024–1033. doi:10.1001/2012.jama.11374

Rizzo, N. S., Jaceldo-Siegl, K., Sabate, J., & Fraser, G. E. (2013). Nutrient profiles of vegetarian and nonvegetarian dietary patterns. *J Acad Nutr Diet, 113*(12), 1610–1619. doi:10.1016/j.jand.2013.06.349

Rizzo, N. S., Sabaté, J., Jaceldo-Siegl, K., & Fraser, G. E. (2011). Vegetarian dietary patterns are associated with a lower risk of metabolic syndrome: The Adventist Health Study 2. *Diabetes Care, 34*(5), 1225–1227. doi:10.2337/dc10-1221

Roberts, W. C. (2010). It's the cholesterol, stupid! *Am J Cardiol, 106*(9), 1364–1366. doi:10.1016/j.amjcard.2010.09.022

Robey, I. F. (2012). Examining the relationship between diet-induced acidosis and cancer. *Nutr Metab (Lond), 9*(1), 72. doi:10.1186/1743-7075-9-72

Rohrmann, S., Linseisen, J., Jakobsen, M. U., Overvad, K., Raaschou-Nielsen, O., Tjonneland, A., . . . Vineis, P. (2011). Consumption of meat and dairy and lymphoma risk in the European Prospective Investigation into Cancer and Nutrition. *Int J Cancer, 128*(3), 623–634. doi:10.1002/ijc.25387

Rohrmann, S., Lukas Jung, S. U., Linseisen, J., & Pfau, W. (2009). Dietary intake of meat and meat-derived heterocyclic aromatic amines and their correlation with DNA adducts in female breast tissue. *Mutagenesis, 24*(2), 127–132. doi:10.1093/mutage/gen058

Rohrmann, S., Overvad, K., Bueno-de-Mesquita, H. B., Jakobsen, M. U., Egeberg, R., Tjønneland, A., . . . Linseisen, J. (2013). Meat consumption and mortality—results from the European Prospective Investigation into Cancer and Nutrition. *BMC Med, 11*, 63. doi:10.1186/1741-7015-11-63

Rollison, D. E., Newschaffer, C. J., Tao, Y., Pollak, M., & Helzlsouer, K. J. (2006). Premenopausal levels of circulating insulin-like growth factor I and the risk of postmenopausal breast cancer. *Int J Cancer, 118*(5), 1279–1284. doi:10.1002/ijc.21471

Rolls, B. J. (2000). The role of energy density in the overconsumption of fat. *J Nutr, 130*(2S Suppl), 268S–271S.

Rolls, B. J., & Bell, E. A. (1999). Intake of fat and carbohydrate: Role of energy density. *Eur J Clin Nutr, 53*, Suppl 1, S166–S173.

Rolls, B. J., Ello-Martin, J. A., & Tohill, B. C. (2004). What can intervention studies tell us about the relationship between fruit and vegetable consumption and weight management? *Nutr Rev, 62*(1), 1–17.

Romaguera, D., Norat, T., Vergnaud, A. C., Mouw, T., May, A. M., Agudo, A., . . . Peeters, P. H. (2010). Mediterranean dietary patterns and prospective weight change in participants of the EPIC-PANACEA project. *Am J Clin Nutr, 92*(4), 912–921. doi:10.3945/ajcn.2010.29482

Romeu, M., Aranda, N., Giralt, M., Ribot, B., Nogues, M. R., & Arija, V. (2013). Diet, iron biomarkers and oxidative stress in a representative sample of Mediterranean population. *Nutr J, 12*(1), 102. doi:10.1186/1475-2891-12-102

Romon, M., Lebel, P., Velly, C., Marecaux, N., Fruchart, J. C., & Dallongeville, J. (1999). Leptin response to carbohydrate or fat meal and association with subsequent satiety and energy intake. *Am J Physiol, 277*(5 Pt 1), E855–E861.

Roncaglioni, M. C., Tombesi, M., Avanzini, F., Barlera, S., Caimi, V., Longoni, P., . . . Risk and Prevention Study Collaborative Group. (2013). n-3 fatty acids in patients with multiple cardiovascular risk factors. *N Engl J Med, 368*(19), 1800–1808. doi:10.1056/NEJMoa1205409

Rong, Y., Chen, L., Zhu, T., Song, Y., Yu, M., Shan, Z., . . . Liu, L. (2013). Egg consumption and risk of coronary heart disease and stroke: Dose-response meta-analysis of prospective cohort studies. *BMJ, 346*, e8539.

Rose, G. (1985). Sick individuals and sick populations. *Int J Epidemiol, 14*(1), 32–38.

Rosell, M., Appleby, P., Spencer, E., & Key, T. (2006). Weight gain over 5 years in 21,966 meat-eating, fish-eating, vegetarian, and vegan men and women in EPIC-Oxford. *Int J Obes (Lond), 30*(9), 1389–1396. doi:10.1038/sj.ijo.0803305

Rosen, J. C., Gross, J., Loew, D., & Sims, E. A. (1985). Mood and appetite during minimal-carbohydrate and carbohydrate-supplemented hypocaloric diets. *Am J Clin Nutr, 42*(3), 371–379.

Rosqvist, F., Iggman, D., Kullberg, J., Jonathan Cedernaes, J., Johansson, H. E., Larsson, A., . . . Risérus, U. (2014). Overfeeding polyunsaturated and saturated fat causes distinct effects on liver and visceral fat accumulation in humans. *Diabetes*. doi:10.2337/db13-1622

Rouse, I. L., Beilin, L. J., Armstrong, B. K., & Vandongen, R. (1983). Blood-pressure-lowering effect of a vegetarian diet: Controlled trial in normotensive subjects. *Lancet, 1*(8314-5), 5–10.

Russell, W. R., Gratz, S. W., Duncan, S. H., Holtrop, G., Ince, J., Scobbie, L., . . . Flint, H. J. (2011). High-protein, reduced-carbohydrate weight-loss diets promote metabolite profiles likely to be detrimental to colonic health. *Am J Clin Nutr, 93*(5), 1062–1072. doi:10.3945/ajcn.110.002188

Sacks, F. M., Bray, G. A., Carey, V. J., Smith, S. R., Ryan, D. H., Anton, S. D., . . . Williamson, D. A. (2009). Comparison of weight-loss diets with different compositions of fat, protein, and carbohydrates. *N Engl J Med, 360*(9), 859–873. doi:10.1056/NEJMoa0804748

Sacks, F. M., Rosner, B., & Kass, E. H. (1974). Blood pressure in vegetarians. *Am J Epidemiol, 100*(5), 390–398.

Saidi, O., Ben Mansour, N., O'Flaherty, M., Capewell, S., Critchley, J. A., & Ben Romdhane, H. (2013). Analyzing recent coronary heart disease mortality trends in Tunisia between 1997 and 2009. *PLoS One, 8*(5), e63202. doi:10.1371/journal.pone.0063202

Samaha, F. F., Iqbal, N., Seshadri, P., Chicano, K. L., Daily, D. A., McGrory, J., . . . Stern, L. (2003). A low-carbohydrate as compared with a low-fat diet in severe obesity. *N Engl J Med, 348*(21), 2074–2081. doi:10.1056/NEJMoa022637

Santesso, N., Akl, E. A., Bianchi, M., Mente, A., Mustafa, R., Heels-Ansdell, D., & Schünemann, H. J. (2012). Effects of higher- versus lower-protein diets on health outcomes: A systematic review and meta-analysis. *Eur J Clin Nutr, 66*(7), 780–788. doi:10.1038/ejcn.2012.37

Schæbel, L. H., Vestergaard, H., Laurberg, P., Rathcke, C. N., & Andersen, S. (2013). Intake of traditional Inuit diet vary in parallel with inflammation as estimated from YKL-40 and hsCRP in Inuit and non-Inuit in Greenland. *Atherosclerosis, 228*(2), 496–501. doi:10.1016/j.atherosclerosis.2013.03.022

Schettler, G. (1983). Atherosclerosis during periods of food deprivation following World Wars I and II. *Prev Med, 12*(1), 75–83.

Schoeller, D. A., & Buchholz, A. C. (2005). Energetics of obesity and weight control: Does diet composition matter? *J Am Diet Assoc, 105*(5 Suppl 1), S24–S28. doi:10.1016/j.jada.2005.02.025

Schoeninger, M. J. (2012). Palaeoanthropology: The ancestral dinner table. *Nature, 487*(7405), 42–43. doi:10.1038/487042a

Schulz, L. O., Bennett, P. H., Ravussin, E., Kidd, J. R., Kidd, K. K., Esparza, J., & Valencia, M. E. (2006). Effects of traditional and western environments on prevalence of type 2 diabetes in Pima Indians in Mexico and the U.S. *Diabetes Care, 29*(8), 1866–1871. doi:10.2337/dc06-0138

Schulz, M., Kroke, A., Liese, A. D., Hoffmann, K., Bergmann, M. M., & Boeing, H. (2002). Food groups as predictors for short-term weight changes in men and women of the EPIC-Potsdam cohort. *J Nutr, 132*(6), 1335–1340.

Schulze, M. B., Hoffmann, K., Manson, J. E., Willett, W. C., Meigs, J. B., Weikert, C., . . . Hu, F. B. (2005). Dietary pattern, inflammation, and incidence of type 2 diabetes in women. *Am J Clin Nutr, 82*(3), 675–684; quiz 714-675.

Schulze, M. B., & Hu, F. B. (2005). Primary prevention of diabetes: what can be done and how much can be prevented? *Annu Rev Public Health, 26*, 445–467. doi:10.1146/annurev.publhealth.26.021304.144532

Schulze, M. B., Manson, J. E., Willett, W. C., & Hu, F. B. (2003). Processed meat intake and incidence of Type 2 diabetes in younger and middle-aged women. *Diabetologia, 46*(11), 1465–1473. doi:10.1007/s00125-003-1220-7

Schwartz, M. W. (2000). Biomedicine. Staying slim with insulin in mind. *Science, 289*(5487), 2066–2067.

Schwartz, M. W., Boyko, E. J., Kahn, S. E., Ravussin, E., & Bogardus, C. (1995). Reduced insulin secretion: An independent predictor of body weight gain. *J Clin Endocrinol Metab, 80*(5), 1571–1576.

Sebastian, A., Frassetto, L. A., Sellmeyer, D. E., Merriam, R. L., & Morris, R. C. (2002). Estimation of the net acid load of the diet of ancestral preagricultural Homo sapiens and their hominid ancestors. *Am J Clin Nutr, 76*(6), 1308–1316.

Select Committee on Nutrition and Human Needs. (1977). *Dietary goals for the United States.* Washington, DC: U.S. Government Printing Office

Sellmeyer, D. E., Stone, K. L., Sebastian, A., & Cummings, S. R. (2001). A high ratio of dietary animal to vegetable protein increases the rate of bone loss and the risk of fracture in post-menopausal women. Study of Osteoporotic Fractures Research Group. *Am J Clin Nutr, 73*(1), 118–122.

Shah, S., Casas, J. P., Drenos, F., Whittaker, J., Deanfield, J., Swerdlow, D. I., . . . Hingorani, A. D. (2013). Causal relevance of blood lipid fractions in the development of carotid atherosclerosis: Mendelian randomization analysis. *Circ Cardiovasc Genet, 6*(1), 63–72. doi:10.1161/CIRCGENETICS.112.963140

Shai, I., Schwarzfuchs, D., Henkin, Y., Shahar, D. R., Witkow, S., Greenberg, I., . . . Group, D. I. R. C. T. D. (2008). Weight loss with a low-carbohydrate, Mediterranean, or low-fat diet. *N Engl J Med, 359*(3), 229–241. doi:10.1056/NEJMoa0708681

Sharman, M. J., Gómez, A. L., Kraemer, W. J., & Volek, J. S. (2004). Very low-carbohydrate and low-fat diets affect fasting lipids and postprandial lipemia differently in overweight men. *J Nutr, 134*(4), 880–885.

Shick, S. M., Wing, R. R., Klem, M. L., McGuire, M. T., Hill, J. O., & Seagle, H. (1998). Persons successful at long-term weight loss and maintenance continue to consume a low-energy, low-fat diet. *J Am Diet Assoc, 98*(4), 408-413. doi:10.1016/S0002-8223(98)00093-5

Shintani, T., Beckham, S., O'Connor, H. K., Hughes, C., & Sato, A. (1994). The Waianae Diet Program: A culturally sensitive, community-based obesity and clinical intervention program for the Native Hawaiian population. *Hawaii Med J, 53*(5), 136–141, 147.

Shintani, T. T., Beckham, S., Brown, A. C., & O'Connor, H. K. (2001). The Hawaii Diet: Ad libitum high carbohydrate, low fat multi-cultural diet for the reduction of chronic disease risk factors: obesity, hypertension, hypercholesterolemia, and hyperglycemia. *Hawaii Med J, 60*(3), 69–73.

Shintani, T. T., Hughes, C. K., Beckham, S., & O'Connor, H. K. (1991). Obesity and cardiovascular risk intervention through the ad libitum feeding of traditional Hawaiian diet. *Am J Clin Nutr, 53*(6 Suppl), 1647S–1651S.

Sho, H. (2001). History and characteristics of Okinawan longevity food. *Asia Pacific J Clin Nutr, 10*(2), 159–164.

Shrapnel, W. S., Calvert, G. D., Nestel, P. J., & Truswell, A. S. (1992). Diet and coronary heart disease. The National Heart Foundation of Australia. *Med J Aust, 156 Suppl,* S9–S16.

Siener, R., & Hesse, A. (2003). The effect of a vegetarian and different omnivorous diets on urinary risk factors for uric acid stone formation. *Eur J Nutr, 42*(6), 332–337. doi:10.1007/s00394-003-0428-0

Simopoulos, A. P. (2006). Evolutionary aspects of diet, the omega-6/omega-3 ratio and genetic variation: nutritional implications for chronic diseases. *Biomed Pharmacother, 60*(9), 502–507. doi:10.1016/j.biopha.2006.07.080

Simpson, S. J., & Raubenheimer, D. (2009). Macronutrient balance and lifespan. *Aging (Albany NY), 1*(10), 875–880.

Singh, P. N., Sabaté, J., & Fraser, G. E. (2003). Does low meat consumption increase life expectancy in humans? *Am J Clin Nutr, 78*(3 Suppl), 526S–532S.

Sinha, R., Cross, A. J., Graubard, B. I., Leitzmann, M. F., & Schatzkin, A. (2009). Meat intake and mortality: A prospective study of over half a million people. *Arch Intern Med, 169*(6), 562–571. doi:10.1001/archinternmed.2009.6

Sinnett, P. F., & Whyte, H. M. (1973). Epidemiological studies in a total highland population, Tukisenta, New Guinea. Cardiovascular disease and relevant clinical, electrocardiographic, radiological and biochemical findings. *J Chronic Dis, 26*(5), 265–290.

Siri-Tarino, P. W., Sun, Q., Hu, F. B., & Krauss, R. M. (2010). Meta-analysis of prospective cohort studies evaluating the association of saturated fat with cardiovascular disease. *Am J Clin Nutr, 91*(3), 535–546. doi:10.3945/ajcn.2009.27725

Sjögren, P., Becker, W., Warensjö, E., Olsson, E., Byberg, L., Gustafsson, I. B., . . . Cederholm, T. (2010). Mediterranean and carbohydrate-restricted diets and mortality among elderly men: a cohort study in Sweden. *Am J Clin Nutr, 92*(4), 967–974. doi:10.3945/ajcn.2010.29345

Skerrett, P. J., & Willett, W. C. (2010). Essentials of healthy eating: a guide. *J Midwifery Womens Health, 55*(6), 492–501. doi:10.1016/j.jmwh.2010.06.019

Slavin, J. (2003). Why whole grains are protective: Biological mechanisms. *Proc Nutr Soc, 62*(1), 129–134. doi:10.1079/PNS2002221

Smith, M., Trexler, E., Sommer, A., Starkoff, B., & Devor, S. (2014). Unrestricted Paleolithic diet is associated with unfavorable changes to blood lipids in healthy subjects. *Int J Exerc Sci, 7*(2), 128–139.

Smith-Warner, S. A., Elmer, P. J., Tharp, T. M., Fosdick, L., Randall, B., Gross, M., . . . Potter, J. D. (2000). Increasing vegetable and fruit intake: Randomized intervention and monitoring in an at-risk population. *Cancer Epidemiol Biomarkers Prev, 9*(3), 307–317.

Snowdon, D. A. (1988). Animal product consumption and mortality because of all causes combined, coronary heart disease, stroke, diabetes, and cancer in Seventh-day Adventists. *Am J Clin Nutr, 48*(3 Suppl), 739–748.

Snowdon, D. A., & Phillips, R. L. (1985). Does a vegetarian diet reduce the occurrence of diabetes? *Am J Public Health, 75*(5), 507–512.

Sofer, S., Eliraz, A., Kaplan, S., Voet, H., Fink, G., Kima, T., & Madar, Z. (2011). Greater weight loss and hormonal changes after 6 months diet with carbohydrates eaten mostly at dinner. *Obesity (Silver Spring), 19*(10), 2006–2014. doi:10.1038/oby.2011.48

Solinger, A. B., & Rothman, S. I. (2013). Risks of mortality associated with common laboratory tests: a novel, simple and meaningful way to set decision limits from data available in the Electronic Medical Record. *Clin Chem Lab Med, 51*(9), 1803–1813. doi:10.1515/cclm-2013-0167

Song, Y., Manson, J. E., Buring, J. E., & Liu, S. (2004). A prospective study of red meat consumption and type 2 diabetes in middle-aged and elderly women: The women's health study. *Diabetes Care, 27*(9), 2108–2115.

Sørensen, L. B., Raben, A., Stender, S., & Astrup, A. (2005). Effect of sucrose on inflammatory markers in overweight humans. *Am J Clin Nutr, 82*(2), 421–427.

Souto, G., Donapetry, C., Calviño, J., & Adeva, M. M. (2011). Metabolic acidosis-induced insulin resistance and cardiovascular risk. *Metab Syndr Relat Disord, 9*(4), 247–253. doi:10.1089/met.2010.0108

Spence, J. D., Jenkins, D. J., & Davignon, J. (2010). Dietary cholesterol and egg yolks: Not for patients at risk of vascular disease. *Can J Cardiol, 26*(9), e336–339.

Spencer, E. A., Appleby, P. N., Davey, G. K., & Key, T. J. (2003). Diet and body mass index in 38000 EPIC-Oxford meat-eaters, fish-eaters, vegetarians and vegans. *Int J Obes Relat Metab Disord, 27*(6), 728–734. doi:10.1038/sj.ijo.0802300

St Jeor, S. T., Howard, B. V., Prewitt, T. E., Bovee, V., Bazzarre, T., Eckel, R. H., & Nutrition Committee of the Council on Nutrition, P. y. A., and Metabolism of the American Heart Association. (2001). Dietary protein and weight reduction: A statement for healthcare professionals from the Nutrition Committee of the Council on Nutrition, Physical Activity, and Metabolism of the American Heart Association. *Circulation, 104*(15), 1869–1874.

Stamler, J. (2010). Diet-heart: A problematic revisit. *Am J Clin Nutr, 91*(3), 497–499. doi:10.3945/ajcn.2010.29216

Stamler, J., Brown, I. J., Daviglus, M. L., Chan, Q., Kesteloot, H., Ueshima, H., . . . INTER-MAP Research Group. (2009). Glutamic acid, the main dietary amino acid, and blood pressure: the INTERMAP Study (International Collaborative Study of Macronutrients, Micronutrients and Blood Pressure). *Circulation, 120*(3), 221–228. doi:10.1161/CIRCU-LATIONAHA.108.839241

Stamler, J., & Dolecek, T. A. (1997). Relation of food and nutrient intakes to body mass in the special intervention and usual care groups in the Multiple Risk Factor Intervention Trial. *Am J Clin Nutr, 65*(1 Suppl), 366S–373S.

Stamler, J., Liu, K., Ruth, K. J., Pryer, J., & Greenland, P. (2002). Eight-year blood pressure change in middle-aged men: Relationship to multiple nutrients. *Hypertension, 39*(5), 1000–1006.

Steck, S. E., Gaudet, M. M., Eng, S. M., Britton, J. A., Teitelbaum, S. L., Neugut, A. I., . . . Gammon, M. D. (2007). Cooked meat and risk of breast cancer—lifetime versus recent dietary intake. *Epidemiology, 18*(3), 373–382. doi:10.1097/01.ede.0000259968.11151.06

Steinberg, D. (2007). *Cholesterol wars.* San Diego, CA: Academic Press.

Steinberg, D., Glass, C. K., & Witztum, J. L. (2008). Evidence mandating earlier and more aggressive treatment of hypercholesterolemia. *Circulation, 118*(6), 672–677. doi:10.1161/CIRCULATIONAHA.107.753152

Steinmetz, K. A., & Potter, J. D. (1991). Vegetables, fruit, and cancer. II. Mechanisms. *Cancer Causes Control, 2*(6), 427–442.

Stephenson, T. J., Setchell, K. D., Kendall, C. W., Jenkins, D. J., Anderson, J. W., & Fanti, P. (2005). Effect of soy protein-rich diet on renal function in young adults with insulin-dependent diabetes mellitus. *Clin Nephrol, 64*(1), 1–11.

Struijk, E. A., May, A. M., Beulens, J. W., van Gils, C. H., Monninkhof, E. M., van der Schouw, Y. T., . . . Peeters, P. H. (2015). Mortality and cancer incidence in the EPIC-NL cohort: impact of the healthy volunteer effect. *Eur J Public Health, 25*(1), 144–149. doi:10.1093/eurpub/cku045

Stuart, C. A., Shangraw, R. E., Peters, E. J., & Wolfe, R. R. (1990). Effect of dietary protein on bed-rest-related changes in whole-body-protein synthesis. *Am J Clin Nutr, 52*(3), 509–514.

Stubbs, R. J., Harbron, C. G., Murgatroyd, P. R., & Prentice, A. M. (1995). Covert manipulation of dietary fat and energy density: Effect on substrate flux and food intake in men eating ad libitum. *Am J Clin Nutr, 62*(2), 316–329.

Stubbs, R. J., Prentice, A. M., & James, W. P. (1997). Carbohydrates and energy balance. *Ann N Y Acad Sci, 819*, 44–69.

Sugimura, T. (1997). Overview of carcinogenic heterocyclic amines. *Mutat Res, 376*(1-2), 211–219.

Sugimura, T. (2000). Nutrition and dietary carcinogens. *Carcinogenesis, 21*(3), 387–395.

Sugiyama, T., Tsugawa, Y., Tseng, C. H., Kobayashi, Y., & Shapiro, M. F. (2014). Different time trends of caloric and fat intake between statin users and nonusers among US adults: Gluttony in the time of statins? *JAMA Intern Med.* doi:10.1001/jamainternmed.2014.1927

Surwit, R. S., Feinglos, M. N., McCaskill, C. C., Clay, S. L., Babyak, M. A., Brownlow, B. S., … Lin, P. H. (1997). Metabolic and behavioral effects of a high-sucrose diet during weight loss. *Am J Clin Nutr, 65*(4), 908–915.

Suzuki, R., Rylander-Rudqvist, T., Ye, W., Saji, S., Adlercreutz, H., & Wolk, A. (2008). Dietary fiber intake and risk of postmenopausal breast cancer defined by estrogen and progesterone receptor status—a prospective cohort study among Swedish women. *Int J Cancer, 122*(2), 403–412. doi:10.1002/ijc.23060

Tang, M., McCabe, G. P., Elango, R., Pencharz, P. B., Ball, R. O., & Campbell, W. W. (2014). Assessment of protein requirement in octogenarian women with use of the indicator amino acid oxidation technique. *Am J Clin Nutr, 99*(4), 891–898. doi:10.3945/ajcn.112.042325

Tang, W., Wang, Z., Fan, Y., Levison, B., Hazen, J., Donahue, L., … Hazen, S. (2014). Prognostic value of elevated levels of intestinal microbe-generated metabolite trimethylamine-n-oxide in patients with heart failure: Refining the gut hypothesis. *J Am College Cardiol, 64*, 1908–1914.

Tang, W. H., Wang, Z., Levison, B. S., Koeth, R. A., Britt, E. B., Fu, X., … Hazen, S. L. (2013). Intestinal microbial metabolism of phosphatidylcholine and cardiovascular risk. *N Engl J Med, 368*(17), 1575–1584. doi:10.1056/NEJMoa1109400

Tangvoranuntakul, P., Gagneux, P., Diaz, S., Bardor, M., Varki, N., Varki, A., & Muchmore, E. (2003). Human uptake and incorporation of an immunogenic nonhuman dietary sialic acid. *Proc Natl Acad Sci U S A, 100*(21), 12045–12050. doi:10.1073/pnas.2131556100

Tantamango-Bartley, Y., Jaceldo-Siegl, K., Fan, J., & Fraser, G. (2013). Vegetarian diets and the incidence of cancer in a low-risk population. *Cancer Epidemiol Biomarkers Prev, 22*(2), 286–294. doi:10.1158/1055-9965.EPI-12-1060

Tarnopolsky, M. A., MacDougall, J. D., & Atkinson, S. A. (1988). Influence of protein intake and training status on nitrogen balance and lean body mass. *J Appl Physiol, 64*(1), 187–193.

Taylor, E. N., Fung, T. T., & Curhan, G. C. (2009). DASH-style diet associates with reduced risk for kidney stones. *J Am Soc Nephrol, 20*(10), 2253–2259. doi:10.1681/ASN.2009030276

Te Morenga, L., Mallard, S., & Mann, J. (2013). Dietary sugars and body weight: systematic review and meta-analyses of randomised controlled trials and cohort studies. *BMJ, 346*, e7492.

Thedford, K., & Raj, S. (2011). A vegetarian diet for weight management. *J Am Diet Assoc, 111*(6), 816–818. doi:10.1016/j.jada.2011.04.014

Thiébaut, A. C., Jiao, L., Silverman, D. T., Cross, A. J., Thompson, F. E., Subar, A. F., … Stolzenberg-Solomon, R. Z. (2009). Dietary fatty acids and pancreatic cancer in the NIH-AARP diet and health study. *J Natl Cancer Inst, 101*(14), 1001–1011. doi:10.1093/jnci/djp168

Thiébaut, A. C., Kipnis, V., Chang, S. C., Subar, A. F., Thompson, F. E., Rosenberg, P. S.,

... Schatzkin, A. (2007). Dietary fat and postmenopausal invasive breast cancer in the National Institutes of Health-AARP Diet and Health Study cohort. *J Natl Cancer Inst, 99*(6), 451–462. doi:10.1093/jnci/djk094

Thomas, D. E., Elliott, E. J., & Baur, L. (2007). Low glycaemic index or low glycaemic load diets for overweight and obesity. *Cochrane Database Syst Rev*(3), CD005105. doi:10.1002/14651858.CD005105.pub2

Thomas, W. A., Davies, J. N., O'Neal, R. M., & Dimakulangan, A. A. (1960). Incidence of myocardial infarction correlated with venous and pulmonary thrombosis and embolism. A geographic study based on autopsies in Uganda. East Africa and St. Louis, U.S.A. *Am J Cardiol, 5*, 41–47.

Thompson, R. C., Allam, A. H., Lombardi, G. P., Wann, L. S., Sutherland, M. L., Sutherland, J. D., ... Thomas, G. S. (2013). Atherosclerosis across 4000 years of human history: The Horus study of four ancient populations. *Lancet, 381*(9873), 1211–1222. doi:10.1016/S0140-6736(13)60598-X

Thorogood, M., Carter, R., Benfield, L., McPherson, K., & Mann, J. I. (1987). Plasma lipids and lipoprotein cholesterol concentrations in people with different diets in Britain. *Br Med J (Clin Res Ed), 295*(6594), 351–353.

Tieland, M., Dirks, M. L., van der Zwaluw, N., Verdijk, L. B., van de Rest, O., de Groot, L. C., & van Loon, L. J. (2012). Protein supplementation increases muscle mass gain during prolonged resistance-type exercise training in frail elderly people: A randomized, double-blind, placebo-controlled trial. *J Am Med Dir Assoc, 13*(8), 713–719. doi:10.1016/j.jamda.2012.05.020

Tipton, K. D., & Wolfe, R. R. (2001). Exercise, protein metabolism, and muscle growth. *Int J Sport Nutr Exerc Metab, 11*(1), 109–132.

Toniolo, P., Bruning, P. F., Akhmedkhanov, A., Bonfrer, J. M., Koenig, K. L., Lukanova, A., ... Zeleniuch-Jacquotte, A. (2000). Serum insulin-like growth factor-I and breast cancer. *Int J Cancer, 88*(5), 828–832.

Tonstad, S., Butler, T., Yan, R., & Fraser, G. E. (2009). Type of vegetarian diet, body weight, and prevalence of type 2 diabetes. *Diabetes Care, 32*(5), 791–796. doi:10.2337/dc08-1886

Tonstad, S., Nathan, E., Oda, K., & Fraser, G. (2013). Vegan diets and hypothyroidism. *Nutrients, 5*(11), 4642–4652. doi:10.3390/nu5114642

Toubro, S., & Astrup, A. (1997). Randomised comparison of diets for maintaining obese subjects' weight after major weight loss: Ad lib, low fat, high carbohydrate diet v fixed energy intake. *BMJ, 314*(7073), 29–34.

Touzeau, A., Amiot, R., Blichert-Toft, J., Flandrois, J.-P., Fourel, F., Grossi, V., ... Lécuyer, C. (2014). Diet of ancient Egyptians inferred from stable isotope systematics. *J Archae Sci, 46*, 114–124.

Trichopoulou, A., Orfanos, P., Norat, T., Bueno-de-Mesquita, B., Ocké, M. C., Peeters, P. H., ... Trichopoulos, D. (2005). Modified Mediterranean diet and survival: EPIC-elderly prospective cohort study. *BMJ, 330*(7498), 991. doi:10.1136/bmj.38415.644155.8F

Trichopoulou, A., Psaltopoulou, T., Orfanos, P., Hsieh, C. C., & Trichopoulos, D. (2007). Low-carbohydrate-high-protein diet and long-term survival in a general population cohort. *Eur J Clin Nutr, 61*(5), 575–581. doi:10.1038/sj.ejcn.1602557

Trock, B. J., Hilakivi-Clarke, L., & Clarke, R. (2006). Meta-analysis of soy intake and breast cancer risk. *J Natl Cancer Inst, 98*(7), 459–471. doi:10.1093/jnci/djj102

Tsai, C. J., Leitzmann, M. F., Willett, W. C., & Giovannucci, E. L. (2004). Dietary protein and the risk of cholecystectomy in a cohort of US women: the Nurses' Health Study. *Am J Epidemiol, 160*(1), 11–18. doi:10.1093/aje/kwh170

Tucker, K. L., Hallfrisch, J., Qiao, N., Muller, D., Andres, R., & Fleg, J. L. (2005). The combination of high fruit and vegetable and low saturated fat intakes is more protective against mortality in aging men than is either alone: The Baltimore Longitudinal Study of Aging. *J Nutr, 135*(3), 556–561.

Tucker, K. L., Rich, S., Rosenberg, I., Jacques, P., Dallal, G., Wilson, P. W., & Selhub, J. (2000). Plasma vitamin B-12 concentrations relate to intake source in the Framingham Offspring study. *Am J Clin Nutr, 71*(2), 514–522.

Turner-McGrievy, G. M., Barnard, N. D., & Scialli, A. R. (2007). A two-year randomized weight loss trial comparing a vegan diet to a more moderate low-fat diet. *Obesity (Silver Spring), 15*(9), 2276–2281. doi:10.1038/oby.2007.270

Turner-McGrievy, G. M., Davidson, C. R., & Wilcox, S. (2014). Does the type of weight loss diet affect who participates in a behavioral weight loss intervention? A comparison of participants for a plant-based diet versus a standard diet trial. *Appetite, 73*, 156–162. doi:10.1016/j.appet.2013.11.008

Turner-McGrievy, G. M., Davidson, C. R., Wingard, E. E., Wilcox, S., & Frongillo, E. A. (2015). Comparative effectiveness of plant-based diets for weight loss: a randomized controlled trial of five different diets. *Nutrition, 31*(2), 350–358. doi:10.1016/j.nut.2014.09.002

Turner-McGrievy, B., Wingard, E., Davidson, C., Taylor, M., & Wilcox S. (2013). How plant-based do we need to be to achieve weight loss? Results of the New Dietary Interventions to Enhance the Treatment for Weight Loss (New DIET) study. *Obesity Week.*

Ullah, M. F., & Khan, M. W. (2008). Food as medicine: Potential therapeutic tendencies of plant derived polyphenolic compounds. *Asian Pac J Cancer Prev, 9*(2), 187–195.

United Nations Environment Programme. (2010). *Assessing the environmental impacts of consumption and production: Priority products and materials.* A Report of the Working Group on the Environmental Impacts of Products and Materials to the International Panel for Sustainable Resource Management.

Valachovicová, M., Krajcovicová-Kudláčková, M., Blazícek, P., & Babinská, K. (2006). No evidence of insulin resistance in normal weight vegetarians. A case control study. *Eur J Nutr, 45*(1), 52–54. doi:10.1007/s00394-005-0563-x

van Dam, R. M., Willett, W. C., Rimm, E. B., Stampfer, M. J., & Hu, F. B. (2002). Dietary fat and meat intake in relation to risk of type 2 diabetes in men. *Diabetes Care, 25*(3), 417–424.

Vang, A., Singh, P. N., Lee, J. W., Haddad, E. H., & Brinegar, C. H. (2008). Meats, processed meats, obesity, weight gain and occurrence of diabetes among adults: Findings from Adventist Health Studies. *Ann Nutr Metab, 52*(2), 96–104. doi:10.1159/000121365

Varki, A. (2008). Sialic acids in human health and disease. *Trends Mol Med, 14*(8), 351–360. doi:10.1016/j.molmed.2008.06.002

Vergnaud, A. C., Norat, T., Mouw, T., Romaguera, D., May, A. M., Bueno-de-Mesquita, H. B., . . . Peeters, P. H. (2013). Macronutrient composition of the diet and prospective weight change in participants of the EPIC-PANACEA study. *PLoS One, 8*(3), e57300. doi:10.1371/journal.pone.0057300

Vergnaud, A. C., Norat, T., Romaguera, D., Mouw, T., May, A. M., Travier, N., . . . Peeters, P.

H. (2010). Meat consumption and prospective weight change in participants of the EPIC-PANACEA study. *Am J Clin Nutr, 92*(2), 398–407. doi:10.3945/ajcn.2009.28713

Vergnaud, A. C., Romaguera, D., Peeters, P. H., van Gils, C. H., Chan, D. S., Romieu, I., . . . Norat, T. (2013). Adherence to the World Cancer Research Fund/American Institute for Cancer Research guidelines and risk of death in Europe: Results from the European Prospective Investigation into Nutrition and Cancer cohort study 1,4. *Am J Clin Nutr, 97*(5), 1107–1120. doi:10.3945/ajcn.112.049569

Verhoef, P., van Vliet, T., Olthof, M. R., & Katan, M. B. (2005). A high-protein diet increases postprandial but not fasting plasma total homocysteine concentrations: a dietary controlled, crossover trial in healthy volunteers. *Am J Clin Nutr, 82*(3), 553–558.

Vogel, R. A., Corretti, M. C., & Plotnick, G. D. (1997). Effect of a single high-fat meal on endothelial function in healthy subjects. *Am J Cardiol, 79*(3), 350–354.

Vogelzangs, N., Beekman, A. T., Milaneschi, Y., Bandinelli, S., Ferrucci, L., & Penninx, B. W. (2010). Urinary cortisol and six-year risk of all-cause and cardiovascular mortality. *J Clin Endocrinol Metab, 95*(11), 4959–4964. doi:10.1210/jc.2010-0192

Voight, B. F., Peloso, G. M., Orho-Melander, M., Frikke-Schmidt, R., Barbalic, M., Jensen, M. K., . . . Kathiresan, S. (2012). Plasma HDL cholesterol and risk of myocardial infarction: A mendelian randomisation study. *Lancet, 380*(9841), 572–580. doi:10.1016/S0140-6736(12)60312-2

Walrand, S., Short, K. R., Bigelow, M. L., Sweatt, A. J., Hutson, S. M., & Nair, K. S. (2008). Functional impact of high protein intake on healthy elderly people. *Am J Physiol Endocrinol Metab, 295*(4), E921–E928. doi:10.1152/ajpendo.90536.2008

Wang, Y., & Beydoun, M. A. (2009). Meat consumption is associated with obesity and central obesity among US adults. *Int J Obes (Lond), 33*(6), 621–628. doi:10.1038/ijo.2009.45

Wang, Y. F., Yancy, W. S., Yu, D., Champagne, C., Appel, L. J., & Lin, P. H. (2008). The relationship between dietary protein intake and blood pressure: Results from the PREMIER study. *J Hum Hypertens, 22*(11), 745–754. doi:10.1038/jhh.2008.64

Wang, Z., Klipfell, E., Bennett, B. J., Koeth, R., Levison, B. S., Dugar, B., . . . Hazen, S. L. (2011). Gut flora metabolism of phosphatidylcholine promotes cardiovascular disease. *Nature, 472*(7341), 57–63. doi:10.1038/nature09922

Watt, M. J., & Hoy, A. J. (2012). Lipid metabolism in skeletal muscle: Generation of adaptive and maladaptive intracellular signals for cellular function. *Am J Physiol Endocrinol Metab, 302*(11), E1315–E1328. doi:10.1152/ajpendo.00561.2011

Watts, G. (2013). Sugar and the heart: Old ideas revisited. *BMJ, 346*, e7800.

Watzl, B. (2008). Anti-inflammatory effects of plant-based foods and of their constituents. *Int J Vitam Nutr Res, 78*(6), 293–298. doi:10.1024/0300-9831.78.6.293

Weaver, C. M., Proulx, W. R., & Heaney, R. (1999). Choices for achieving adequate dietary calcium with a vegetarian diet. *Am J Clin Nutr, 70*(3 Suppl), 543S–548S.

Weigle, D. S., Breen, P. A., Matthys, C. C., Callahan, H. S., Meeuws, K. E., Burden, V. R., & Purnell, J. Q. (2005). A high-protein diet induces sustained reductions in appetite, ad libitum caloric intake, and body weight despite compensatory changes in diurnal plasma leptin and ghrelin concentrations. *Am J Clin Nutr, 82*(1), 41–48.

Welch, A. A., Shakya-Shrestha, S., Lentjes, M. A., Wareham, N. J., & Khaw, K. T. (2010). Dietary intake and status of n-3 polyunsaturated fatty acids in a population of fish-eating and non-fish-eating meat-eaters, vegetarians, and vegans and the product-precursor ratio [corrected] of á-linolenic acid to long-chain n-3 polyunsaturated fatty acids: results from the EPIC-Norfolk cohort. *Am J Clin Nutr, 92*(5), 1040–1051. doi:10.3945/ajcn.2010.29457

Welle, S., & Thornton, C. A. (1998). High-protein meals do not enhance myofibrillar synthesis after resistance exercise in 62- to 75-yr-old men and women. *Am J Physiol, 274*(4 Pt 1), E677–E683.

Whelton, S. P., Hyre, A. D., Pedersen, B., Yi, Y., Whelton, P. K., & He, J. (2005). Effect of dietary fiber intake on blood pressure: a meta-analysis of randomized, controlled clinical trials. *J Hypertens, 23*(3), 475–481.

Wiedermann, C. J., Kiechl, S., Dunzendorfer, S., Schratzberger, P., Egger, G., Oberhollenzer, F., & Willeit, J. (1999). Association of endotoxemia with carotid atherosclerosis and cardiovascular disease: Prospective results from the Bruneck Study. *J Am Coll Cardiol, 34*(7), 1975–1981.

Willcox, B. J., Willcox, D. C., Todoriki, H., Fujiyoshi, A., Yano, K., He, Q., . . . Suzuki, M. (2007). Caloric restriction, the traditional Okinawan diet, and healthy aging: The diet of the world's longest-lived people and its potential impact on morbidity and life span. *Ann N Y Acad Sci, 1114*, 434–455. doi:10.1196/annals.1396.037

Willcox, D. C., Willcox, B. J., Todoriki, H., & Suzuki, M. (2009). The Okinawan diet: Health implications of a low-calorie, nutrient-dense, antioxidant-rich dietary pattern low in glycemic load. *J Am Coll Nutr, 28*(Suppl), 500S–516S.

Willett, W. (2003). Lessons from dietary studies in Adventists and questions for the future. *Am J Clin Nutr, 78*(3 Suppl), 539S–543S.

Willett, W. C. (2010). The WHI joins MRFIT: A revealing look beneath the covers. *Am J Clin Nutr, 91*(4), 829–830. doi:10.3945/ajcn.2010.29347

Willett, W. C., & Stampfer, M. J. (2013). Current evidence on healthy eating. *Annu Rev Public Health, 34*, 77–95. doi:10.1146/annurev-publhealth-031811-124646

Wing, R. R., Vazquez, J. A., & Ryan, C. M. (1995). Cognitive effects of ketogenic weight-reducing diets. *Int J Obes Relat Metab Disord, 19*(11), 811–816.

Witard, O. C., Jackman, S. R., Breen, L., Smith, K., Selby, A., & Tipton, K. D. (2013). Myofibrillar muscle protein synthesis rates subsequent to a meal in response to increasing doses of whey protein at rest and after resistance exercise. *Am J Clin Nutr.* doi:10.3945/ajcn.112.055517

Wolever, T. M., Jenkins, D. J., Ocana, A. M., Rao, V. A., & Collier, G. R. (1988). Second-meal effect: Low-glycemic-index foods eaten at dinner improve subsequent breakfast glycemic response. *Am J Clin Nutr, 48*(4), 1041–1047.

Wolk, A., Manson, J. E., Stampfer, M. J., Colditz, G. A., Hu, F. B., Speizer, F. E., . . . Willett, W. C. (1999). Long-term intake of dietary fiber and decreased risk of coronary heart disease among women. *JAMA, 281*(21), 1998–2004.

Woolf, S., & Aron, L. (Eds.). (2013). *U.S. health in international perspective: Shorter lives, poorer health.* Washington, DC: National Academies Press.

World Cancer Research Fund/American Insitute for Cancer Research. (2007). *Food, nutrition, physical activity, and the prevention of cancer: A global perspective.* Washington, DC: AICR.

Wynn, E., Krieg, M. A., Lanham-New, S. A., & Burckhardt, P. (2010). Postgraduate Symposium: Positive influence of nutritional alkalinity on bone health. *Proc Nutr Soc, 69*(1), 166–173. doi:10.1017/S002966510999173X

Yang, D., Liu, Z., Yang, H., & Jue, Y. (2013). Acute effects of high-protein versus normal-protein isocaloric meals on satiety and ghrelin. *Eur J Nutr*. doi:10.1007/s00394-013-0552-4

Yang, W., Li, B., Dong, X., Zhang, X. Q., Zeng, Y., Zhou, J. L., . . . Xu, J. J. (2013). Is heme iron intake associated with risk of coronary heart disease? A meta-analysis of prospective studies. *Eur J Nutr*. doi:10.1007/s00394-013-0535-5

Yao, X. G., Frommlet, F., Zhou, L., Zu, F., Wang, H. M., Yan, Z. T., . . . Li, N. F. (2010). The prevalence of hypertension, obesity and dyslipidemia in individuals of over 30 years of age belonging to minorities from the pasture area of Xinjiang. *BMC Public Health, 10,* 91. doi:10.1186/1471-2458-10-91

Ye, E. Q., Chacko, S. A., Chou, E. L., Kugizaki, M., & Liu, S. (2012). Greater whole-grain intake is associated with lower risk of type 2 diabetes, cardiovascular disease, and weight gain. *J Nutr, 142*(7), 1304–1313. doi:10.3945/jn.111.155325

Yerushalmy, J., & Hilleboe, H. E. (1957). Fat in the diet and mortality from heart disease; a methodologic note. *N Y State J Med, 57*(14), 2343–2354.

Young, V. R. Long term nitrogen balance studies and other criteria for protein requirement estimations. In W. Rand (Ed.).

Young, V. R. (1991). Soy protein in relation to human protein and amino acid nutrition. *J Am Diet Assoc, 91*(7), 828–835.

Young, V. R., & Borgonha, S. (2000). Nitrogen and amino acid requirements: The Massachusetts Institute of Technology amino acid requirement pattern. *J Nutr, 130*(7), 1841S–1849S.

Young, V. R., El-Khoury, A. E., Raguso, C. A., Forslund, A. H., & Hambraeus, L. (2000). Rates of urea production and hydrolysis and leucine oxidation change linearly over widely varying protein intakes in healthy adults. *J Nutr, 130*(4), 761–766.

Young, V. R., & Pellett, P. L. (1994). Plant proteins in relation to human protein and amino acid nutrition. *Am J Clin Nutr, 59*(5 Suppl), 1203S–1212S.

Zamora-Ros, R., Agudo, A., Luján-Barroso, L., Romieu, I., Ferrari, P., Knaze, V., . . . González, C. A. (2012). Dietary flavonoid and lignan intake and gastric adenocarcinoma risk in the European Prospective Investigation into Cancer and Nutrition (EPIC) study. *Am J Clin Nutr, 96*(6), 1398–1408. doi:10.3945/ajcn.112.037358

Zhang, C., Schulze, M. B., Solomon, C. G., & Hu, F. B. (2006). A prospective study of dietary patterns, meat intake and the risk of gestational diabetes mellitus. *Diabetologia, 49*(11), 2604–2613. doi:10.1007/s00125-006-0422-1

Zimmerman, M. R. (1977). An experimental study of mummification pertinent to the antiquity of cancer. *Cancer, 40*(3), 1358–1362.

zur Hausen, H. (2012). Red meat consumption and cancer: Reasons to suspect involvement of bovine infectious factors in colorectal cancer. *Int J Cancer, 130*(11), 2475–2483. doi:10.1002/ijc.27413

Index

About the Author

DR. GARTH DAVIS is a leader in the field of bariatric medicine and the medical director of bariatric surgery at Memorial Hermann Memorial City Medical Center and the Davis Clinic for surgical and medical weight management. He attended medical school at Baylor College of Medicine and was inducted into the Alpha Omega Alpha Honor Medical Society. Dr. Davis is certified by the American Board of Surgery and is a Fellow of the American Society for Metabolic and Bariatric Surgery. He starred on the hit TLC show *Big Medicine*. Dr. Davis lives in Houston with his family.